Master Techniques in Orthopaedic Surgery®

The
Spine

Third Edition

Master Techniques in Orthopaedic Surgery®

Editor-in-Chief
Bernard F. Morrey, MD

Founding Editor
Roby C. Thompson, MD

Volume Editors

Fractures
Donald A. Wiss, MD

Knee Arthroplasty
Paul Lotke, MD
Jess H. Lonner, MD

Orthopaedic Oncology and Complex Reconstruction
Franklin H. Sim, MD
Peter F.M. Choong, MD
Kristy L. Weber, MD

Pediatrics
Vernon T. Tolo, MD
David L. Skaggs, MD

Relevant Surgical Exposures
Bernard F. Morrey, MD
Matthew C. Morrey, MD

Reconstructive Knee Surgery
Douglas W. Jackson, MD

Soft Tissue Surgery
Steven L. Moran, MD
William P. Cooney III, MD

Sports Medicine
Freddie H. Fu, MD

The Elbow
Bernard F. Morrey, MD

The Foot and Ankle
Harold B. Kitaoka, MD

The Hand
James Strickland, MD
Thomas Graham, MD

The Hip
Robert L. Barrack, MD

The Foot and Ankle
Harold B. Kitaoka, MD

The Shoulder
Edward V. Craig, MD

The Spine
Thomas A. Zdeblick, MD
Todd J. Albert, MD

The Wrist
Richard H. Gelberman, MD

Master Techniques in Orthopaedic Surgery®

The Spine

Third Edition

Thomas A. Zdeblick, M.D.

AA McBeath Professor and Chairman
Department of Orthopedics and Rehabilitation
University of Wisconsin
Madison, Wisconsin

Todd J. Albert, M.D.

Richard H. Rothman Professor and Chairman
Department of Orthopaedic Surgery
Professor of Neurosurgery
Thomas Jefferson University and Hospitals
President
The Rothman Institute
Philadelphia, Pennsylvania

. Wolters Kluwer | Lippincott Williams & Wilkins
Health

Philadelphia • Baltimore • New York • London
Buenos Aires • Hong Kong • Sydney • Tokyo

Acquisitions Editor: Brian Brown
Product Manager: David Murphy
Production Project Manager: David Saltzberg
Design Manager: Doug Smock
Manufacturing Manager: Beth Welsh
Production Services: SPi Global

Printed in China

Library of Congress Cataloging-in-Publication Data
Spine (Zdeblick : 2013)
   The spine / edited by Thomas A. Zdeblick and Todd J. Albert. — Third edition.
        p. ; cm. — (Master techniques in orthopaedic surgery)
   Includes bibliographical references and index.
   ISBN 978-1-4511-7361-1 (alk. paper)
   I. Zdeblick, Thomas A., editor of compilation. II. Albert, Todd J., editor of compilation. III. Title.
IV. Series: Master techniques in orthopaedic surgery.
   [DNLM: 1. Spine—surgery. 2. Orthopedic Procedures—methods. WE 725]
   RD768
   617.5'6059—dc23
                                                                                         2013031362

Care has been taken to confirm the accuracy of the information presented and to describe generally accepted practices. However, the authors, editors, and publisher are not responsible for errors or omissions or for any consequences from application of the information in this book and make no warranty, expressed or implied, with respect to the currency, completeness, or accuracy of the contents of the publication. Application of the information in a particular situation remains the professional responsibility of the practitioner.

   The authors, editors, and publisher have exerted every effort to ensure that drug selection and dosage set forth in this text are in accordance with current recommendations and practice at the time of publication. However, in view of ongoing research, changes in government regulations, and the constant flow of information relating to drug therapy and drug reactions, the reader is urged to check the package insert for each drug for any change in indications and dosage and for added warnings and precautions. This is particularly important when the recommended agent is a new or infrequently employed drug.

   Some drugs and medical devices presented in the publication have Food and Drug Administration (FDA) clearance for limited use in restricted research settings. It is the responsibility of the health care provider to ascertain the FDA status of each drug or device planned for use in their clinical practice.

To purchase additional copies of this book, call our customer service department at (800) 638-3030 or fax orders to (301) 223-2320. International customers should call (301) 223-2300.

Visit Lippincott Williams & Wilkins on the Internet: at LWW.com. Lippincott Williams & Wilkins customer service representatives are available from 8:30 am to 6 pm, EST.

10 9 8 7 6 5 4 3 2 1

To our families, including our larger family—the residents and fellows we have trained—who inspire our daily work and the work of educating and of caring for patients.

Contributors

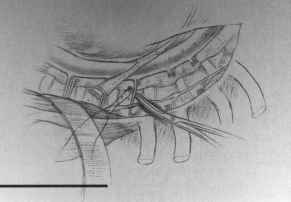

Todd J. Albert, M.D.
Richard H. Rothman Professor and Chairman
Department of Orthopaedic Surgery
Professor of Neurosurgery
Thomas Jefferson University and Hospitals
President
The Rothman Institute
Philadelphia, Pennsylvania

D. Greg Anderson, M.D.
Professor
Department of Orthopaedic Surgery
    and Neurological Surgery
Thomas Jefferson University
Rothman Institute
Philadelphia, Pennsylvania

Paul A. Anderson, M.D.
Professor
Department of Orthopedics and Rehabilitation
University of Wisconsin
Madison, Wisconsin

Ronald I. Apfelbaum, M.D.
Professor Emeritus
Department of Neurosurgery
University of Utah
Salt Lake City, Utah

Neil Badlani, M.D., M.B.A.
Fellow
Department of Orthopaedic Surgery
Rush University Medical Center
Chicago, Illinois

Carlo Bellabarba, M.D.
Professor
Joint Professor of Neurological Surgery
Orthopedics and Sports Medicine
University of Washington
Spine Surgeon
Orthopaedics and Sports Medicine
UW Medicine
Seattle, Washington

Sigurd H. Berven, M.D.
Professor of Orthopaedic Surgery
Director of Spine Fellowship
Department of Orthopaedic Surgery
University of California, San Francisco
San Francisco, California

David S. Bradford, M.D.
Department of Orthopaedic Surgery
University of California, San Francisco
Moffitt-Long Hospital
San Francisco, California

Keith H. Bridwell, M.D.
J. Albert Key Distinguished Professor of Orthopaedic Surgery
Professor of Neurological Surgery
Department of Orthopaedic Surgery
Barnes-Jewish Hospital
Washington University in St. Louis
St. Louis, Missouri

Darrel S. Brodke, M.D.
Professor
Department of Orthopaedics
University of Utah School of Medicine
Department of Orthopaedic Surgery
University of Utah Medical Center
Salt Lake City, Utah

Frank P. Cammisa Jr, M.D.
Associate Professor of Clinical Surgery
Department of Orthopedic Surgery
Weill Medical College of Cornell University
Chief
Spinal Surgical Service
Hospital for Special Surgery
New York, New York

Jens R. Chapman, M.D.
Hansjöerg Wyss Professor and Chair
Joint Professor of Neurological Surgery
Orthopaedics and Sports Medicine
University of Washington
Director, Spine Service
Orthopaedics and Sports Medicine
UW Medicine
Seattle, Washington

Zachary Child, M.D.
Fellow
Department of Orthopedic Spine Surgery
Orthopedics and Sports Medicine
University of Washington
Clinical Instructor
Department of Orthopaedic Surgery
Harborview Medical Center
Seattle, Washington

Bradford L. Currier, M.D.
Professor of Orthopedics
Director, Mayo Spine Fellowship
Department of Orthopedic Surgery
Mayo Clinic
St. Mary's Hospital
Rochester, Minnesota

Mathias Daniels, M.D.
Clinical Instructor in Orthopaedics
Department of Orthopaedics
University of Washington
Fellow in Spine Surgery
Department of Orthopedics
Harborview Medical Center
Seattle, Washington

Bruce V. Darden II, M.D.
Fellowship Director
Othocarolina Spine Center
Charlotte, North Carolina

Mark B. Dekutoski, M.D.
The CORE Institute
Phoenix, Arizona

Sanford E. Emery, M.D., M.B.A.
Professor and Chairman
Department of Orthopedics
West Virginia University
Morgantown, West Virginia

Mark S. Eskander, M.D.
Spine Surgeon
Department of Orthopaedics
Christiana Hospital
Newark, Delaware

Jesse L. Even, M.D.
Spine Fellow
Department of Orthopaedic Surgery
University of Pittsburgh
Pittsburgh, Pennsylvania

Naderafshar Fereydonyan, M.D.
Assistant Professor
Department of Neurosurgery
Tehran University of Medical Science
Neurosurgeon
Department of Neurosurgery
Rasool Akram Hospital
Tehran, Iran

Michael A. Finn, M.D.
Assistant Professor
Department of Neurosugery
University of Colorado
Aurora, Colorado

Jeremy L. Fogelson, M.D.
Instructor of Neurologic Surgery
Mayo Clinic
Rochester, Minnesota

Sapan D. Gandhi, B.S.
Medical Student
Drexel University College of Medicine
Philadelphia, Pennsylvania

Federico P. Girardi, M.D.
Associate Professor of Clinical Surgery
Department of Orthopedic Surgery
Weill Medical College of Cornell University
Associate Attending Orthopaedic Surgeon
Spinal Surgical Service
Hospital for Special Surgery
New York, New York

Christine L. Hammer, M.D.
Resident
Department of Neurosurgery
Thomas Jefferson University Hospital
Philadelphia, Pennsylvania

C. Chambliss Harrod, M.D.
Attending Spine Surgeon
Bone & Joint Clinic—The Spine Center
Baton Rouge, Louisiana

James S. Harrop, M.D.
Professor of Neurosurgery
Department of Neurosurgery
Jefferson Medical College
Thomas Jefferson University Hospital
Philadelphia, Pennsylvania

John G. Heller, M.D.
Baur Professor of Orthopaedic Surgery
Department of Orthopaedic Surgery
Emory University School of Medicine
Atlanta, Georgia

Alan S. Hilibrand, M.D.
Professor of Orthopaedic Surgery
Rothman Institute
Jefferson Medical College
Attending
Department of Orthopaedic Surgery
Jefferson University Hospital
Philadelphia, Pennsylvania

Serena S. Hu, M.D.
David S. Bradford Chair of Spine Surgery
Department of Orthopedic Surgery
University of California, San Francisco
Chief, Spine Service
Department of Orthopedic Surgery
Moffitt-Long Hospital UCSF
San Francisco, California

Alexander P. Hughes, M.D.
Assistant Profesor of Clinical Surgery
Department of Orthopedic Surgery
Weill Medical Collge of Cornell University
Assistant Attending Orthopaedic Surgeon
Spinal Surgical Service
Hospital for Special Surgery
New York, New York

Siddharth B. Joglekar, M.D.
Clinical Instructor
Department of Orthopedic Surgery
UCSF Fresno
Orthopedic Staff Surgeon
Department of Surgery
VA Medical Center Fresno
Fresno, California

James D. Kang, M.D.
Professor
Vice Chair
Department of Orthopedic Surgery
Univeristy of Pittsburgh
Univeristy of Pittsburgh Medical Center
Pittsburgh, Pennsylvania

Michael P. Kelly, M.D.
Assistant Professor
Department of Orthopedic Surgery
Department of Neurological Surgery
Washington University
St. Louis, Missouri

Christopher K. Kepler, M.D., M.B.A.
Assistant Professor
Department of Orthopedic Surgery
Thomas Jefferson University
Rothman Institute
Philadelphia, Pennsylvania

Thomas J. Kesman, M.D., M.B.A.
Orthopedic Spine Surgeon
Department of Orthopedic Surgery
Reliant Medical Group
Worcester, Massachusetts

Yongjung J. Kim, M.D.
Associate Professor
Department of Orthopedic Surgery
Columbia University, College of Physicians and Surgeons
Chief, Spinal Deformity Surgery
Department of Orthopedic Surgery
New York Presbyterian Hospital
New York, New York

Han Jo Kim, M.D.
Fellow in Adult and Pediatric Spinal Deformity and
    Reconstruction
Department of Orthopedic Surgery
Washington University in St. Louis
Barnes-Jewish Hospital
St. Louis, Missouri

Christian Klare, M.D.
Resident
Department of Orthopedic Surgery
Dartmouth-Hitchcock Medical Center
Lebanon, New Hampshire

Darren R. Lebl, M.D.
Clinical Instructor
Department of Orthopedic Surgery
Weill Medical College of Cornell University
Assistant Attending Orthopaedic Surgeon
Spinal Surgical Service
Hospital for Special Surgery
New York, New York

Lawrence G. Lenke, M.D.
The Jermoe J. Gilden Distinguished Professor
    of Orthopaedic Surgery, Chief of Service
Department of Orthopaedic Surgery
Washington University School of Medicine
Co-director, Adult/Pediatric Scoliosis and
    Reconstructive Spinal Surgery
Department of Orthopedic Surgery
Barnes-Jewish Hospital and St. Louis Children's Hospital
Saint Louis, Missouri

Robert A. McGuire Jr, M.D.
Professor and Chairman
Spine Surgeon
Department of Orthopedic and Rehabilitation
University of Mississippi Health Care
Jackson, Mississippi

Justin W. Miller, M.D.
Spine Surgeon
Department of Surgery
Indiana Spine Group
Indianapolis, Indiana

Charbel D. Moussallem, M.D.
Clincal Spine Fellow
Department of Orthopedic Surgery
Mayo Clinic
St. Mary's Hospital
Rochester, Minnesota

Praveen Mummaneni, M.D.
Professor and Vice Chair of Neurological Surgery
Director of Minimally Invasive and Cervical Spine Surgery
Director, Minimally Invasive and Complex Spine
    Fellowship Program
Co-director, Spinal Surgery and UCSF Spine Center
University of San Francisco
San Francisco, California

Ahmad Nassr, M.D.
Department of Orthopedic Surgery
Mayo Clinic
St. Mary's Hospital
Rochester, Minnesota

Shyam A. Patel, B.S.
Medical Student
Drexel University College of Medicine
Hahnemann University Hospital
Philadelphia, Pennsylvania

Mark Pichlemann, M.D.
Assistant Professor of Neurologic Surgery
Mayo Clinic College of Medicine
Jacksonville, Florida

Frank M. Phillips, M.D.
Professor
Head, Section of Minimally Invasive Spine Surgery
Department of Orthopedic Surgery
Rush University Medical Center
Chicago, Illinois

Kris Radcliff, M.D.
Assistant Professor
Department of Orthopedic Surgery
Thomas Jefferson University
Philadelphia, Pennsylvania
Spine Surgeon
Rothman Institute
Egg Harbor, New Jersey

K. Daniel Riew, M.D.
Mildred B. Simon Distinguished Professor
 of Orthopaedic Surgery
Chief, Cervical Spine Service
Department of Orthopaedic Surgery
Washington University School of Medicine
Barnes-Jewish Hospital
St. Louis, Missouri

Jeffrey A. Rihn, M.D.
Assistant Professor
Department of Orthopedic Surgery
Thomas Jefferson University Hospital
Rothman Institute
Philadelphia, Pennsylvania

Anthony S. Rinella, M.D.
Founder, Illinois Spine & Scoliosis Center
Spine and Scoliosis Surgeon
Homer Glen, Illinois

Rick C. Sasso, M.D.
Professor
Chief of Spine Surgery
Clinical Orthopedics Surgery
Indiana University, School of Medicine
Indiana Spine Group
Indianapolis, Indiana

James D. Schwender, M.D.
Staff Surgeon
Orthopaedic Surgery of the Spine
Twin Cities Spine Center
Minneapolis, Minnesota

William Ryan Spiker, M.D.
Resident
Department of Orthopaedics
University of Utah School of Medicine
Department of Orthopaedic Surgery
University of Utah Medical Center
Salt Lake City, Utah

Nikhil A. Thakur, M.D.
Assistant Professor
Upstate Bone and Joint Center
Department of Orthopaedics
Upstate Medical University—SUNY
Upstate University Hospital at Community General
Syracuse, New York

Clifford B. Tribus, M.D.
Professor
Department of Orthopedic and Rehabilitative Medicine
University of Wisconsin-Madison
Madison, Wisconsin

Roman Trimba, M.S.
Resident Physician
Department of Orthopaedic Surgery
Wright State University Boonshoft School of Medicine
Miami Valley Hospital
Dayton, Ohio

Alexander R. Vaccaro, M.D., Ph.D.
Professor
Department of Orthopedic Surgery
Thomas Jefferson University
Vice Chair
Department of Orthopedic Surgery
Thomas Jefferson University Hospital
Philadelphia, Pennsylvania

Sanjay Yadla, M.D.
Neurosurgeon
Neurosciences Institute
Alexian Brothers Medical Center
Elk Grove Village, Illinois

Thomas A. Zdeblick, M.D.
AA McBeath Professor and Chairman
Department of Orthopedics and Rehabilitation
University of Wisconsin
Madison, Wisconsin

Series Preface

Since its inception in 1994, the *Master Techniques in Orthopaedic Surgery* series has become the gold standard for both physicians in training and experienced surgeons. Its exceptional success may be traced to the leadership of the original series editor, Roby Thompson, whose clarity of thought and focused vision sought "to provide direct, detailed access to techniques preferred by orthopaedic surgeons who are recognized by their colleagues as 'masters' in their specialty," as he stated in his series preface. It is personally very rewarding to hear testimonials from both residents and practicing orthopaedic surgeons on the value of these volumes to their training and practice.

A key element of the success of the series is its format. The effectiveness of the format is reflected by the fact that it is now being replicated by others. An essential feature is the standardized presentation of information replete with tips and pearls shared by experts with years of experience.

Abundant color photographs and drawings guide the reader through the procedures step-by-step.

The second key to the success of the *Master Techniques* series rests in the reputation and experience of our volume editors. The editors are truly dedicated "masters" with a commitment to share their rich experience through these texts. We feel a great debt of gratitude to them and a real responsibility to maintain and enhance the reputation of the *Master Techniques* series that has developed over the years. We are proud of the progress made in formulating the third edition volumes and are particularly pleased with the expanded content of this series. Six new volumes will soon be available covering topics that are exciting and relevant to a broad cross section of our profession. While we are in the process of carefully expanding *Master Techniques* topics and editors, we are committed to the now-classic format.

The first of the new volumes is *Relevant Surgical Exposures,* which I have had the honor of editing. The second new volume is *Essential Procedures in Pediatrics.* Subsequent new topics to be introduced are *Soft Tissue Reconstruction, Management of Peripheral Nerve Dysfunction, Advanced Reconstructive Techniques in the Joint,* and finally *Essential Procedures in Sports Medicine.* The full library thus will consist of 16 useful and relevant titles.

I am pleased to have accepted the position of series editor, feeling so strongly about the value of this series to educate the orthopaedic surgeon in the full array of expert surgical procedures. The true worth of this endeavor will continue to be measured by the ever-increasing success and critical acceptance of the series. I remain indebted to Dr. Thompson for his inaugural vision and leadership, as well as to the *Master Techniques* volume editors and numerous contributors who have been true to the series style and vision. As I indicated in the preface to the second edition of *The Hip* volume, the words of William Mayo are especially relevant to characterize the ultimate goal of this endeavor: "The best interest of the patient is the only interest to be considered." We are confident that the information in the expanded *Master Techniques* offers the surgeon an opportunity to realize the patient-centric view of our surgical practice.

Bernard F. Morrey, M.D.

Preface

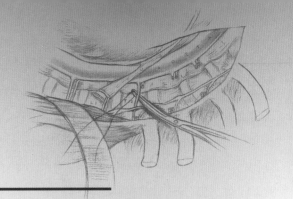

Welcome to the third edition of *Master Techniques in Orthopaedic Surgery: The Spine*. Since publication of the first edition in 1997, the field of spinal surgery has moved forward at a dizzying pace. Perhaps in no other branch of orthopaedic surgery has technology so radically changed surgical treatment.

We sought out those master surgeons whom we believe to be leaders in the discipline and asked them to present their material in a concise and logical manner, stressing the important points and making clear the steps involved in performing each procedure. The techniques are well illustrated, and complications and pitfalls to be avoided are outlined.

As in prior editions, we think readers will benefit greatly from this edition. Indeed, we ourselves picked up many pearls from putting this together and are impressed with the expertise shown and the richness of this format. We hope you find it equally useful.

Thomas A. Zdeblick, M.D.
Todd J. Albert, M.D.

Contents

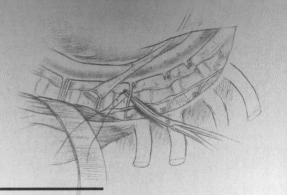

PART IV Tumor Resection 385

PART I
CERVICAL SPINE

1 Anterior Cervical Approach

Sanford E. Emery

Since the 1950s, the anterior approach to the cervical spine has become the approach of choice for many operative procedures performed today. Much of the pathoanatomy necessitating surgery is located in the anterior column of the spine, which lends itself to the direct anterior approach in treating degenerative, traumatic, neoplastic, infectious, and deformity conditions. Knowledge of the anatomy and respecting tissue planes allows the spine surgeon anterior access from C1 to the cervicothoracic junction. We will review the approach to the midcervical spine since it is by far the most common approach utilized, followed by the less common techniques for the upper cervical spine and the cervicothoracic junction.

ANTERIOR APPROACH TO THE CERVICAL SPINE (C3–C7)

Indications/Contraindications

The goals of most operative spine procedures are decompression of the spinal canal, arthrodesis, or both. Because much of the pathology requiring operative intervention involves the disc space or vertebral bodies, the anterior approach is indicated for many disorders using decompression and fusion techniques. Disc herniations or spondylosis changes with cord or root compression are easily accessed from the anterior approach. Larger procedures such as cervical corpectomies to decompress longer areas of the spinal canal or to correct deformity will require the anterior approach in most instances. Reconstruction of the anterior column following fractures, neoplasms, or severe infections utilizes the same operative approach.

Contraindications to the anterior approach are uncommon. Multiple prior anterior surgeries, skin changes from radiation, or at times, severe obesity may lead the surgeon to opt for posterior approach options to treat certain conditions. It should be noted that in patients with prior anterior approaches, any suspicion of a recurrent laryngeal nerve (RLN) palsy with unilateral vocal cord paralysis should be identified before other anterior procedures are performed, since the uninjured side should not be used so as to avoid potential bilateral vocal cord paralysis.

Preoperative Preparation

In preparing for an anterior operative procedure, the surgeon should palpate the skin and soft tissues of the patient's neck looking for an enlarged thyroid gland that could be problematic for exposure of the lower cervical spine. Some retraction on the carotid arteries during the anterior approach is unavoidable, so patients with known or suspected carotid artery disease should be evaluated pre-operatively, though in this author's opinion the risk of neurologic sequelae from retraction of the carotid artery is extremely rare. Identification of an existing unilateral vocal cord paralysis is mentioned above and would dictate approaching the spine anteriorly from the same side as the injured RLN so as not to create a bilateral injury and thus an inability to protect the airway.

The course of the vertebral artery should be checked preoperatively using routine magnetic resonance imaging or occasionally computed tomography angiography or magnetic resonance angiography. Aberrant medialization of vertebral arteries is uncommon though well described (5) and creates a high risk for vertebral artery injury in even routine cases.

Technique

Positioning of the patient for the anterior approach is important in facilitating exposure of the spine. For patients without severe cord compression, a roll can be placed between the shoulder blades allowing for neck extension and retraction of the shoulders. A general-use radiolucent table with a rectangular extension will allow raising or lowering of the head into more or less extension as needed during the case such as to compress the bone graft before plating. For discectomy and one-level corpectomy procedures, traction is not needed since screw-post–type retractors can easily distract discs or one-level corpectomy distances. For two or more level corpectomy procedures, intraoperative traction can be helpful. Both neck extension and the amount of weights must be used with extreme care or not at all in patients with spinal cord compression so as not to create spinal cord injury. Taping down of the shoulders or using wrist restraints with light traction can help with fluoroscopic or radiographic visualization of the lower cervical spine. Over pulling should be avoided so as not to create a brachial plexus injury. Rotation of the head 10 to 15 degrees away from the side of the operative approach will help with exposure.

The superficial anatomy enables placement of a transverse incision at the appropriate level for the indicated procedure. The hyoid bone is at C3, the thyroid cartilage at C4 and C5, and the cricoid cartilage is at C6. The carotid tubercle is often palpable as a prominence of the transverse process of C6. Practically speaking, an incision for a C5–C6 discectomy and fusion procedure is typically three finger breadths above the clavicle and two finger breadths for a C6–C7 level. Fluoroscopic or radiographic confirmation intraoperatively is, of course, required to ensure the appropriate level. The typical sizing of the transverse incision starts approximately a centimeter on the other side of midline coming over to just past the border of the sternocleidomastoid on the surgeon's side. Cephalad and caudad incision of the fascial planes will allow for easy retraction and a surprisingly extensile approach over many vertebral levels. A longitudinal incision can be made along the border of the sternocleidomastoid for a more extensile approach, though it is much less cosmetic and rarely required. Two transverse incisions at distinct levels for long reconstruction constructs is also an option.

After appropriate prepping and draping, the skin incision is made transversely at the chosen level for the classic Smith-Robinson anterior approach to the midcervical spine (24) (Fig. 1-1). Skin and subcutaneous tissue are incised with a knife blade, and any bleeding is controlled with cautery. Below the subcutaneous tissue is the platysma with vertical fibers. This author divides the platysma sharply the length of the incision, although it can be split vertically and retracted. There is a thin superficial cervical fascial layer that is incised transversely. This layer usually exposes branches of the external jugular system, which at times can be large. Tying and dividing these branches is sometimes prudent, although often they can simply be retracted with the deeper tissues. At this point, the deep cervical fascial layer is incised superiorly and inferiorly just medial to the border of the sternocleidomastoid (Fig. 1-2). This layer is the fascia that envelops the sternocleidomastoid and continues medially to envelop the strap muscles (10). Identifying and incising this fascial layer allows for extensile retraction up and down the anterior spine. The carotid artery is then palpated with an index finger and held laterally (Fig. 1-3). An appendicial-type retractor is placed medial to the surgeon's index finger deeply and retracts the trachea and esophagus medially. This retraction allows for a combination of blunt and sharp dissection of the pretracheal or alar fascia, which overlies the prevertebral fascia. At this point, the discs and vertebral bodies should be easily palpable and visible. The prevertebral fascia (11) can be lifted with forceps and dissected with a pair of Metzenbaum scissors to expose the anterior longitudinal ligament, discs, and vertebral bodies. A peanut-type dissector is useful for sweeping away the thin fascial layers off of the spine superiorly and inferiorly, and the deep retractors can be placed. The longus colli muscles run along each side

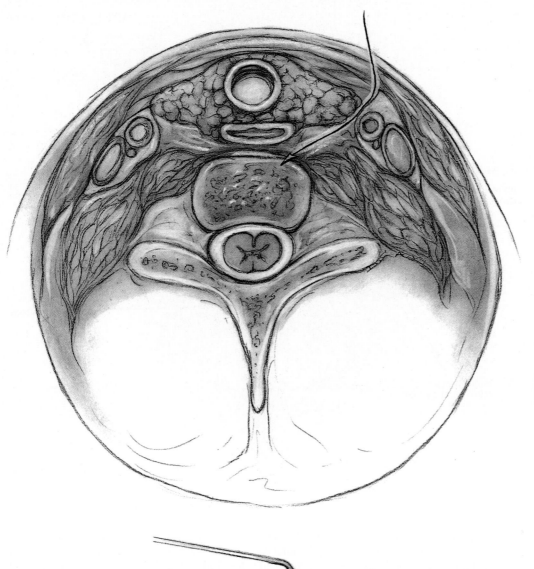

FIGURE 1-1

Superficially, the anterior approach to the subaxial spine utilizes the interval between the sternocleidomastoid muscle (lateral) and trachea/strap muscles (medial). Deep to this, the interval is between the carotid sheath and the esophagus.

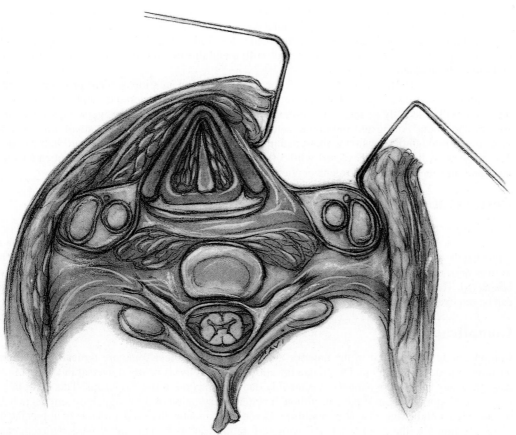

FIGURE 1-2

The muscles are contained within an investing fascial layer (superficial to the individual muscle encapsulating fascia). An interfascial dissection between the strap muscles and the sternocleidomastoid is developed bluntly by spreading with a clamp or Metzenbaum scissors. Once through this layer, finger dissection continues in a posteromedial direction toward the spine.

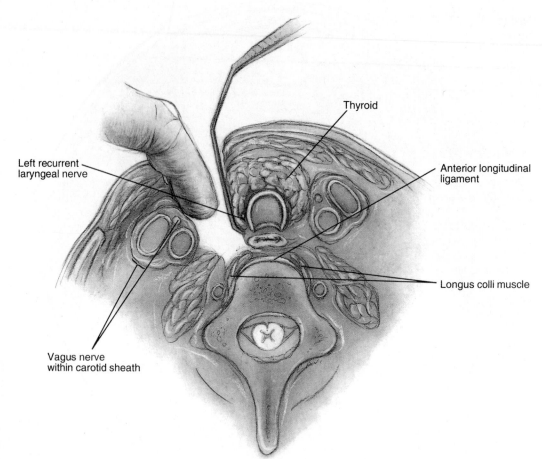

Left recurrent
laryngeal nerve

Thyroid

Anterior longitudinal
ligament

Longus colli muscle

Vagus nerve
within carotid sheath

FIGURE 1-3
The carotid pulse can be palpated and the artery displaced laterally at all times, which ensures that the dissection is medial to the carotid sheath. With a finger palpating the pulse laterally, a handheld retractor is placed medially to retract the trachea and esophagus.

of the spine and will actually converge toward the tubercle of C1 if the exposure is extended cephalad. The medial border of the longus colli along each side is typically elevated for 3 to 4 mm using cautery. This dissection allows deep retractor blades to grip better and minimizes dislodgement of the retractors. Overzealous elevation of longus colli could threaten the vertebral arteries, however, and should be avoided.

Self-retaining retractors have been used for many years for anterior cervical procedures and, with careful use, are very safe. Handheld retractors are possibly easier on the esophagus since the retraction will inherently be more intermittent, but this method requires more personnel. After the surgery, the wound is irrigated and the retractors removed. Many surgeons use a small drain that is brought out through the incision without making a cosmetically unacceptable separate stab wound. The platysma is the first layer closed with 3-0 Vicryl followed by 4-0 Vicryl in the subcutaneous layer and often a subcuticular Prolene or Vicryl layer for cosmetic skin closure.

Postoperative Management

Elevating the patient's head of the bed approximately 30 to 40 degrees may mitigate postoperative swelling. Most patients undergoing the common anterior cervical procedures can be extubated immediately after surgery. Larger multilevel corpectomy cases or more complex conditions such as tumors or deformity corrections may warrant a delayed extubation primarily to monitor airway edema (8). There is very little tension on the anterior cervical tissues, and typically the skin sutures can be removed in days rather than weeks.

Complications

Complications encountered in the anterior approach to the cervical spine are typically based on anatomy unique to this region. Dysphagia (swallowing difficulty) is nearly universal in the first few days after surgery in these patients, presumably due to retraction of the esophagus. This complication recovers quickly in most patients although better investigation of dysphagia in recent years has documented a higher increase at 6 months and even at 12 months than was previously appreciated (3,15,22). Injury to the esophageal wall with perforation can also occur and, if unrecognized, can lead to a life-threatening postoperative mediastinitis. Intraoperative indigo carmine can be injected by the anesthesiologist into the esophagus via a nasogastric tube to try and detect any perforations though this technique has not been proven to be reliable. If any are noted, then otolaryngologic or thoracic consultation is recommended for closure and no oral intake is allowed for a period postoperatively to allow the injury to seal over.

Dysphonia (hoarseness or voice changes) can arise from injury to either the RLN or the superior laryngeal nerve. The RLN supplies all the intrinsic muscles of the larynx with the exception of cricothyroid, which is supplied by the superior laryngeal nerve. An RLN palsy leaves the vocal cord in an open or semiopen position on that side, causing difficulty with phonation and even protection of the airway. The left RLN branches off the vagus and loops under the arch of the aorta and returns cephalad in the tracheal esophageal groove up to the larynx. The path of the right RLN is slightly more variable (Fig. 1-4). It loops under the right subclavian artery and travels up to the larynx with a slightly less predictable course. Rarely, the nerve will descend directly into the larynx without looping as a recurrent structure (21). Because of these anatomic findings, some surgeons prefer a left-sided approach believing it will decrease the incidence of RLN injury. This opinion has been difficult to prove in the literature with any statistical validity (4), however, and both right-sided and left-sided approaches are commonly utilized. Suggested techniques to decrease RLN palsy such as deflating and reinflating the endotracheal tube cuff, which may allow the tube to adjust itself within the larynx after the retractors are placed, is believed to be effective by some authors and not by others (1,2). Most recurrent nerve palsies recover over time, but can take up to a year postoperatively (29). Typically, the superior laryngeal nerve is at risk for exposure at the C3–C4 level. Small traversing nerves should be protected and retracted rather than simply transected. Superior laryngeal nerve injury results in weak phonation and voice fatigue, which can be a major disability for singing.

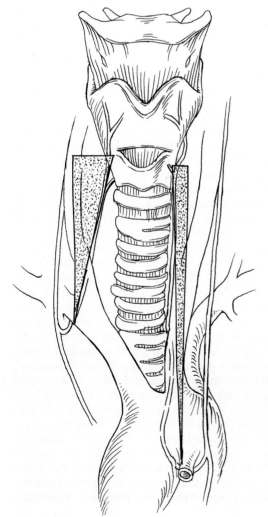

FIGURE 1-4

On the left side, the RLN is more consistently located within the carotid sheath and has less medial-lateral variability than on the right side. On the right side, there is much more medial-lateral variability in its location. (Adapted from Netterville JL, Koriwchak MJ, Winkle M, et al.: Vocal fold paralysis following the anterior approach to the cervical spine. *Ann Otol Rhinol Laryngol* 105: 85–91, 1996.)

Vertebral artery injury, though more at risk during discectomy or corpectomy procedures, can be injured during the approach as well. As mentioned above, preoperative identification of aberrant vertebral arteries is important to avoid an artery looping more medially under the longus colli. Though possible, injury of the carotid artery is notably rare in anterior approaches to the cervical spine.

Horner syndrome has been described as a complication of the anterior approach. This complication results from an injury to the sympathetic plexus that descends lateral to the longus colli muscle on each side. The sympathetic plexus courses more medially near the carotid tubercle at C6. Clinical features of Horner syndrome are ptosis (drooping eyelid), miosis (pupillary constriction), and anhidrosis (dry eye) (7).

TRANSORAL APPROACH TO THE UPPER CERVICAL SPINE

Indications/Contraindications

This operative approach allows direct visualization of the anterior arch of C1 and the body of C2. It is used for removal of the odontoid and pannus in rheumatoid arthritis patients when indicated, for debridement of infection, and decompression for tumor. Because the incision is transmucosal in the posterior pharynx, there is theoretically a higher infection rate with this approach given oral-pharyngeal flora. Thus the most common indications for transoral approaches are for debridement or decompression and more limited for bone graft reconstruction or instrumentation. Other authors have described a tongue and mandible splitting technique for a more extensile approach (25,28) or endoscopic endonasal odontoidectomy (16,20), but other alternatives such as the high retropharyngeal approach are more common.

Preoperative Preparation

Close examination of the oral-pharyngeal cavity should be done preoperatively, looking for any dental caries or active infections that might need treatment preoperatively. This approach does require the patient to be able to open the jaw an adequate amount (typically 3 to 4 cm) for placement of retractors and visualization.

Technique

Position of the patient and setup are very important for transoral techniques. Oral rather than nasotracheal intubation should be performed so the endotracheal tube is not in the operative field. The patient should be placed in slight Trendelenburg to prevent fluids from entering the trachea and pulmonary tree. A well-functioning endotracheal tube cuff is essential. Sterile gauze should be packed into the hypopharynx to help prevent leakage into the airway tree. The nares are draped out of the operative field with plastic drapes. A red rubber or Foley catheter can be placed through the nose into the hypopharynx, and the uvula can be tied to the tip of the catheter with a simple stitch. The tube is then pulled back, which retracts the uvula out of the operative field without injuring it. The oral cavity is then prepped with Betadine; some surgeons fill the whole oral cavity with Betadine and let it sit for minutes to minimize bacteria in the field. A microscope and C-arm are highly recommended.

Special transoral retractors with a broad tongue blade are available and are commonly used by otolaryngologists (Fig. 1-5). The anterior tubercle of the ring of C1 can typically be palpated in the posterior pharynx and should be confirmed by radiograph with needle localization. A vertical incision approximately 2 to 3 cm in length is made in the posterior pharynx (Fig. 1-6). This incision can be made in the midline, and a full-thickness soft tissue flap is elevated off the bone and retracted laterally. An alternative is a more lateral incision and raising one large flap in the opposite direction. There are four layers of tissue incised to access the spine: the pharyngeal mucosa, the pharyngeal constrictor muscles, the buccopharyngeal fascia, and the prevertebral fascia. These layers are not dissected out but rather kept in one full-thickness flap to maximize the blood supply and healing potential. A knife is easier on the tissue edges than cautery and may facilitate the best closure.

Retraction of the soft tissue flaps can be aided using stay sutures on each edge. Subperiosteal dissection on the anterior arch of C1 is performed until the lateral masses of the C1–C2 joints are exposed. If removing the odontoid, a burr is utilized to resect the anterior arch of C1. The burr can then be used to thin the dens, hollowing it out to protect the soft tissues. When the dens is thin enough, it can be elevated off of the transverse ligament and tectorial membrane with curettes and pituitary rongeurs. Initially removing the base of the dens makes the operation more difficult as the odontoid becomes movable and thus more difficult to excise. The wound is vigorously irrigated to minimize the infection rate. Closure is very important, again to prevent infection. A two-layer closure is recommended with the deep muscle layer closed snugly with resorbable

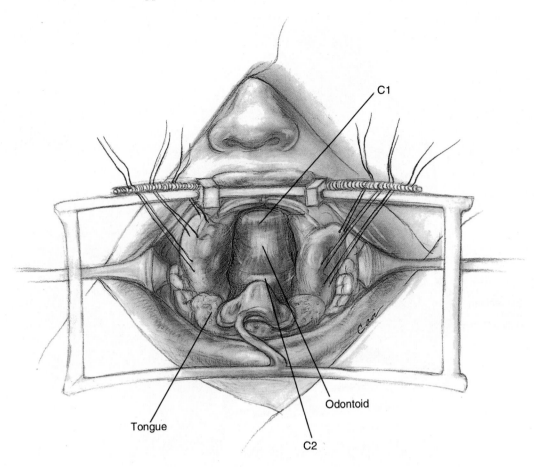

C1

Odontoid

Tongue

C2

FIGURE 1-5
Rectangular-shaped self-retaining retractors should be used for transoral exposure. A broad tongue blade with a suction device offers retraction inferiorly, whereas the superior aspect of the retractor rests on upper teeth, which must be padded to prevent injury to the teeth. A cut portion of a Foley catheter can be used for this padding.

suture such as 3-0 Vicryl with mattress sutures. The mucosa is then closed loosely with simple resorbable sutures.

Postoperative Management

Perioperative antibiotics are always utilized, and anaerobic coverage is recommended. Upper oral-pharyngeal swelling can compromise the airway, and extubation decisions should be made by the surgeon and anesthesiologist with this potential complication in mind. Delay of oral intake is recommended for a couple of days until the wound is sealed and the patient upright and preferably mobile.

Complications

Infection risk with the transoral approach has actually decreased substantially over many years, with rates documented between 0% and 3% in contemporary series (17,19,29). This change is most likely due to better prophylactic antibiotics, improved surgical technique including careful closure, and perhaps patient selection. Protection of the airway intraoperatively from fluids draining down into the trachea and pulmonary tree is very important for these patients. Postoperative airway management is also critical to avoid swelling complications and airway compromise. Other complications include iatrogenic instability from removal of the dens in certain patients, most of which will require concomitant posterior stabilization either at the same sitting or in a staged fashion. If a cerebrospinal fluid leak occurs during the procedure, then meningitis is of concern as a potential complication as well.

HIGH ANTERIOR RETROPHARYNGEAL APPROACH TO THE UPPER CERVICAL SPINE

Indications/Contraindications

The high retropharyngeal approach to the upper cervical spine is an alternative to the transoral approach in many patients. It allows exposure from the clivus down to the midcervical spine and is

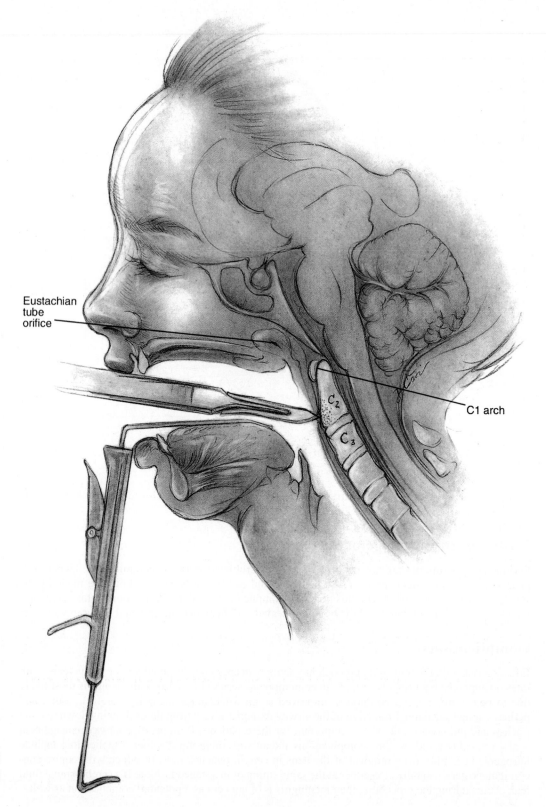

Eustachian
tube
orifice

C1 arch

FIGURE 1-6

The knife blade should
incise through the
anterior longitudinal
ligament down to the
bone. The entire soft
tissue layer is then
subperiosteally stripped
as a unit of tissue using
a periosteal elevator.

extensile. It is a retropharyngeal dissection and thus theoretically offers a lower infection rate than
transoral procedures. The approach for spine procedures is well described by McAfee et al. (18)
and others (14,27) and is typically indicated for high cervical tumors, infections, and even fractures. Anterior reconstruction and instrumentation is facilitated with this approach. Contraindications would be soft tissue concerns such as postradiation contractures. It is also very helpful if not
necessary for the patient to have some neck extension and rotation to allow for adequate exposure
of the highest levels.

Preoperative Preparation

As mentioned, the patient should be evaluated for the ability to extend and rotate the neck to allow for easier retraction and visibility at the uppermost levels. A short Kirschner wire (K-wire) placed directly into the anterior mandible in the midline can be bent at the tip and umbilical tape tied to this K-wire. A 1-pound weight can then be suspended off the end of the table, which retracts the jaw cephalad to help with exposure. Normal or abnormal function of the facial nerve and hypoglossal nerve should be noted as these structures are at risk during the approach. Injury or ischemia from retraction of the carotid artery is exceedingly rare in anterior cervical approaches, but preoperative evaluation of the carotids should be considered.

Technique

Positioning with a Mayfield rigid headholder versus tong-type traction depends on the particular case and the preference of the surgeon. A nasotracheal tube is preferred so as to allow better closure of the jaw with the K-wire plus umbilical tape in the step mentioned above. The head is extended as much as safely possible and rotated to the opposite side. Left- or right-sided approaches are based on surgeon preference since the RLN is not at risk this high in the neck. A transverse incision is made below the mandible at the level of the hyoid bone. Most pathologic entities requiring this approach warrant a several-centimeter transverse incision beginning past the midline on the opposite side of the cervical spine and ending on the surgeon's side at the anterior border of the sternocleidomastoid. The incision can become extensile distally with a "T" distal extension along the anterior border of the sternocleidomastoid (Fig. 1-7).

The transverse incision is carried down through subcutaneous fat. The platysma is usually quite thin and incised transversely. A submandibular gland is often visualized near the posterior angle of the jaw. This gland can be resected with attention paid to ligating the duct to avoid a postoperative fistula. The digastric muscle and the tiny stylohyoid muscle are visible in this layer. The digastric muscle has two bellies (Fig. 1-8), with the anterior belly descending from the floor of the mandible to the hyoid where a 90-degree sling or pulley structure turns the tendon laterally to form the posterior belly, which then attaches to the mastoid process. The digastric can be divided and tagged, which exposes the hypoglossal nerve that is fairly large in diameter (Fig. 1-9). The mandibular branch of the facial nerve, which controls motor to the lower lip, is a smaller diameter structure located higher in the field near the mandible and may not be easily visualized (Fig. 1-10). Vessels in this region from superior to inferior include the facial arteries and veins, the ascending pharyngeal arteries and veins, the lingual arteries and veins, and the superior thyroid vessels (Fig. 1-11). The superior laryngeal nerve may be visible in the lower aspect of the field. Ligation of these vessels may or may not be necessary for any given patient. Dissection along the anterior border of the sternocleidomastoid and incising the deep cervical fascia will facilitate a deeper dissection medial to the carotid sheath and posterior to the pharynx toward the spine (Fig. 1-12). The hypoglossal nerve should be dissected free as needed to allow for safe superior retraction. A nerve stimulator may be helpful to identify the hypoglossal nerve and/or the mandibular branch of the facial nerve. For visualization to the highest levels in the cervical spine, this author recommends two assistants with handheld retractors. Using handheld retractors not only allows for better visualization but also gives the soft tissue frequent breaks with intermittent relaxation of the assistants.

As the dissection is carried deeper, ligation of the small vessels mentioned above may be needed to allow for appropriate retraction. Blunt dissection is carried down to the alar fascia, and the spine is palpable. This layer is dissected superiorly and inferiorly, and the prevertebral fascia can be swept off of the vertebrae with a peanut dissector on a long clamp exposing the desired levels. Deep retractors are then placed as in the standard midcervical Smith-Robinson type of approach. The longus colli muscles converge to the anterior tubercle of the ring of C1 and thus will cover more of these upper cervical vertebrae. Cautery can be used to elevate off longus colli on each side for exposure as needed.

Closure of the wound is straightforward with 3-0 interrupted absorbable sutures in the platysma, 4-0 absorbable sutures in the subcutaneous layer, and a final skin suture with a running nylon suture or vertical mattress sutures.

Postoperative Management

Often this approach is utilized for significant pathology such as tumors or severe infection, and drains are usually warranted. Perioperative antibiotics are given per the normal routine. Airway issues are of paramount importance given the ability of the soft hypopharyngeal tissues to swell

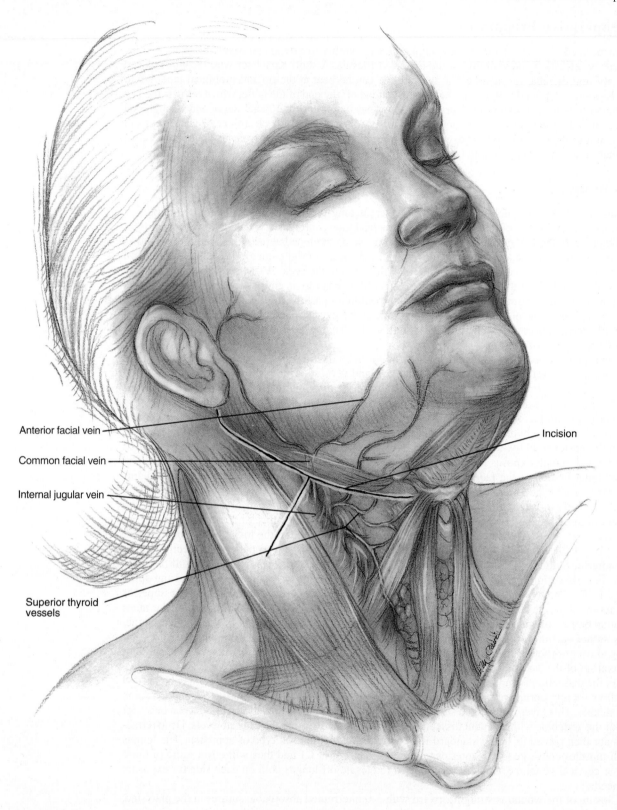

Anterior facial vein

Common facial vein

Internal jugular vein

Superior thyroid vessels

Incision

FIGURE 1-7

The hyoid bone is palpated along the anterior neck midline just below the jaw. This represents the medial extent of the incision. The incision can optionally be "T-ed" at its midaspect, approximately at the anterior border of the sternocleidomastoid muscle. Carried distally along the muscle border, this limb of the incision can be used for extensile exposure of the entire cervical spine.

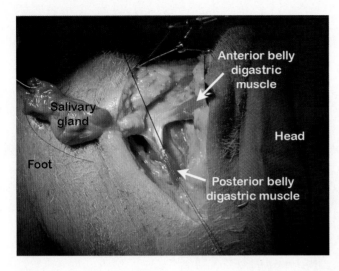

FIGURE 1-8

This cadaver dissection demonstrates a left-sided high retropharyngeal approach to the upper cervical spine. Note the salivary gland retracted out of the way, and the boomerang shape of the digastric muscle and its tendinous middle section.

from long periods of retraction. An extubation strategy should be determined by the surgeon and anesthesiologist.

Complications

Airway swelling after complex procedures poses a threat for prolonged intubation on a case by case basis. Esophageal or hypopharyngeal injury is possible and should be suspected with any wound infection or fevers postoperatively. Injury to the mandibular branch of the facial nerve can produce facial nerve palsy of the lower lip area. Injury of the hypoglossal nerve will affect motor function of the tongue. A superior laryngeal nerve palsy will result in voice changes and voice fatigue.

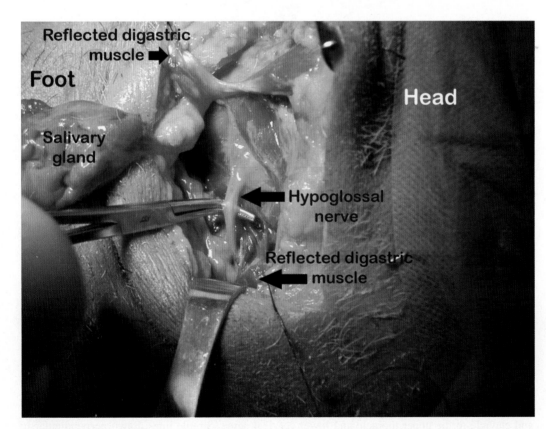

FIGURE 1-9

After the digastric muscle has been divided and retracted, hypoglossal nerve is identified.

FIGURE 1-10

The retromandibular vein crosses the parotid gland in its approximate midaspect. The common facial vein crosses the anterior aspect of the masseter muscle along the inferior angle of the jaw. These two veins should be dissected free and ligated near their junctions with the internal jugular vein, allowing the soft tissue flaps to be retracted proximally and distally. Keeping the dissection deep to and inferior to these ligated veins helps protect the facial nerve branch from injury.

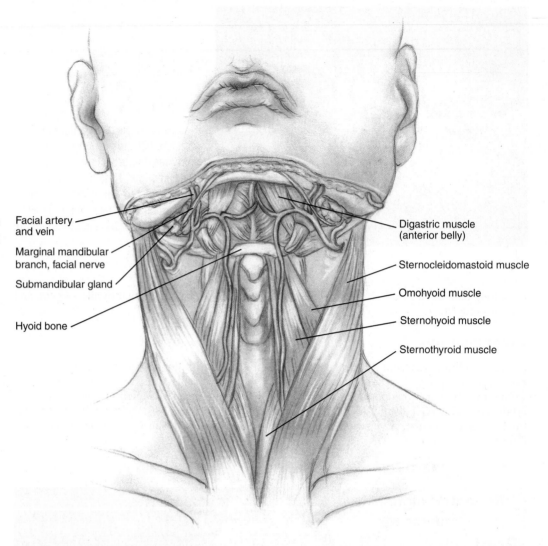

Facial artery and vein

Marginal mandibular branch, facial nerve

Submandibular gland

Hyoid bone

Digastric muscle (anterior belly)

Sternocleidomastoid muscle

Omohyoid muscle

Sternohyoid muscle

Sternothyroid muscle

ANTERIOR APPROACH TO THE CERVICOTHORACIC JUNCTION (C7–T3)

Indications/Contraindications

The anterior approach to the cervicothoracic junction is limited by the manubrium, sternum, and great vessels of the mediastinum. Neoplastic or infectious disorders often destroy the anterior column of the spine, so this approach may be useful in addressing those pathologic entities. Anterior reconstruction techniques as well as instrumentation can be utilized within the limits for distal fixation afforded by the anatomy. Because the cervicothoracic junction is normally kyphotic, the use of additional posterior instrumentation is often recommended. Degenerative conditions, primarily affecting the C7–T1 level, are often best approached via this low cervical anterior approach. To get at the posterior pathoanatomy at C7–T1 or T1–T2, it may be necessary to perform a corpectomy so as to visualize and resect the pertinent problem areas, rather than to try to visualize the posterior portion of the disc level with a difficult line of sight for discectomy alone.

Preoperative Preparation

Imaging studies must be carefully examined to predict what is achievable with this low anterior cervicothoracic approach (9). Sagittal images show the relationship of the manubrium, sternum, and clavicle to the upper thoracic and lower cervical spine. Simple lines drawn perpendicular to the manubrium at its uppermost border simulates a surgeon's line of sight to the upper thoracic vertebrae. This line usually lands at the T2–T3 disc space but can be variable depending on body

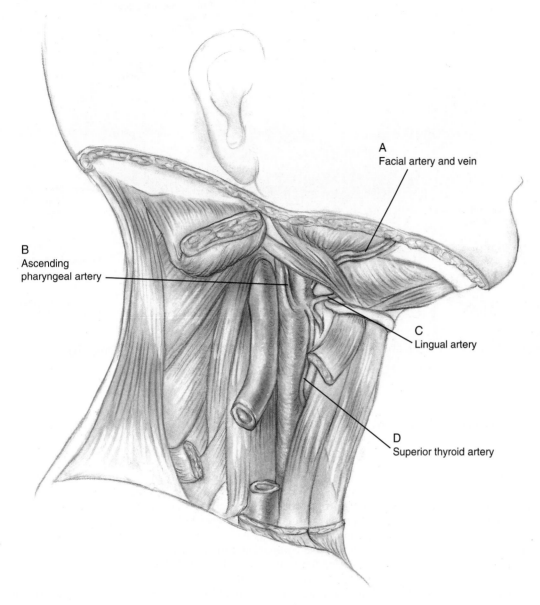

A
Facial artery and vein

B
Ascending
pharyngeal artery

C
Lingual artery

D
Superior thyroid artery

FIGURE 1-11

The plane of dissection progresses between the carotid sheath and the esophagus/ larynx medially, just as in the lower cervical approach. The difference is that numerous anteriorly projecting branch vessels from the carotid and internal jugular must be ligated before this plane can be adequately developed. These include, from cranial to caudad, the (*A*) facial artery and vein, (*B*) ascending pharyngeal artery and vein, (*C*) lingual artery and vein, and (*D*) superior thyroid artery and vein.

habitus. Preoperative planning should suggest whether partial manubriectomy or a sternal splitting approach would be preferable to a low anterior transverse incision alone. If removal of the manubrium or the medial clavicle is a possibility, then prudence would warrant a cardiothoracic surgeon to be available.

Technique

Positioning on the operating table is the same as the standard anterior approach to the cervical spine. A roll is typically placed in between the shoulder blades to help the shoulders retract. The head is placed in slight extension and rotated away from the surgeons if there is not severe cervical stenosis that would make this positioning dangerous. Prepping of the surgical field is obviously larger if a manubriectomy or sternal splitting approach is possible. Three different incisions can be utilized depending on the particular case. A low transverse incision immediately above the clavicle can provide excellent access to C7 and T1 in most patients. The dissection here is the same as for the approach in the midcervical spine. If exposure from C7 to T3 is needed, then an L-shaped incision can be used. A midline vertical incision from the midsternum or manubrium is made to 1 cm above the sternal notch and then is carried laterally, along a line in 1 cm proximal to the clavicle. This transverse limb is carried past the border of the sternocleidomastoid to the midclavicle if needed. If extensile exposure to the middle and upper cervical spine is necessary, then a full-length longitudinal incision along the medial border of the sternocleidomastoid, starting from the upper cervical

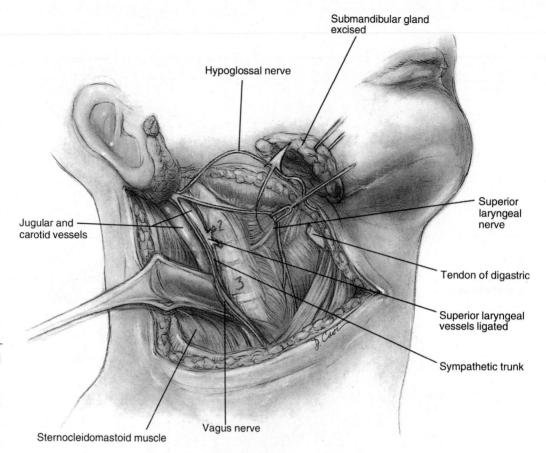

Submandibular gland
excised

Hypoglossal nerve

Superior
laryngeal
nerve

Jugular and
carotid vessels

Tendon of digastric

Superior laryngeal
vessels ligated

Sympathetic trunk

Sternocleidomastoid muscle

Vagus nerve

FIGURE 1-12

The hypoglossal nerve lies deep to the stylo-hyoid and digastric muscles and emerges from the carotid sheath deep to the internal jugular vein but superficial to the carotid artery. It must be dissected free along its path to allow it to be safely retracted superiorly.

spine, can be carried all the way down to the sternal notch and distally in the midline of the sternum (Fig. 1-13).

For the L-shaped incision, the vertical component over the sternum and manubrium will cut through skin, subcutaneous tissue, and fascia over the bone. Subperiosteal dissection along the anterior surface of the manubrium and sternum is carried lateral enough to expose the sterno-clavicular joints. The L-shaped transverse component will be carried through skin, subcutaneous tissue, and platysma as in the standard Smith-Robinson dissection. The superficial cervical fascia is incised transversely and the deep cervical fascia incised superiorly and inferiorly. Dissection medial to the sternocleidomastoid and lateral to the trachea and esophagus is carried deeper to the alar fascia. Continued dissection will expose the prevertebral fascia and the anterior cervico-thoracic spine.

As its name implies, the sternocleidomastoid has one head that inserts in the proximal manu-brium and the more lateral head directly into the medial clavicle. These tendons are released with electrocautery, being careful to avoid external jugular veins, which may be ligated as needed. The sternohyoid and sternothyroid muscles insert into the deep surface of the manubrium, which are also carefully released and tagged (Fig. 1-14).

If the medial portion of the clavicle is to be removed (13,26) (Fig. 1-15), the anterior periosteum is dissected with cautery to the junction of the medial and middle thirds. Subperiosteal posterior dissection should be done with a small Cobb elevator with great care since the subclavian artery and vein are immediately deep to the clavicle. If this circumferential subperiosteal dissection is first done at the clavicular osteotomy site, then the medial portion of the clavicle can be gently elevated to assist in further posterior subperiosteal dissection toward the sternoclavicular joint, which aids in visualization. The clavicle can then be sharply disarticulated from the manubrium.

Resection of the manubrium can leave both sternoclavicular joints or, if a partial medial resection of the clavicle is preferred, then the opposite sternoclavicular joint should be maintained. The anterior cortex and cancellous bone of the manubrium can be removed with a high-speed burr. This process makes subperiosteal dissection of the posterior cortex easier, and it can be removed with Kerrison

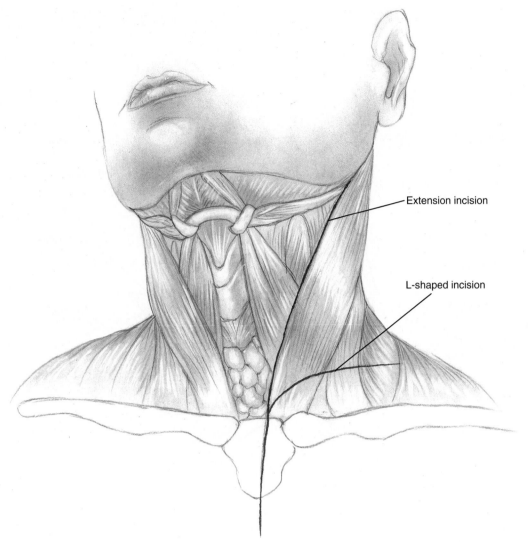

Extension incision

L-shaped incision

FIGURE 1-13

Two different incisions can be made. If extensile exposure of the entire cervical spine down to the upper thoracic spine is necessary, then an incision is made along the medial border of the sternocleidomastoid muscle down to its insertion into the clavicle. This then joins a midline incision along the midsternum up to 1 cm proximal to the sternal notch. If exposure of only C7–T3 is necessary, then an L-shaped incision is made.

rongeurs. The posterior periosteum ideally is left intact to protect the great vessels and thymus. Dissection to the spine is now similar to that performed in the midcervical area, with incising the deep cervical fascia, dissecting between the carotid sheath and the trachea/esophagus, through the alar fascia to the prevertebral fascia and to the spine. Long, thin Deaver-type or Wiley-type handheld retractors are utilized to achieve and maintain exposure of these cervicothoracic vertebrae (Fig. 1-16). Longus colli is dissected subperiosteally with cautery exposing the lateral aspects of the anterior vertebral bodies. After the operative procedure is performed, the strap muscles and heads of the sternocleidomastoids are reapproximated to the thick periosteal sleeve deep to the manubrium and clavicle. A small drain is typically used and the layers are closed as described earlier for the standard midcervical approach.

The options for the specific anterior approach to the cervicothoracic junction are as follows: (a) low transverse cervical (standard Smith-Robinson), (b) sternal splitting, (c) partial removal of the manubrium, (d) removal of medial clavicle, (e) removal of medial clavicle and partial manubriectomy, and (f) transthoracic approach (12).

Which of these specific approaches are utilized will depend on the pathoanatomy of the patient's problem and the patient's body habitus. In this author's experience, most pathology requiring removal of the T1 body with reconstruction and fixation into T2 is achievable through a low transverse incision. The benefits of this incision and dissection are that it is comparable to the midcervical approach and is thus familiar to spine surgeons. The advantages of the sternal splitting approach is that it is fast and routine for cardiothoracic surgeons and provides a maximum expo-

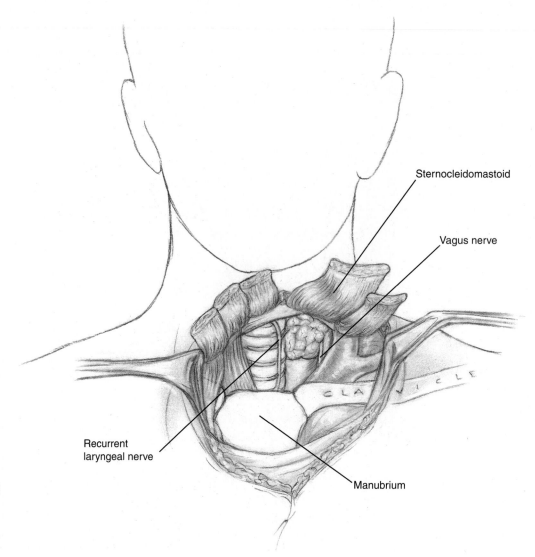

Sternocleidomastoid

Vagus nerve

Recurrent
laryngeal nerve

Manubrium

FIGURE 1-14

The plane deep to the platysma is developed above and below, creating generous flaps. These are then reflected proximally and distally and tagged with suture to the opposing skin to maintain retraction.

sure down to T4. A partial median sternotomy (of the manubrium) and a transverse osteotomy through the synostosis of the manubrium and sternum have also been described (6). Removal of the medial portion of the clavicle creates adequate exposure but has a potential downside of shoulder instability and pain. Authors have described raising a flap of the medial clavicle and manubrium for exposure and replacing the bone flap and using K-wires for stabilization (23). This technique is certainly an option but seems more complex than partial manubriectomy or median sternotomy in this author's opinion. The lateral transthoracic approach should not be forgotten as it is familiar to most spine surgeons and certainly to thoracic surgeons. Removal of the third rib and retraction of the scapula cephalad, which may require release of some rhomboid attachments, allows for visualization up to T1 and down into the midthoracic spine. Body habitus plays a role in the ease of this approach. Though not described in this chapter, posterolateral techniques with wide costotransversectomies and lateral extracavitary approaches have become more popular over the past decade to treat conditions that may be difficult to approach anteriorly at the cervicothoracic levels.

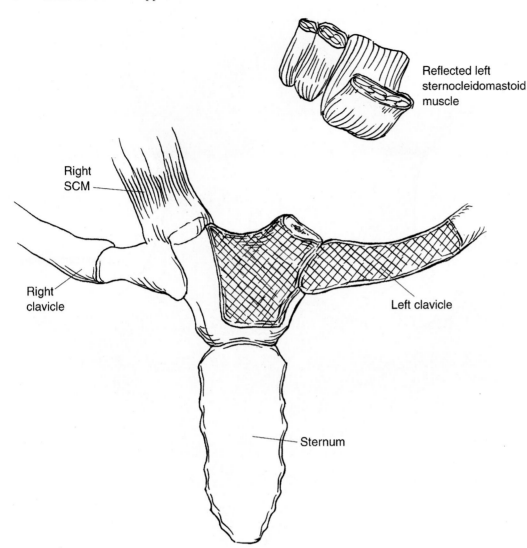

Reflected left
sternocleidomastoid
muscle

Right
SCM

Right
clavicle

Left clavicle

Sternum

FIGURE 1-15
The manubrium is
marked for resection as
necessary, which should
leave the contralateral
sternoclavicular joint
and a thin border of
bone on that side intact.
Distally, the cut should
extend approximately
3 to 4 cm, essentially
removing a rectangle of
bone from the proximal
sternum.

Postoperative Management

Prophylactic antibiotic usage and drain management are similar to other anterior cervical procedures and vary per surgeon preference. Postoperative airway management is also similar to midcervical spine procedures. Whether bracing or adjunct posterior cervicothoracic stabilization is needed
will depend on the individual case and surgeon preference.

Complications

Injury to the great vessels, particularly the venous structures behind the manubrium and sternum, is
an unavoidable risk. Meticulous subperiosteal dissection can minimize this risk. As stated earlier,
available backup with cardiothoracic surgical expertise should be arranged preoperatively. The RLN
can be stretched from retractors on either side. From a left-sided approach, the thoracic duct can be
injured, which if not recognized could lead to development of chylothorax. Injury to the esophagus
and complaints of dysphagia postoperatively are possible as with the standard anterior midcervical
approach.

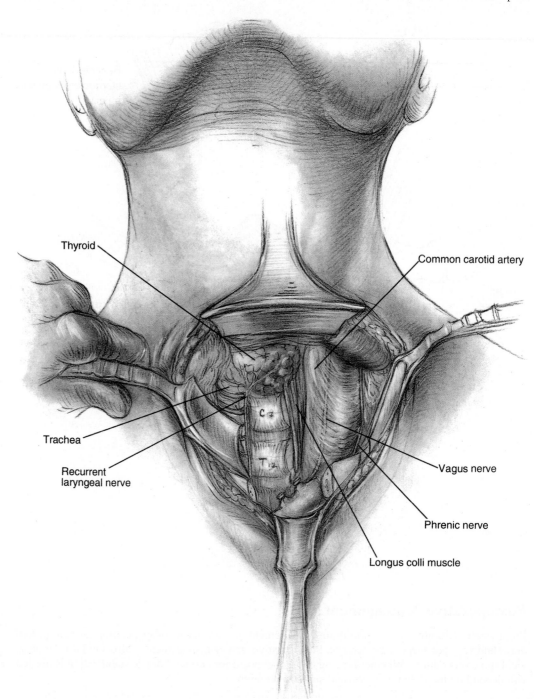

Thyroid

Common carotid artery

Trachea

Recurrent
laryngeal nerve

Vagus nerve

Phrenic nerve

Longus colli muscle

FIGURE 1-16

Handheld retractors
can be used for medial-
lateral retraction. A disc
space is identified and
marked with a spinal
needle. Subperiosteal
dissection is continued
as described previously
to elevate the longus
colli off the anterior
surface of the vertebral
bodies.

RECOMMENDED READING

1. Apfelbaum RI, Kriskovich MD, Haller JR: On the incidence, cause, and prevention of recurrent laryngeal nerve palsies during anterior cervical spine surgery. *Spine* 25: 2906–2912, 2000.
2. Audu P, Artz G, Scheid S, et al.: Recurrent laryngeal nerve palsy after anterior cervical spine surgery: the impact of endotracheal tube cuff deflation, reinflation, and pressure adjustment. *Anesthesiology* 105: 898–901, 2006.
3. Bazaz R, Lee MJ, Yoo JU: Incidence of dysphagia after cervical spine surgery: a prospective study. *Spine* 27: 2453–2458, 2002.
4. Beutler WJ, Sweeney CA, Connollt PJ: Recurrent laryngeal nerve injury with anterior cervical spine surgery: risk with laterality of surgical approach. *Spine* 26: 1337–1342, 2001.
5. Curylo LJ, Mason HC, Bohlman HH, et al.: Tortuous course of the vertebral artery and anterior cervical decompression: a cadaveric and clinical case study. *Spine* 25: 2860–2864, 2000.
6. Darling G, McBroom R, Perrin R: Modified anterior approach to the cervicothoracic junction. *Spine* 20: 1519–1521, 1995.
7. Ebrahein NA, Lu J, Yang H, et al.: Vulnerability of the sympathetic trunk during the anterior approach to the lower cervical spine. *Spine* 13: 1603–1606, 2000.

8. Emery SE, Akhavan S, Miller P, et al.: Steroids and risk factors for airway compromise in multilevel cervical corpectomy patients: a prospective, randomized, double-blind study. *Spine* 34: 229–232, 2009.
9. Fraser J, Diwan A, Peterson M, et al.: Preoperative magnetic resonance imaging screening for a surgical decision regarding the approach for the anterior spine fusion at the cervicothoracic junction. *Spine* 27: 675–681, 2002.
10. Goss CM, ed. *Gray's anatomy*, 29th ed. Philadelphia, PA: Lea & Febiger, 1973.
11. Hoppenfeld S, deBoer P: *Surgical exposures in orthopaedics: the anatomic approach*. Philadelphia, PA: JB Lippincott Company, 1984.
12. Kaya R, Turkmenoglu O, Kic O, et al.: A perspective for the selection of surgical approaches in patients with upper thoracic and cervicothoracic junction instabilities. *Surg Neurol* 65: 454–463, 2006.
13. Kurz L, Pursel S, Herkowitz H: Modified anterior approach to the cervicothoracic junction. *Spine* 16: S542–S547, 1991.
14. Laus M, Pignatti G, Malaguti MC, et al.: Anterior extraoral surgery to the upper cervical spine. *Spine* 21: 1687–1693, 1996.
15. Lee MJ, Bazaz R, Furey CG, et al.: Risk factors for dysphagia after anterior cervical spine surgery: a two-year prospective cohort study. *Spine J* 7: 141–147, 2007.
16. Leng LZ, Anand VK, Hartl R, et al.: Endonasal endoscopic resection of an os odontoideum to decompress the cervico-medullary junction: minimal access surgical technique. *Spine* 34: E139–E143, 2009.
17. Louis R: Anterior surgery of the upper cervical spine. *Chir Organi Mov* 77: 75–80, 1992.
18. McAfee PC, Bohlman HH, Riley LH, et al.: The anterior retropharyngeal approach to the upper part of the cervical spine. *J Bone Joint Surg Am* 69: 1371–1383, 1987.
19. Merwin G, Post J, Sypert G: Transoral approach to the upper cervical spine. *Laryngoscope* 101: 780–784, 1991.
20. Messina A, Bruno MC, Decq P, et al.: Pure endoscopic endonasal odontoidectomy: anatomical study. *Neurosurg Rev* 30: 189–194, 2007.
21. Netterville JL, Koriwchak MJ, Winkle M, et al.: Vocal fold paralysis following the anterior approach to the cervical spine. *Ann Otol Rhinol Laryngol* 105: 85–91, 1996.
22. Riley LH III, Skolasky RL, Albert TJ, et al.: Dysphagia after anterior cervical decompression and fusion: prevalence and risk factors from a longitudinal cohort study. *Spine* 30: 2564–2569, 2005.
23. Sar C, Hamzaoglu A, Talu U, et al.: An anterior approach to the cervicothoracic junction of the spine (modified osteotomy of manubrium sterni and clavicle). *J Spinal Disorders* 12: 102–106, 1999.
24. Smith GW, Robinson RA: The treatment of certain cervical-spine disorders by anterior removal of the intervertebral disc and interbody fusion. *J Bone Joint Surg Am* 40: 607–624, 1958.
25. Succo G, Solini A, Crosetti E, et al.: Enlarged approach to the anterior cervical spine. *J Laryngol Otol* 115: 994–997, 2001.
26. Sundaresan N, Shah J, Foley K, et al.: An anterior surgical approach to the upper thoracic vertebrae. *J Neurosurg* 61: 686–690, 1984.
27. Vender JR, Harrison SJ, McDonnell DE: Fusion and instrumentation at C1-3 via the high anterior cervical approach. *J Neurosurg (Spine)* 92: 24–29, 2000.
28. Vishteh AG, Beals SP, Joganic EF, et al.: Bilateral sagittal split mandibular osteotomies as an adjunct to the transoral approach to the anterior craniovertebral junction. [Technical note]. *J Neurosurg* 90: 267–270, 1999.
29. Winslow CP, Meyers AD: Otolaryngologic complications of the anterior approach to the cervical spine. *Am J Otolaryngol* 20: 16–27, 1999.

2 Anterior Cervical Discectomy and Fusion

Christopher K. Kepler and Todd J. Albert

INDICATIONS/CONTRAINDICATIONS

Anterior cervical discectomy and fusion (ACDF) is indicated to relieve anterior-based compression of either the spinal cord or nerve roots causing (a) cervical radiculopathy unresponsive to 8 to 12 weeks of nonoperative treatment; (b) cervical radiculopathy with a progressive neurologic deficit; or (c) cervical myelopathy. Prior to any surgical procedure, appropriate imaging studies must be obtained that demonstrate neural element compression that is consistent with the patient's clinical presentation. Although expectant management is sometimes employed by spine surgeons in the treatment of cervical myelopathy, it is our practice to operate on patients with myelopathy in a relatively expedient manner given the relative frequency of progression of symptoms and the uncertain recovery of function. Additionally, ACDF may be performed to treat certain traumatic injuries including central cord syndrome and some types of extension-distraction injuries.

Contraindications to ACDF include (a) anterior compression that is not confined to the disc space or the area immediately adjacent to the disc space and (b) anatomic or approach-related concerns that preclude anterior surgery. A relative contraindication is the requirement for decompression at more than three levels because of the increasing risk of nonunion with more operative levels.

PREOPERATIVE PLANNING

Prior to indicating patients for surgery, the surgeon must take a careful history and perform a physical examination with the goal of determining what spinal levels are likely to be causing the patient's presenting signs and symptoms. Concordance between the patient's presentation and imaging findings is increasingly important as improvements in magnetic resonance imaging (MRI) allows detailed anatomic visualization and frequently identifies spine pathology in asymptomatic individuals (1).

Disc herniation or spondylosis at the C2–C3 level leads to compression of the C3 nerve root, which does not have a motor component. C3 radiculopathy is most often manifested as pain but is rare, in part due to the relative capaciousness of the spinal canal at this level. C3–C4 disease causing C4 radiculopathy also lacks a motor component but typically results in pain along the top of the shoulder or trapezius region. C4–C5 disc herniation or spondylosis causes C5 radiculopathy which is most often associated with weakness of the deltoid and pain/numbness in the upper arm that may radiate into the radial aspect of the forearm. Disc herniation or spondylosis at C5–C6 leads to a C6 radiculopathy. Patients with C6 radiculopathy present with weakness in the biceps or wrist extensors, decreased or absent biceps tendon reflex, and forearm and hand pain/numbness, classically including the thumb and forefinger. C6–C7 is the most commonly affected cervical level and causes a C7 radiculopathy that most commonly leads to triceps or wrist flexion weakness, diminished triceps reflexes, and forearm or hand pain/numbness affecting the long finger. Finally, C8 radiculopathy is caused by either disc herniation or spondylosis at the C7–T1 level and results in finger flexion weakness and pain/numbness in the forearm extending into the ring and small fingers.

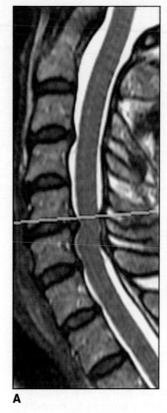

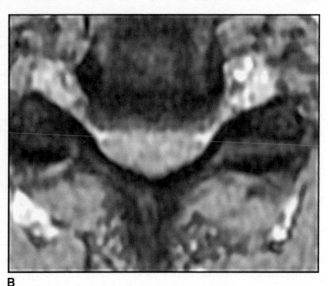

A　　　　　　　　　B

FIGURE 2-1

Sagittal **(A)** and axial **(B)** T2-weighted MRI images demonstrating large herniated disc at C5–C6 causing spinal cord compression.

Patient with cervical myelopathy may or may not also complain of symptoms of cervical radiculopathy in which case localization of levels may be done as described above. Common presenting symptoms of patients with cervical myelopathy include imbalance, difficulty with fine motor tasks, generalized bilateral hand numbness, and difficulty holding objects. More rarely, patients complain of urinary or bowel symptoms. Pertinent exam findings include the presence of pathologic reflexes such as Hoffmann sign or Babinski sign, diminished upper extremity reflexes and enhanced lower extremity reflexes, or ankle clonus.

All patients should initially undergo anteroposterior, neutral lateral, flexion lateral, and extension lateral radiographs. Plain radiographs are essential to evaluate the standing alignment of the cervical spine, identify levels of dynamic instability, and evaluate for the presence of congenital stenosis. Patients who cannot extend to at least neutral cervical alignment must undergo anterior column reconstruction and should not be treated solely via posterior-approach surgery as laminectomy will not decompress the spinal cord in a kyphotic spine. MRI is most commonly used to evaluate the degree and location of neural element compression (Fig. 2-1), but computed tomography scan may be used in those patients with contraindications to MRI, preferably after myelogram to improve identification of sites with compressive lesions.

Surgical levels for patients being treated for radiculopathy should be selected based on concordance between presenting symptoms and imaging findings. When patients are being treated for myelopathy, all levels causing spinal cord compression should be addressed to offer the best chance to arrest symptoms. Finally, it is our practice to carefully consider inclusion of adjacent levels with advanced degeneration that are indeterminate with regard to contribution to radiculopathic symptoms. Hilibrand et al. demonstrated that such levels in the adjacent cervical spine are likely to continue to degenerate, resulting in adjacent-level disease (2).

TECHNIQUE

General anesthesia is administered, and the endotracheal tube is taped at the corner of the patient's mouth and retracted contralaterally and superiorly. The authors' preference for primary ACDF is to tape the tube in the right corner of the mouth to facilitate a left-sided approach in order to minimize the risk of injury to the recurrent laryngeal nerve as this structure is more reliably protected within the tracheoesophageal interval on the left side. Care should be taken that a line connecting the bottom lip and the inferior aspect of the ear is free of tape as this will define the superior border of the surgical field. Next, bony prominences and any intravenous lines are padded, and

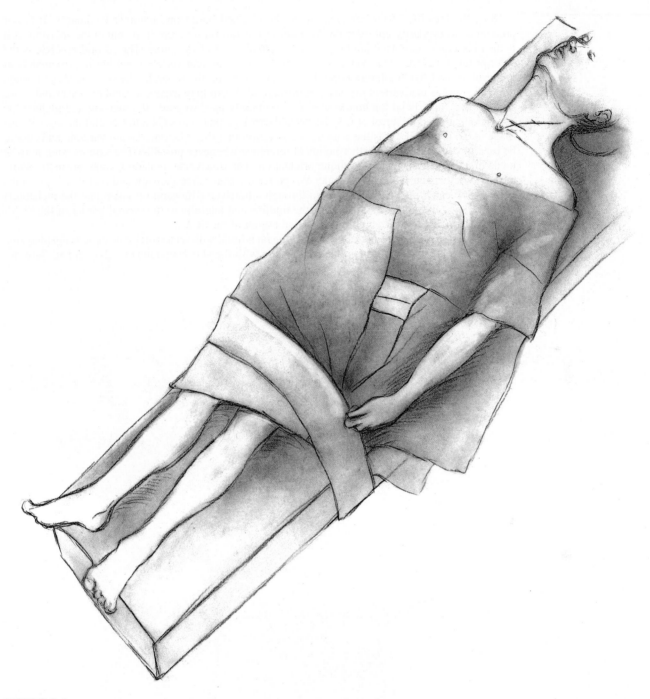

FIGURE 2-2

Position for a left-sided anterior approach. Note that the neck is extended, the arms are tucked at the side, and the ipsilateral iliac crest can be draped out if necessary. Wide tape can be used to depress the shoulders to facilitate visualization of lower cervical levels for identification using an intraoperative radiograph.

the arms are tucked at the sides. The neuromonitoring personnel should obtain a postintubation, prepositioning set of motor evoked potentials to establish baseline readings. Next the shoulders are retracted inferiorly using tape to optimize visualization on the localization radiograph. The neck is extended to open the disc spaces anteriorly via increased lordosis (Fig. 2-2). This maneuver, however, slightly decreases the cross-sectional area of the central canal, so a set of motor evoked potentials should be obtained after final positioning. If there is any decrease in signal amplitude, the neck position is adjusted into less or no extension and the motor evoked potentials are rechecked. The draping should include both sternocleidomastoid (SCM) muscles and the sternal notch in the surgical field, and the iliac crest should also be prepped and draped if autograft bone is to be used.

Next, the location of the incision should be planned based on anatomic landmarks. It is our preference to primarily consider the location of the carotid tubercle in planning the incision as it is the only commonly used landmark that is actually part of the spine. The carotid tubercle is the anterior tubercle of the transverse process of the sixth cervical vertebra and lies approximately at the level of the C5–C6 intervertebral disc. While palpating the tubercle, the surgeon should watch the vital signs as inadvertent pressure on the carotid sheath may trigger a vagal response and cause bradycardia. Superficial landmarks are also commonly used to guide the incision and include the hyoid bone around the level of C3, the thyroid cartilage that spans C4 and C5, and the cricoid cartilage at C6 (Fig. 2-3). It is the authors' observation that these landmarks are variable and should be used in conjunction with other points of reference whenever possible. The skin incision may be made in either a transverse or oblique orientation. The transverse incision is more cosmetic while the oblique incision is more extensile. We prefer the transverse incision and feel that up to four-level ACDF can typically be performed through a transverse incision provided that the incision is carried a few millimeters medially past the midline and laterally to the medial border of the SCM. An oblique incision is made along the medial border of the SCM.

After the skin incision is made, the underlying fat is bluntly dissected off of the underlying platysma muscle. We prefer to divide the platysma in line with the skin incision (Fig. 2-4). Small flaps are

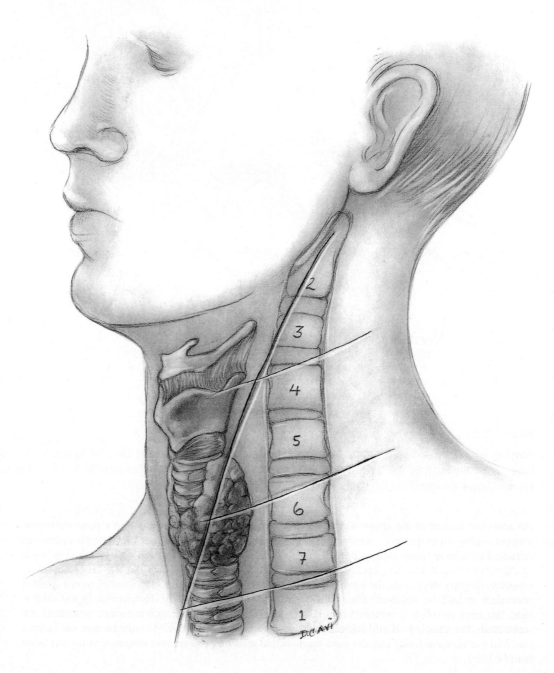

FIGURE 2-3

Superficial landmarks are helpful in planning the skin incision but should be used in conjunction with the carotid tubercle, which is the anterior tubercle of the transverse process of C6. The hyoid bone is approximately at the level of C3, the thyroid cartilage spans C4–C5, and the cricoid cartilage lies at approximately C6.

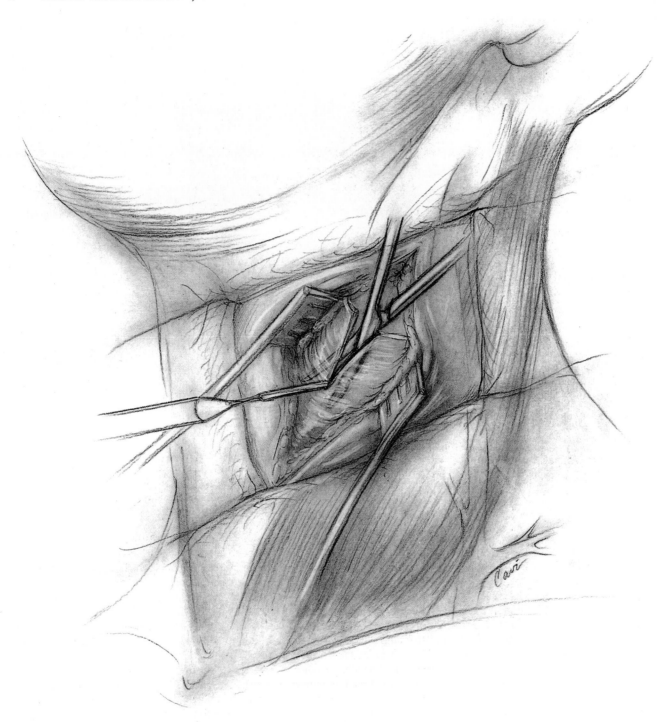

FIGURE 2-4

Transverse skin incision exposing the platysma muscle, which is incised transversely with electrocautery.

raised above and below the platysma to assist in identification of this layer during closure. Next the interval between the strap muscles medially and the SCM laterally is identified by dissecting using Metzenbaum scissors (Fig. 2-5). Release of connective tissue that overlies the interval between the strap muscles and the SCM is critical when utilizing a transverse incision for more than two-level ACDF. Surgeons performing procedures in the lower cervical spine may encounter the omohyoid muscle belly passing obliquely from superomedial to inferolateral across the surgical field—this muscle may be transected using electrocautery to provide greater visualization (usually we do not find this necessary) of the spine but should be the only muscle transected beside the platysma. The carotid sheath is identified through gentle palpation of the patient's pulse along the medial border of the SCM, and the anterior border of the spine can also be palpated medial to the carotid sheath. The interval between the medial border of the carotid sheath and the lateral border of the strap muscles

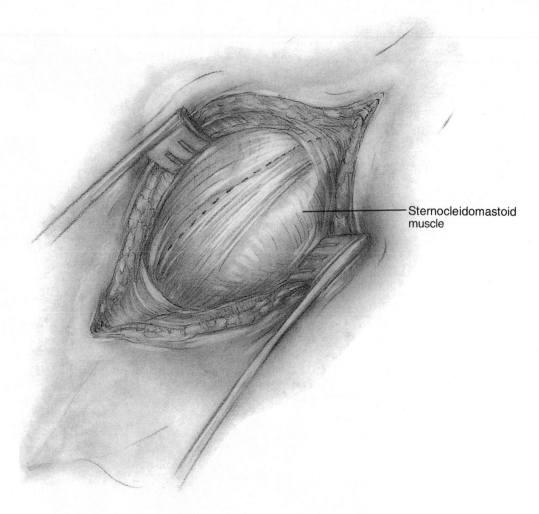

Sternocleidomastoid
muscle

FIGURE 2-5

The superficial cervical
fascia is incised medial
to the SCM muscle.

should be freed throughout the entire extent of the incision to facilitate an extensile exposure of the spine (Fig. 2-6).

Next, an appendiceal retractor is used to retract the trachea and esophagus and strap muscles medially. The spine is again palpated directly through the prevertebral fascia to identify the midline, and Metzenbaum scissors are used to incise the prevertebral fascia in the midline. Next, we use a Kittner dissector to clear the prevertebral fascia from the midline and identify the disc spaces. Careful study of the preoperative lateral radiograph is often useful to use unique osteophyte geography in identification of the surgical level(s). Care should be taken not to disrupt the disc space during this initial dissection as it can lead to subsequent disc degeneration if a nonoperative level is injured. Next, we place a bent spinal needle into the disc space and perform an intraoperative lateral radiograph to identify levels (Fig. 2-7). It is important to use all available information to place the needle into a disc space that is to be fused; iatrogenic annulotomy by spinal needles placed at the wrong level has been suggested to contribute to early disc degeneration (4).

After identification of the correct level(s), the prevertebral fascia is elevated off the vertebral bodies using electrocautery, taking care not to disrupt the cranial and caudal disc spaces, which are not to be included in the fusion. The longus colli is similarly elevated off the vertebral bodies and disc spaces. The longus colli should be elevated in a single flap to provide a location to place side-to-side retractors and should not be elevated past the lateral border of the vertebral bodies and disc spaces to avoid injury to the sympathetic chain. Once this exposure is completed, side-to-side self-retaining retractors are placed.

Next, the discectomy is performed. First, a rectangular annulotomy is made with a no. 15 scalpel blade on a long handle (Fig. 2-8). Using a pituitary rongeur and no. 3 Kerrison rongeur, the majority of the disc can be removed (Fig. 2-9A). The Kerrison rongeur is particularly helpful for cleaning out superficial to the uncovertebral joints, an essential step for identification of the midline. A cervical Cobb elevator is inserted into the disc space and rotated against the endplates to loosen up levels stiffened by advanced spondylosis. After the uncovertebral joint away from the primary surgeon has been cleaned of all disc material, a small intervertebral spreader is placed to the far lateral aspect of the uncovertebral joint and opened to improve visualization of the posterior disc

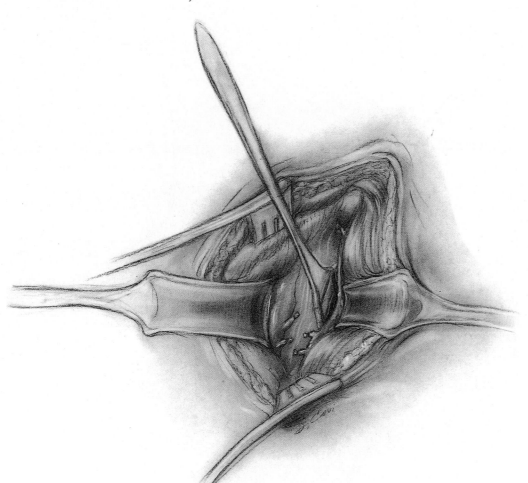

FIGURE 2-6

The carotid sheath is retracted laterally while the esophagus and trachea are retracted medially, and a subperiosteal dissection of the prevertebral and longus colli is completed using both blunt dissection and electrocautery.

space. Caspar retractors are equally helpful for this purpose. Straight and curved curettes are used to remove residual disc and the cartilaginous portion of the endplates, taking care not to disrupt the bony endplate (Figs. 2-9 and 2-10). A burr is usually used to very gently decorticate but not disrupt the bony endplate. Often, we use a burr before removal of the posteriormost aspects of the disc in order to eliminate posterior osteophytes that protrude into the disc space, obscure the true posterior border of the vertebral bodies, and inhibit access to the neural canal. Particular care must be taken to resect uncovertebral osteophytes that may compress exiting nerves in the neural foramen, being wary that excessive lateral resection can endanger the vertebral artery. We routinely resect both the posterior annulus and posterior longitudinal ligament (PLL) in order to directly visualize decompression of the dura and spinal cord. The annulus and PLL are sometimes already disrupted, in which case a 1- or 2-mm Kerrison rongeur can be used to remove these structures. If the annulus and PLL are intact, a small curved curette is used to create a vertical rent in both the residual annulus and PLL. A blunt nerve hook helps to define this interval, and a 1- or 2-mm Kerrison rongeur is then used to remove the annulus and PLL. The nerve hook is carefully passed behind the cranial and caudal vertebral bodies to evaluate whether disc material or posterior osteophytes continue to cause spinal cord compression. Disc material behind the body can usually be delivered into the disc space and removed using a nerve hood while posterior osteophytes causing significant compression may require more aggressive resection of the posterior vertebral margins to remove the compressive portions via partial corpectomy. At the lateral border of each disc space, a 2-mm Kerrison rongeur is used to ensure an adequate foraminal decompression, and we use a blunt nerve hook to palpate each neural foramen. A brief rush of blood when the nerve hook is passed into the foramen is an indication that the decompression has extended to the lateral vascular leash and has adequately freed the exiting nerve root.

With the decompression performed and the endplates prepared to accept a graft, we use trial rasps to determine the appropriate size graft. Depending on surgeon preference, either lordotic or parallel grafts can be placed and the corresponding rasps should be used. Beginning with a 6-mm trial rasp, we sequentially rasp until the rasp fits snugly within the disc space. The disc space

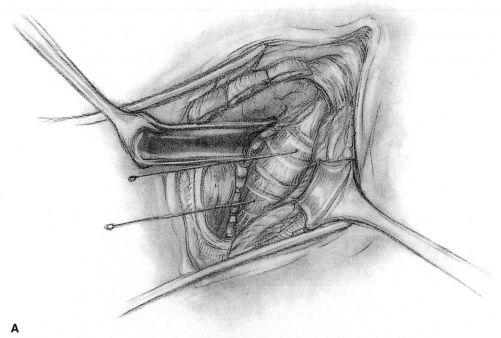

A

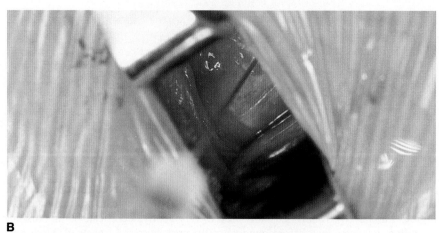

B

FIGURE 2-7

A,B: A spinal needle is placed into the disc space at the level thought to be the operative level before taking a lateral radiograph to confirm the correct level.

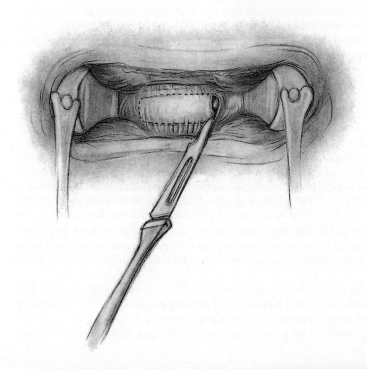

FIGURE 2-8

Exposure of the disc space is complete, and a scalpel is used to initiate disc removal.

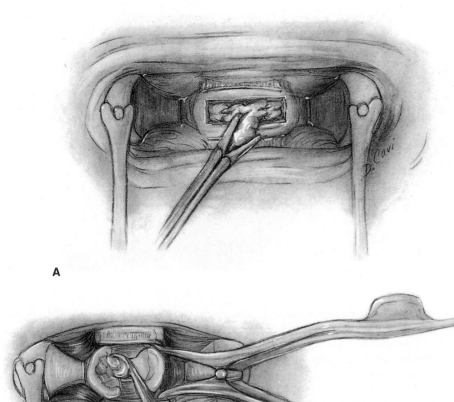

A

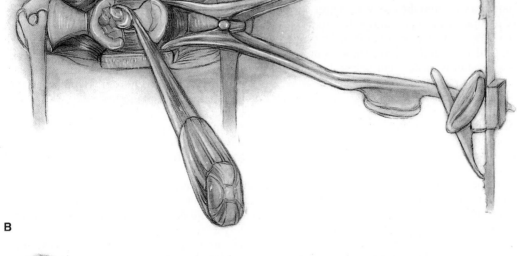

B

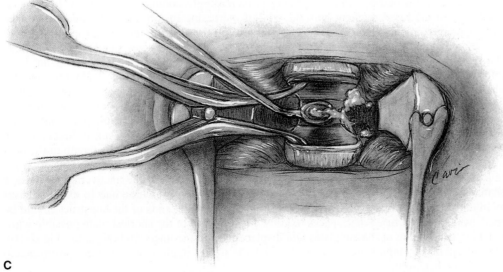

C

FIGURE 2-9

A–C: The disc and cartilaginous endplates are removed with a combination of pituitary rongeurs and curettes. A small lamina spreader improves the exposure and access to the neural canal.

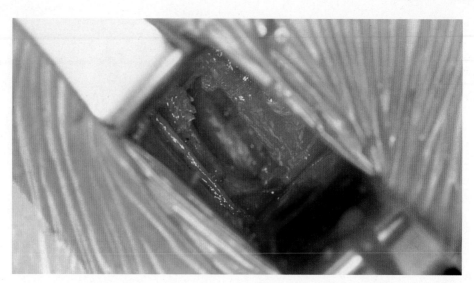

FIGURE 2-10

Surgical view of Figure 2-8.

depth should be measured using depth gauge. If allograft is to be used, the graft size is selected and the graft customized if necessary using a burr or sagittal saw. Intervertebral spacers were classically fashioned from autologous iliac crest that was cut to fit the disc space. Although we have moved away from the use of autograft due to concerns over donor site morbidity, the availability of accurately machined allograft, and increasing evidence that there is no difference in outcome, the harvest of iliac crest autograft is simple, yields excellent intervertebral spacers, and may be particularly useful in heavy smokers in whom concern about nonunion is heightened (Fig. 2-11). An incision is made 1 cm below the anterior iliac crest, taking care to begin the incision 3 cm posterior to the anterior-superior iliac spine in order to avoid injuring the lateral femoral cutaneous nerve. The fascia overlying the crest is incised longitudinally with electrocautery and fascial flaps raised in a subcutaneous manner to expose the inner and outer tables of the crest. Using an oscillating saw, a wedge approximately 2 mm wider than the size needed is harvested using vertical cuts approximately 20 mm deep. After the transverse cut is made to complete the harvest, bone wax is applied to the cut cancellous surfaces to stop bony bleeding and the wound is closed in layers.

We prefer a lordotic graft as the wedged shape facilitates insertion (Fig. 2-12). An upward force on the patient's chin will typically provide enough distraction to allow graft insertion. The graft is seated to its final position using a tamp and mallet and should be countersunk beyond the natural anterior border of the vertebral bodies by approximately 2 mm (Fig. 2-13), taking care to consider anterior osteophytes that must be removed if using an anterior plate to allow the plate to sit flush against the vertebral bodies. Anterior plating is increasingly common after ACDF to increase the stiffness of the fused segment with the goal of increasing fusion rate and reducing reliance on postoperative bracing (Fig. 2-14) (8,9). After seating the graft(s), the shortest plate that will span the cranial and caudal disc spaces is selected so as to keep the screws and ends of the plate as far from the preserved disc spaces as possible as plate proximity to adjacent levels has been implicated in the development of adjacent-level ossification disease (5) (Fig. 2-15). Osteophytes at the vertebral margins must be removed using a burr to create a flat surface to receive the plate. Although there are many plate designs available, one principal decision the surgeon must make is whether to use a static or dynamic plate. If possible, we prefer to use a dynamic plate that allows load sharing with the intervertebral graft to encourage loading and may result in higher fusion rates. Screw length can be estimated based on the localization radiograph if the length of the bent portion of the spinal needle is known; the goal is to select the longest unicortical screw possible. The plate should be centered on the vertebral body—visualization of the uncovertebral joints is essential for centering the plate. Lateral screws may have poor purchase and in extreme cases may injury the vertebral artery. Screws at the cranial and caudal ends of the construct should be angled away from the fused disc spaces to allow for selection of the shortest plate possible without risking penetration of the endplates and displacement of the intervertebral grafts (Fig. 2-16). Many current plates employ mechanisms that lock the screws in place once they are positioned to prevent screw back-out.

Intraoperative anteroposterior and lateral radiographs are then obtained to ensure correct placement of the grafts and plate. The wound is copiously irrigated although infection rates for ACDF are very low. A drain is placed and the platysma as well as a layered skin closure is performed.

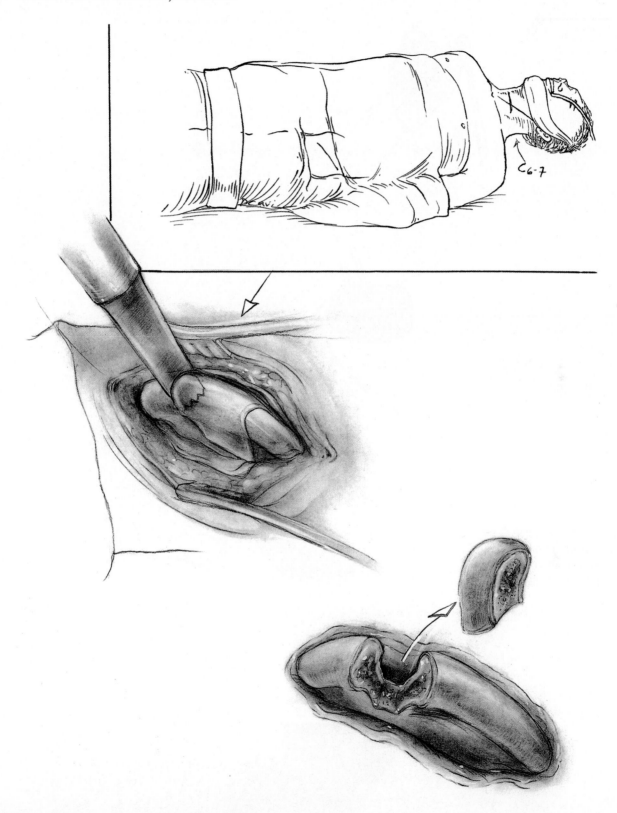

FIGURE 2-11

A tricortical iliac crest bone graft. The graft should be harvested at least 3 cm posterior to the anterior superior iliac spine to avoid injury to the lateral femoral cutaneous nerve.

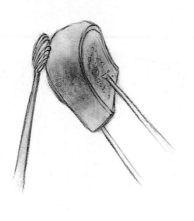

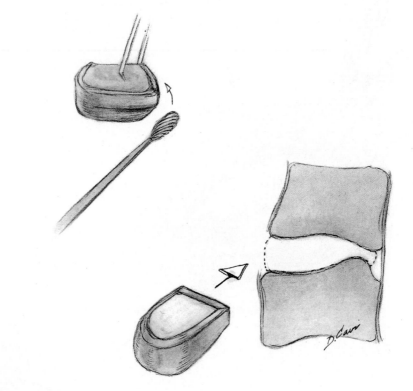

FIGURE 2-12

When a graft is either harvested from the iliac crest or fashioned out of a larger piece of allograft bone, we prefer to bevel the posterior aspect of the graft to make a lordotic-shaped graft.

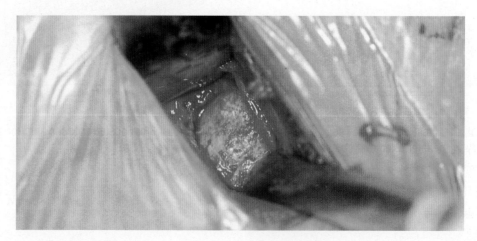

FIGURE 2-13

The graft is inserted into the disc space; when using iliac crest autograft, the iliac crest cortex is positioned anteriorly.

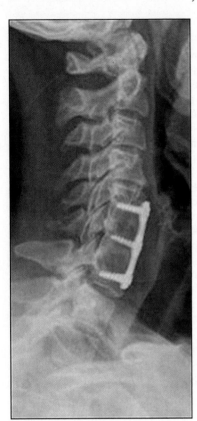

FIGURE 2-14

Lateral radiograph demonstrating anterior cervical plate with evidence of solid fusion across C5–C7.

POSTOPERATIVE MANAGEMENT

After surgery, the patient is placed in a cervical collar. For one- and two-level surgeries, we utilize a soft foam collar. For patients who undergo ACDF at more than two levels, we utilize a hard collar. Patients are started on soft/dysphagia diets initially although this is advanced if they do not have difficulty swallowing after surgery. Ambulation is encouraged on the day of surgery. Drains are typically removed the day after surgery, and most patients are also discharged home on the first day after surgery. We have found that no strict postoperative rehabilitation regimen is necessary other than aggressive mobilization to prevent the development of thromboembolic disease. Isometric neck strengthening begins coincident with the removal of the collar. Most patients can return to work within 6 weeks and often earlier depending on the demands of their occupation. By 3 months, most patients are cleared to return to full activity although postoperative radiographs must be carefully followed to ensure that fusion is achieved.

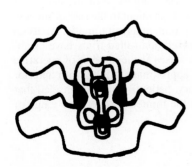

FIGURE 2-15

Schematic demonstrating proper position of cervical plate.

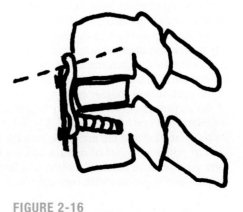

FIGURE 2-16

Angulation of the proximal and distal screws will enable the surgeon to keep the ends of the plate itself as far from the adjacent disc spaces as possible.

COMPLICATIONS

As surgeons have to use less autograft bone due to concerns over donor site morbidity, associated complications such as hematoma, infection, meralgia paresthetica (due to lateral femoral nerve injury), and chronic donor site pain are more uncommonly seen. The most common complication after ACDF is dysphagia. While most patients will have minor pain and/or difficulty with swallowing for the 1st weeks after surgery, this will resolve in 90% or more of patients by the 6 week mark. In patients with persistent dysphagia, a wide variety in residual symptoms are seen ranging from difficulty with certain foods to severe dysfunction requiring feeding tube placement in extreme cases. Another complication likely related to retraction during surgery is recurrent laryngeal nerve injury. Although this remains a subject of debate, many surgeons feel that a left-sided approach reduces the risk of recurrent laryngeal nerve injury due to the more protected location of the nerve. Patients who require revision anterior cervical surgery should undergo evaluation prior to surgery by an otolaryngologist; patients with full functional vocal folds can undergo surgery using a contralateral approach while those with evidence of recurrent nerve palsy should have surgery using the same side approach as the first operation to avoid injury to both recurrent laryngeal nerves.

Significant neurologic injury during ACDF is exceedingly rare. A recent survey of Scoliosis Research Society members reported acute neurologic injury after surgery in only 0.28% of cases, although this number may underreport the true incidence due to the need for self-reporting in this database (6). Spinal cord injury is even rarer as the majority of the deficits in this survey were related to isolated nerve root injuries that improved in the postoperative period.

Fear of vertebral artery injury should motivate careful analysis of the location of the vertebral arteries on preoperative imaging. Occasionally, anomalous vertebral pathways will place these structures at risk as the arteries curve into the disc space where they could be injured during discectomy. The pathway of each vertebral artery should be traced on preoperative MRI as a part of routine preoperative planning.

Although the incidence of graft extrusion has been curtailed by increasing use of anterior cervical plating, backing out of screws is occasionally seen and places the esophagus at risk. In addition to raising the specter of nonunion as screw movement is associated with instability, screws that are backing out should be removed in an expedient manner in order to preserve cervical structures.

As described above, the incidence of nonunion increases as more levels are grafted. The use of anterior cervical plating has decreased but not eliminated this problem. While patients with cervical nonunion must be monitored carefully for the development of associated symptoms, many patients with radiographic nonunion continue to enjoy excellent results and no intervention is necessary. Patients with risk factors for the development of nonunion such as diabetes or tobacco use should be counseled preoperatively about this risk, and consideration should be given to the use of autograft or a postoperative bone stimulator. Firm counseling about the benefits of smoking cessation will benefit patients in terms of both their likelihood of successful spine fusion and their general medical health.

RESULTS

ACDF is an effective treatment for the symptoms of cervical radiculopathy. Inasmuch as patients with myelopathy may have concomitant radicular symptoms, patients may note significant improvement in symptoms after ACDF for myelopathy, but patients must be reminded that the purpose of operating on patients with myelopathy is to halt progression of the disease with uncertain relief of any symptoms attributable to spinal cord compression. With regard to relief of arm pain, it is our experience that approximately 90% of patients will be satisfied after surgery with the degree of improvement in their symptoms. The rate of successful fusion is not equivalent to the rate of success of the operation as roughly half of patients who develop nonunion remain asymptomatic. Analysis of the control groups from recent total disc replacement randomized controlled trials have established a union rate of 95% for single-level ACDF (7); this rate decreases as the number of operative levels increases, and the nonunion rate for three-level ACDF is approximately 20% with anterior plating. Although range of motion will not be normal after surgery, patients can be counseled that their postoperative range of motion will improve compared with the limited preoperative range of motion seen in patients with cervical spondylosis (3).

RECOMMENDED READING

1. Boden SD, McCowin PR, Davis DO, et al.: Abnormal magnetic-resonance scans of the cervical spine in asymptomatic subjects. A prospective investigation. *J Bone Joint Surg Am* 72: 1178–1184, 1990.
2. Hilibrand AS, Carlson GD, Palumbo MA, et al.: Radiculopathy and myelopathy at segments adjacent to the site of a previous anterior cervical arthrodesis. *J Bone Joint Surg Am* 81: 519–528, 1999.

3. Hilibrand AS, Balasubramanian K, Eichenbaum M, et al.: The effect of anterior cervical fusion on neck motion. *Spine (Phila Pa 1976)* 31: 1688–1692, 2006.
4. Nassr A, Lee JY, Bashir RS, et al.: Does incorrect level needle localization during anterior cervical discectomy and fusion lead to accelerated disc degeneration? *Spine (Phila Pa 1976)* 34: 189–192, 2009.
5. Park JB, Cho YS, Riew KD: Development of adjacent-level ossification in patients with an anterior cervical plate. *J Bone Joint Surg Am* 87: 558–563, 2005.
6. Smith JS, Fu KM, Polly DW Jr, et al.: Complication rates of three common spine procedures and rates of thromboembolism following spine surgery based on 108,419 procedures: a report from the Scoliosis Research Society Morbidity and Mortality Committee. *Spine (Phila Pa 1976)* 35: 2140–2149, 2010.
7. Upadhyaya CD, Wu JC, Trost G, et al.: Analysis of the three United States Food and Drug Administration investigational device exemption cervical arthroplasty trials. *J Neurosurg Spine* 16: 216–228, 2012.
8. Wang JC, McDonough PW, Endow KK, et al.: Increased fusion rates with cervical plating for two-level anterior cervical discectomy and fusion. *Spine (Phila Pa 1976)* 25: 41–45, 2000.
9. Wang JC, McDonough PW, Kanim LE, et al.: Increased fusion rates with cervical plating for three-level anterior cervical discectomy and fusion. *Spine (Phila Pa 1976)* 26: 643–646, 2001; discussion 646–647.

3 Anterior Cervical Arthroplasty

Thomas J. Kesman and Bruce V. Darden II

INDICATIONS/CONTRAINDICATIONS

Anterior cervical discectomy and fusion (ACDF) has developed into the primary operation for treating symptomatic cervical disc disease over the past several decades (1). While ACDF is reliable at treating the arm pain associated with radiculopathy and the spinal cord compression associated with myelopathy, there are lingering questions regarding the loss of motion and potential adjacent segment degeneration (ASD) over long-term follow-up as a result of the procedure (2,3,5).

Anterior cervical arthroplasty (ACA) was developed with these issues in mind. The goal of ACA is to not only relieve the radiculopathic or myelopathic symptoms but also preserve motion and decrease the likelihood of ASD. Initially, some surgeons had concerns about ongoing motion and potential repetitive microtrauma with the use of arthroplasty in myelopathy; however, studies have shown that patients do no worse with arthroplasty than fusion with single-level myelopathic disease (11).

Indications for ACA are similar to those of ACDF:

Single-level symptomatic cervical disc disease (radiculopathy and/or myelopathy) between C3 and C7 in a skeletally mature patient

Disc herniation, osteophyte formation, and/or loss of disc height on imaging studies

Functional deficit (pain) or neurologic deficit in a distribution consistent with findings on imaging (MRI or CT/CT Myelogram)

Failure of nonoperative treatments for at least 6 weeks in the absence of progressive neurologic deficits

Contraindications for ACA include

Allergy to any component, metal or plastic, appearing in the desired implant

Active local or systemic infection

Osteoporosis with T score <-2.5

Moderate to advanced spondylosis with bridging osteophytes

Disc collapse greater than 50% of its normal height

Absence of motion at desired level of implantation

Marked cervical instability defined by greater than 3 mm of translation on flexion/extension radiographs and/or more than 11 degrees of angulation at the disc space as compared to adjacent levels

Significant kyphotic deformity

Multiple levels requiring treatment

With the above guidelines in mind, it is up to the individual surgeon to determine the appropriate indication for surgery.

PREOPERATIVE PREPARATION

The most important part of preoperative planning is making an accurate diagnosis. A detailed history and physical exam are essential to planning an appropriate surgery.

The patient should be examined for signs of radiculopathy as exhibited in Table 3-1. Findings consistent with myelopathy including a positive Hoffmann reflex, positive Babinski sign,

TABLE 3-1	Radicular Patterns			
Disc Level	Nerve Root	Reflex Abnormality	Motor Weakness	Sensory Deficit/Pain Distribution
C3–C4	C4			Supraclavicular region
C4–C5	C5		Deltoid	Lateral aspect of the arm
C5–C6	C6	Diminished biceps reflex	Wrist extensors	Index finger and thumb
C6–C7	C7	Diminished triceps reflex	Triceps	Middle finger

spasticity, clonus, gait instability as well as motor weakness, sensory deficits, and bowel and bladder dysfunction should also be noted.

Baseline anteroposterior (AP) and lateral x-rays can be helpful in identifying overall alignment as well as instability or spondylosis. For those patients contemplating a possible surgical intervention, advanced imaging with CT/CT myelogram or MRI is required (Fig. 3-1).

Careful review of diagnostic information including history, physical exam, and electrodiagnostics (as applicable), in conjunction with advanced imaging is key. An appropriate diagnosis and good surgical technique will yield a superior outcome to a technically perfect surgery for the wrong indication.

Once the decision for surgery has been made, further preoperative planning should occur. The surgeon should measure the width and depth of the disc space endplates to allow for appropriate implant sizing. Some companies have templates available to size their proprietary implant.

TECHNIQUE

The majority of the initial steps in ACA are similar to ACDF. General endotracheal anesthesia is induced with the endotracheal tube taped in the corner of the mouth away from the approach side of the neck. The patient is transferred supine on the radiolucent portion of an operating table. The radiolucency of the operating table is essential in ACA since both AP and lateral x-rays must be obtained using C-arm fluoroscopy. For those surgeons who prefer intraoperative electrophysiologic monitoring, electrodes can be placed once the patient is transferred to the operating table. Support the natural/neutral position of the neck using a small neck roll or towel beneath the posterior neck

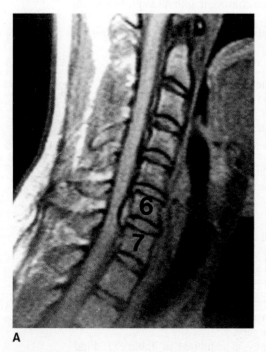
A

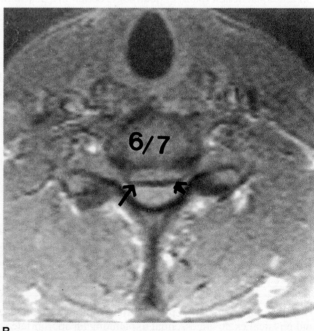
B

FIGURE 3-1

MRI images revealing a large central herniated disc at C6–C7 level (*arrows*) with minimal degeneration at other levels in sagittal **(A)** and axial **(B)** images.

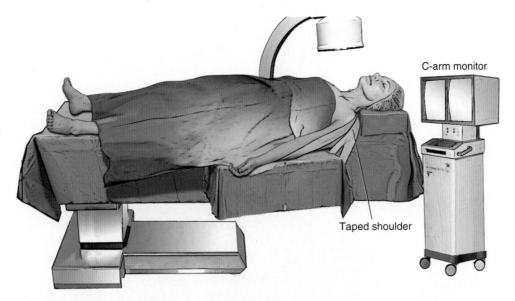

C-arm monitor

Taped shoulder

FIGURE 3-2

Positioning for surgery
for a left-sided anterior
approach.

and shoulders. The additional support will help to minimize any potential movement during the procedure. The overall position of the head and neck is important, verifying correct neutral position in all planes (flexion/extension, lateral bending, rotation) (Fig. 3-2). An AP fluoroscopic image is obtained at this point to verify that the patient is rotationally neutral. Once the position of the head/neck has been optimized, the head is secured to the table using a strap or tape. Traction is not recommended as it will provide a distracting force on the neck that may cause the surgeon to oversize the implant.

AP and lateral fluoroscopic images should be obtained after securing the head position to verify that the disc space of interest and the respective vertebral bodies are clearly visible on both projections and that the head has not moved. If the shoulders are obscuring the lateral view, traction can be applied to the shoulders using wide tape or other devices to pull the shoulders more distally and out of the view of the lateral image. Any time additional traction is placed on the arms, caution must be exercised to avoid undue pressure on the brachial plexus, especially if the head is already secured.

The patient is then prepped and draped in the usual sterile fashion. Either a standard left-sided approach or right-sided approach is acceptable. We prefer the left-side approach where the anatomy of the recurrent laryngeal nerve is more predictable. The transverse incision, curved in line with Langer's lines, can be placed via common landmarks (Table 3-2) or by taking a fluoroscopic lateral image with a radiopaque object (Kelly clamp) placed on the skin. Once the incision is localized, the skin is incised with a knife. An insulated monopolar electrocautery is then used to cauterize through the fat to reach the underlying platysma. The platysma is incised with electrocautery in line with the incision. The surgeon then must identify the medial border of the sternocleidomastoid muscle and proceed medial to it. The carotid sheath is palpated with a finger to feel the carotid pulse and the sheath retracted laterally. Medially, the esophagus and trachea are pulled across the midline using blunt handheld retractors (Fig. 3-3). The prevertebral fascia and longus colli overlying the anterior cervical spine are identified. Once the anticipated disc level is identified, a small disc marker is inserted into the disc. A lateral radiograph is then taken to verify the appropriate level. The surgeon can adjust proximally or distally as need be to be operating on the correct level disc. Once the correct disc is identified on x-ray, the disc is marked with the electrocautery or knife to remove a small portion of that disc. If crossing vessels are encountered (superior or inferior thyroid), they may be cauterized carefully using bipolar electrocautery and divided.

The above procedure is universal to all major cervical disc arthroplasties in the United States. Below we will describe the procedure for the Synthes ProDisc-C (Synthes USA, Inc., West Chester, PA)

TABLE 3-2 **Anatomic Landmarks**	
Disc Level	**Anatomic Landmark**
C3	Hyoid bone
C4–C5	Thyroid cartilage
C6	Cricoid cartilage

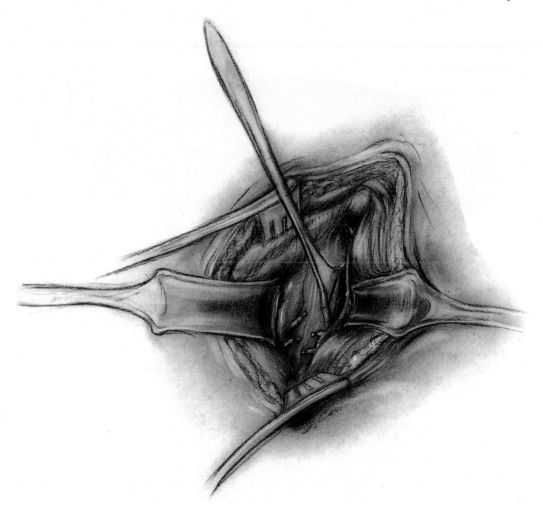

FIGURE 3-3

Handheld retractors are used to retract and protect the trachea and esophagus medially and the carotid sheath laterally. The prevertebral fascia and longus colli muscles can then be elevated in the midline.

implant as an example (10) (Fig. 3-4), but other popular arthroplasty devices such as the BRYAN Cervical Disc System (Fig. 3-5) or the Prestige Cervical Disc (Fig. 3-6) (Medtronic, Inc., Minneapolis, MN) will have similar procedures and their individual technique manuals should be consulted for specific details.

The prevertebral fascia and longus colli overlying the disc of interest are elevated. Elevation of the longus colli allows for improved visualization and protection of more lateral structures. A Cloward-type self-retaining retractor is placed beneath each of the longus colli in a medial/lateral fashion. The retractor is then assembled to hold the blades in place.

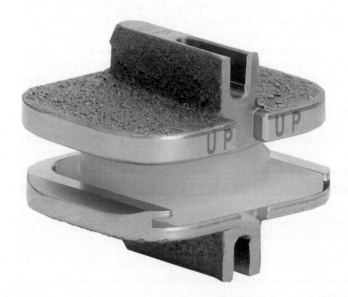

FIGURE 3-4

ProDisc-C implant. (© 2012 Synthes, Inc. or its affiliates. All rights reserved.)

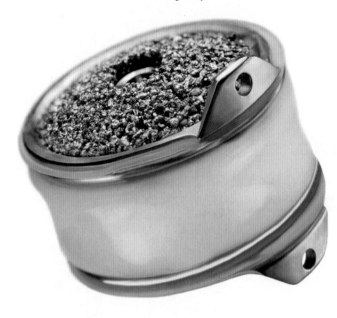

FIGURE 3-5
BRYAN Cervical Disc. (Images provided by Medtronic, Inc.)

AP fluoroscopy is then brought in to identify the precise midline of the spine. A mark is placed on the superior and inferior vertebral bodies, which will remain in place throughout the operation.

Retainer screws are placed in the midline using lateral fluoroscopy to keep the screws parallel to the operative disc space. The retainer screw in the superior body should be placed in the superior one-third of the superior body, and the inferior screw should be placed in the inferior one-third of the inferior vertebral body. This will allow for adequate working room for milling at the disc level later in the operation. The trajectory of the screw is determined by the starter awl that is used to perforate the anterior cortex and create the trajectory of the screw using fluoroscopy. Once the path has been created, a 3.5-mm retainer screw can be inserted under fluoroscopy to a depth where the posterior cortex is engaged. The process is repeated for the screw in the inferior vertebral body. The retainer is then placed over the two screws and locked into place using set screws on the top of the retainer (Fig. 3-7). The disc space can be pretensioned using the retainer but should not be distracted. The retainer is not intended to distract the disc space.

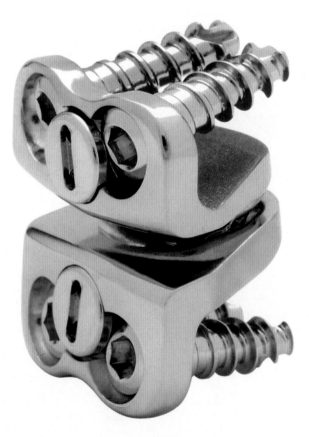

FIGURE 3-6
Prestige implant. (Images provided by Medtronic, Inc.)

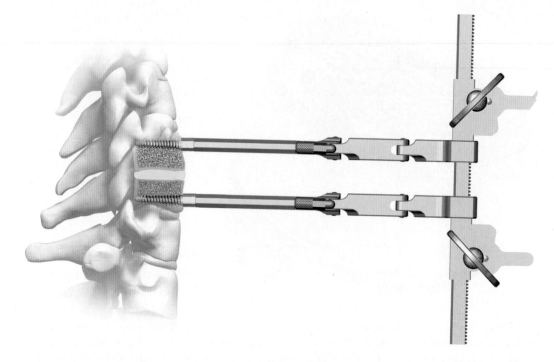

FIGURE 3-7

Artist's representation of lateral view with retainer in place.

The surgeon now completes a preliminary discectomy in the usual fashion by creating an annulotomy with a knife and using small curettes, Kerrison punches, to remove the disc material (Fig. 3-8). Once the disc space is relatively clear, the vertebral distractor is inserted to the back of the vertebral bodies. The disc space is now distracted using this tool and the retainer locked in place to hold this distraction. With the disc space distracted, the discectomy can be fully completed posteriorly, the segment mobilized, and foramen decompressed. A micro nerve hook can be used to ensure that no disc fragments are behind either of the two vertebral bodies or in the foramina. The posterior longitudinal ligament may be removed if the pathology necessitates this step. Care should be taken to not disrupt the endplates as exposure of bleeding cancellous bone will make the disc space more osteogenic and possibly may increase the risk of heterotopic ossification.

With the discectomy complete, implant trials are inserted after which any tension on the retainer is released. The size of the implant can be estimated from preoperative CT or MRI images, or using

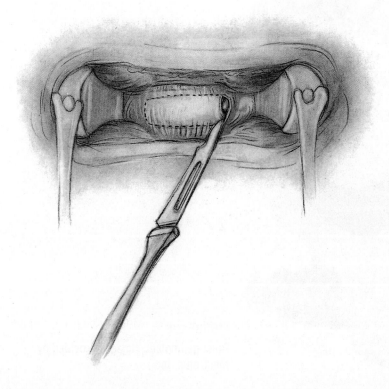

FIGURE 3-8

With the self-retaining retractor in place, a standard discectomy can be performed.

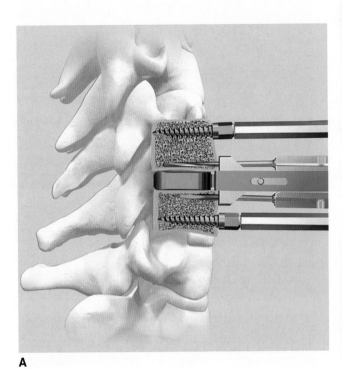

A

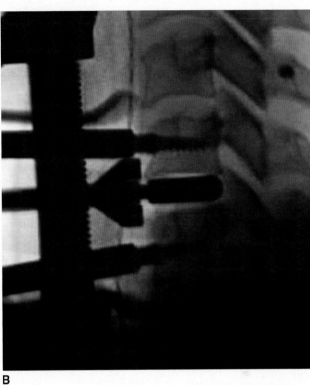

B

FIGURE 3-9

A: Artist's representation of ProDisc-C trial in place. **B:** Fluoroscopic images of ProDisc-C trial in place. (© 2012 Synthes, Inc. or its affiliates. All rights reserved.)

intraoperative calipers. These measurements are only guidelines, and an intraoperative trial should be completed. The trial should cover as much of the smaller vertebral body as possible and have a height consistent with adjacent unaffected levels. Implant sizing should be checked on AP and lateral fluoroscopy to verify that the posterior portion of the trial is flush with the posterior vertebral bodies (Fig. 3-9).

Keel cuts may be created in the vertebral bodies using either a chisel or a powered mill. We prefer the mill as it applies less force to the spine to make the keel cut and reduces the risk of posterior vertebral body fractures while using the chisel. The milling guide is seated over the trial and tightened into place. The surgeon should verify that the trial and milling guide are in the precise midline on an AP fluoroscopic image. Once verified, a sharp retaining pin should be placed in the inferior hole of the milling guide for additional stability. The powered mill can be then inserted into the superior hole. Once the mill bit reaches the anterior cortex, power is given to the device and the mill is plunged until it stops into the vertebral body toward the disc space as much as the guide will allow. The mill is then angled away from the disc space and then retracted slowly to cut the channel in the bone (Fig. 3-10). The temporary sharp pin is removed from the lower portion of the guide and a blunt retaining pin is placed to the channel just created superiorly, and the milling process is repeated through the inferior hole in the guide.

Once both channels have been cut, lateral fluoroscopy is used with the keel cut cleaners to remove any additional bone from the channel and to also verify depth of the keel cut (Fig. 3-11). Irrigate the disc space to wash out any bone shavings or residual soft tissue from the discectomy.

The appropriately sized implant as determined by the trial is opened and attached to the inserter (Fig. 3-12). The implant is moved into place, making sure to line up the keels on the implant with the keel cuts in the bone. Also, care must be taken to put the implant in the correct orientation with the word "UP" on the superior portion of the disc space. The implant should be impacted until it is flush with the posterior vertebral body on a lateral fluoroscopic image (Fig. 3-13). The implant should not be placed past the posterior extent of the keel cut. Once the surgeon is satisfied with the lateral image, a final AP image is taken to confirm placement in the midline (Fig. 3-14).

The retainer screws are removed, and bone wax is placed in the holes. Any bleeding cancellous surfaces should be covered with bone wax to create an environment less amenable to bone formation. The wound should be copiously irrigated to decrease the risk of infection and heterotopic ossification. The Cloward-type retractors are then removed and exchanged for handheld right-angled

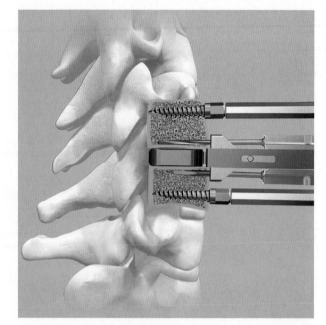

FIGURE 3-10

Keel cut with mill in superior vertebral body and stabilizing pin in inferior vertebral body. (2012 Synthes, Inc. or its affiliates. All rights reserved.)

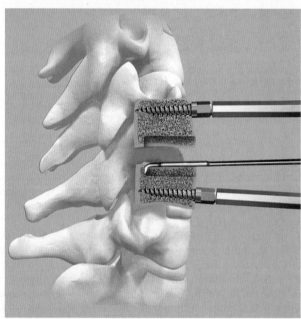

FIGURE 3-11

Verify keel depths and clean the keel cuts using the keel cut cleaner. (2012 Synthes, Inc. or its affiliates. All rights reserved.)

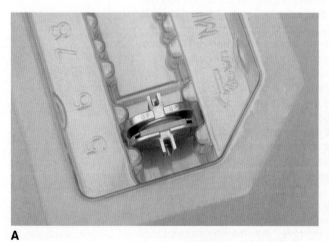

A

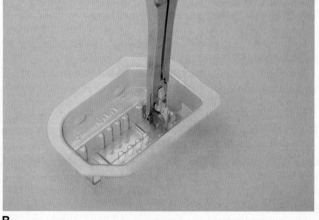

B

FIGURE 3-12

A: Verify that "UP" on the ProDisc-C implant is placed into the superior vertebral body. **B:** ProDisc-C implant loaded on inserter. (2012 Synthes, Inc. or its affiliates. All rights reserved.)

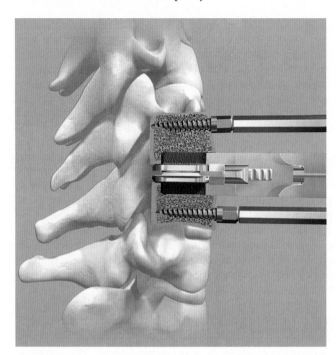

retractors. The esophagus must be inspected for any injury and the entire surgical field evaluated for adequate hemostasis.

A drain may be placed at the surgeon's discretion. The wound is then closed by closing the platysma with absorbable sutures followed by routine subcutaneous and skin closure.

PEARLS AND PITFALLS

The most important factor in placing a cervical arthroplasty is the ability to image the operative segment with a C-arm and image intensifier. If this is not feasible to visualize the superior endplate of the proximal vertebrae and the inferior endplate of the inferior vertebrae, then the cervical arthroplasty should be aborted and an anterior cervical fusion performed. To optimally place the implant, it is important to make sure that a true AP and lateral C-arm images are obtained. This is best done by looking at the uncovertebral joints bilaterally and centering these as opposed to a

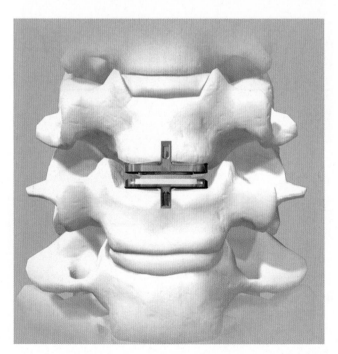

spinous process that might not be completely in the midline, on the AP view. The lateral view should also be meticulously aligned. If the operative segment has anterior or posterior osteophytes that have to be removed with a high-speed burr, it is again best to abort the total disc arthroplasty and proceed to fusion. The bone dust created by the burr may be a factor in development of heterotopic ossification. Also, if the space is narrowed enough to require a burr to widen out the endplates, then there is not enough room to allow for placement of a cervical arthroplasty. If the two operative endplates cannot be adequately placed parallel one to another, then the arthroplasty may end up being placed in a "fish-mouthed" position. This then places the prosthesis in extension and may limit both the flexion and extension of the arthroplasty. It is important to have an adequate size footplate to cover the cortical rim of the vertebral bodies. If too small an implant is placed, this may allow for subsidence. When the surgeon is faced with deciding between two sizes of an arthroplasty as far as height is concerned, it is prudent to choose the smaller size. Placing an arthroplasty that is "too tight" in height will limit range of motion. It is also important to restore the center of rotation of the vertebral segment. This requires that the arthroplasty be placed as posteriorly as possible. In the case of the ProDisc-C cervical disc arthroplasty, the footplate needs to be placed to the posterior cortical rim. This prevents the center of rotation being placed too far anteriorly and therefore overloading the facet joints. At the end of the procedure, it is imperative to obtain meticulous hemostasis, to minimize the risk of heterotopic ossification. This requires extensive use of bone wax applied to all bony surfaces and use of any other hemostatic agents as determined by the surgeon.

POSTOPERATIVE MANAGEMENT

If a drain was placed, it is usually removed the morning of postoperative day 1. The patient is instructed in basic neck exercises to promote motion and reduce stiffness. A soft collar can be worn for comfort. No strenuous activity should be undertaken before follow-up in 2 to 3 weeks for suture removal and wound check. Additionally, prophylaxis for heterotopic ossification is reasonable if feasible. We give our patients without risk factors for intolerance to nonsteroidal anti-inflammatory medications indomethacin sustained-release 75 mg PO b.i.d. for 3 weeks.

Routine follow-up radiographs are taken at 6 weeks, 3 months, and 1 year to verify position of the implant (Fig. 3-15).

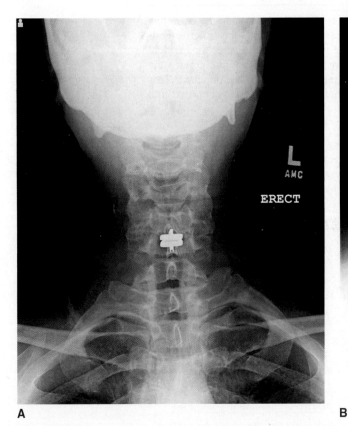

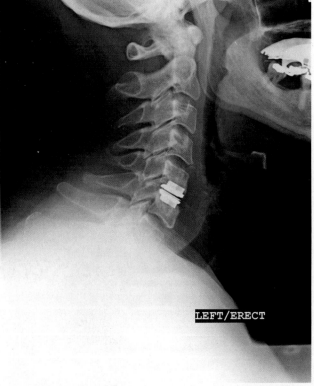

A   B

FIGURE 3-15

A: Post-op AP x-ray. **B:** Post-op lateral x-ray.

COMPLICATIONS

Anterior cervical arthroplasty has the same intraoperative risks as does anterior cervical discectomy and fusion. The FDA investigational device exemption (IDE) studies of Prestige, Bryan, and ProDisc-C arthroplasties did not show any different complication profiles for arthroplasties versus the control fusion patients (4,8,9). There were neither any major neurologic complications among the arthroplasty patients nor any problems specific to the device insertion. There is the potential risk of accelerated wear of the arthroplasty secondary to malpositioning. Due to the overall short follow-up period of these studies, wear problems have not been proven. There have been case reports of early osteolysis of the vertebrae adjacent to the implant. One patient had an early explanation and fusion due to osteolysis. When no significant wear debris was found, speculation to the cause centered on an immune-mediated response (13).

The risk of dysphagia in arthroplasty patients has been shown to be lower than in fusion patients (12). Heterotopic ossification has been reported in all arthroplasty studies, with the rates of heterotopic ossification (HO) occurring in up to 71.4% of cases (6,7,14). While HO occurs, over 90% of patients maintain at least 3 degrees of motion at the operative site. There also have been no adverse effects on the clinical outcomes in patients who develop HO.

RESULTS

The clinical results of anterior cervical arthroplasty come primarily from the US FDA IDE trials; these randomized multicenter studies were designed as noninferiority studies. The trials of Prestige ST, Bryan Cervical Disc Replacement, and ProDisc-C represent level 1 clinical data. Mummaneni et al. reported on the Prestige ST trial. All clinically evaluated parameters in Short Form 36 (SF-36), Visual Analogue Scale (VAS), and Neck Disability Index (NDI), improved from baseline and comparably to fusion. Overall success (NDI improvement greater than 15 points, maintenance of neurologic status, and absence of implant-related adverse events) occurred in 79.3% of the arthroplasty patients versus 67.8% in fusion patients (8) ProDisc-C IDE results were evaluated in a paper by Murrey et al. Both the arthroplasty patients and the fusion patients improved similarly; the ProDisc-C patients showed a much lower reoperation rate (1.8%) versus fusion (8.5%), ($p = 0.033$) (9). Bryan Cervical Disc Replacement IDE results reported by Heller et al. (4) demonstrated statistically significant improvement in the VAS and NDI scales as well as overall success at 2-year follow-up in the arthroplasty group (4).

The early overall clinical results of anterior cervical arthroplasty are promising. Whether cervical arthroplasty can diminish adjacent segment degeneration and have acceptable rates of wear long-term are questions to be answered by future studies.

ACKNOWLEDGMENTS

Images of the ProDisc-C implant and technique guide images provided by Synthes, Inc. Images of the BRYAN implant and Prestige implants provided by Medtronic, Inc. The BRYAN Cervical Disc System incorporates technology developed by Gary K. Michelson, MD.

RECOMMENDED READING

1. Bradford DS, Zdeblick TA, Thompson RC, eds.: *Master techniques in orthopaedic surgery: the spine*. 2nd ed. Philadelphia, PA: Lippincott Williams & Wilkins, 2004.
2. Goffin J, Geusens E, Vantomme N, et al.: Long-term follow-up after interbody fusion of the cervical spine. *J Spinal Disord Tech* 17(2): 79–85, 2004.
3. Gore DR, Sepic SB: Anterior discectomy and fusion for painful cervical disc disease: a report of 50 patients with an average follow-up of 21 years. *Spine* 23: 2047–2051, 1998.
4. Heller JG, Sasso RC, Papadopoulos SM, et al.: Comparison of Bryan cervical disc arthroplasty with anterior cervical decompression and fusion: clinical and radiographic results of a randomized, controlled, clinical trial. *Spine* 34: 101–107, 2009.
5. Hilibrand AS, Carlson GD, Palumbo MA, et al.: Radiculopathy and myelopathy at segments adjacent to the site of a previous anterior cervical arthrodesis. *J Bone Joint Surg Am* 81: 519–528, 1999.
6. Leung C, Casey AT, Goffin J, et al.: Clinical significance of heterotopic ossification in cervical disc replacement: a prospective, multicenter clinical trial. *Neurosurgery* 57: 759–763, 2005.
7. Mehren C, Suchomel P, Grochulla F, et al.: Heterotopic ossification in total cervical disc replacement. *Spine* 31: 2802–2806, 2006.
8. Mummaneni PV, Burkus JK, Haid RW, et al.: Clinical and radiographic analysis of cervical disc arthroplasty compared with allograft fusion: a randomized controlled clinical trial. *J Neurosurg Spine* 6: 198–209, 2007.
9. Murrey DB, Janssen M, Delamarter R, et al.: Results of the prospective, randomized multicenter Food and Drug Administration investigational device exemption study of the ProDisc C total disc replacement versus anterior discectomy and fusion for the treatment of 1-level symptomatic cervical disc disease. *Spine J* 9: 275–286, 2009.

10. Pro-Disc-C Total Disc Replacement, Technique Guide. Synthes, Inc, 2008.
11. Riew DK, Buchowski JM, Sasso R, et al.: Cervical disc arthroplasty compared with arthrodesis for the treatment of myelopathy. *J Bone Joint Surg Am* 90: 2354–2364, 2008.
12. Segebarth PB, Datta J, Darden BV, et al.: Incidence of dysphagia comparing cervical disc arthroplasty and ACDF. *SAS J* 4(1): 3–8, 2010.
13. Tumialan LM, Gluf WM: Progressive vertebral body osteolysis after cervical arthroplasty. *Spine* 36(14): 973–978, 2011.
14. Yi S, Kim KN, Yang MS, et al.: Difference in occurrence of heterotopic ossification according to prosthesis type in the cervical artificial disc replacement. *Spine* 35(16): 1556–1561, 2010.

4 Cervical Vertebrectomy and Plating

William Ryan Spiker and Darrel S. Brodke

INDICATIONS

Cervical vertebrectomy (also known as corpectomy) and plating is indicated for patients with anterior compression of the cervical spinal cord and exiting cervical nerve roots. It is an alternative to multiple level discectomy and interbody fusion and is uniquely well suited to relieve cord compression occurring not only at the disc level but also behind the vertebral bodies (e.g., disc herniation fragment). Common indications for vertebrectomy and plating of the cervical spine include degenerative cervical spondylotic myelopathy (without hyperlordosis), traumatic fractures and dislocations, congenital cervical stenosis, ossification of the posterior longitudinal ligament (OPLL), tumors, and infections.

CONTRAINDICATIONS

Anterior cervical exposures should not be attempted in the face of severe anterior neck trauma with tracheal or esophageal injury that precludes safe access to the spine. Similarly, careful consideration is necessary when placing hardware in the infected patient. Anterior surgery should be avoided when in the setting of posterior sources of neural compression such as hyperlordosis or ligamentous infolding. Diminished bone quality from osteoporosis or metastatic disease may lead to graft failure, subsidence, migration, or kyphotic collapse. Relative contraindications that carry increased risk of complications include poor nutrition (albumin and prealbumin levels), bleeding disorder, aberrant vertebral artery anatomy, smoking, history of previous nonunion, advanced age, and inability to follow postoperative activity restrictions. Additionally, anterior corpectomy of more than two vertebral bodies with a strut graft (with or without plate) has a high nonunion rate with increased risk of graft or plate dislodgement and often necessitates additional posterior stabilization (9).

PREOPERATIVE PREPARATION

History and Physical

As always, preoperative preparation begins with an accurate and thorough history and physical examination.

- Key historical facts include duration, severity and timing of symptoms, symptoms of myelopathy/radiculopathy, exacerbating and mitigating factors, and results of previous treatments.
- Key physical examination findings include inspection of cervical alignment (lordosis vs kyphosis), evaluation for anterior neck scars, upper extremity examination to rule out peripheral causes of symptoms, cervical spine range of motion, and detailed neurovascular exam of upper and lower extremities including strength, sensation, reflexes, and assessment of long-tract signs.

Patient Education

Patients should be extensively counseled regarding the goals of surgery and the specific risks of surgical intervention. Managing postoperative infections, persistent pain, numbness or weakness, decreased range of motion, and other complications are made easier when these topics have been broached preoperatively.

Radiology

Radiographic evaluation begins with plain radiographs, including flexion and extension views and a long spine film in patients with a deformity on examination or initial radiographic views. MRI provides excellent visualization of the soft tissues, including the spinal cord and exiting nerve roots. The course of the vertebral arteries should be confirmed on every preoperative MRI to minimize risk of intraoperative injury. In cases with severe deformity, tumor resection, or difficult revisions, angiography can be used to more clearly understand the course of the vertebral arteries and their branches. Preoperative occlusion of the artery may be beneficial in specific patients. CT myelography can also be used to identify neural structure impingement with the advantage of improved visualization of bony structures (important in OPLL) and decreased scatter from previously placed hardware.

Graft Choices

Preoperative planning for vertebrectomy includes determination of the size and type of bone graft to be used for anterior column reconstruction. Autologous iliac crest bone graft is an option for one or sometimes two-level vertebral body resections, while auto or allograft fibula grafts are usually preferred for larger reconstructions. Consideration for supplemental posterior fixation is important in three-level vertebrectomies and high-risk patients (history of smoking, osteoporosis, kyphotic deformity, etc.) to minimize risk of pseudarthrosis. Due to the high union rates in circumferential (anterior and posterior) fusions, allograft is often used for anterior column support in these cases.

An alternative to allograft bone for anterior column support after vertebrectomy is the placement of a cage or spacer made of titanium, ceramic, carbon fiber, or poly-ether-ether-ketone (PEEK). These have the advantage of strength and easy of placement, while potentially adding significant cost to the case.

TECHNIQUE

(Fig. 4-1)

- Large fluoroscope—off of the upper right hand corner of the OR table
- Surgical microscope—off of the lower right hand corner of the OR table
- High-speed air drill—at foot of OR table—opposite of scrub tech
- Skin preparation: chlorhexidine (+/– alcohol pre-prep)
- +/– Loupe versus microscope

Positioning

- Know preoperative cervical range of motion—discuss possible nasotracheal/fiberoptic intubation if poor range of motion
- Discuss role of total IV anesthesia to allow measurement of somatosensory and motor evoked potentials.
- Supine position, arms tucked to side
- Head straight or rotated slightly away from side of surgical approach
- Pad between scapula to obtain desired extension. Care must be taken to avoid hyperextension in the myelopathic patient.
- Wide cloth tape can be used to pull down on the shoulders to increase fluoroscopic visualization of the caudal cervical spine (C6–T1). Care should be taken to avoid overly aggressive retraction and brachial plexus injury
- Mark desired level of incision with fluoroscopic guidance prior to skin preparation

Traction

- Intraoperative traction to stabilize spine during vertebrectomy is particularly important in patients with myelopathy and unstable fractures. This may also limit Ligamentum Flavum infolding and cord compression with positioning.
- Head halter traction can be used for single-level resections
- Gardner-Wells tongs can be used with single- or multilevel resections

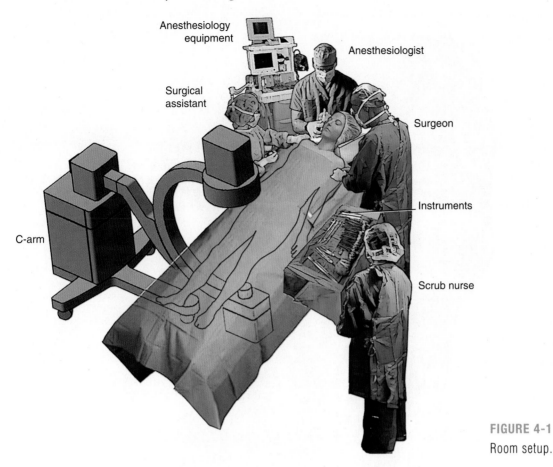

Anesthesiology
equipment

Anesthesiologist

Surgical
assistant

Surgeon

Instruments

C-arm

Scrub nurse

FIGURE 4-1
Room setup.

- Halo ring traction can be used if the patient is going to be in halo-vest immobilization postoperatively (attach the vest at the conclusion of surgery)
- 10 to 15 pounds of traction is used to stabilize the spine, can be increased as necessary during placement of the graft

Graft Harvest

- Iliac crest: small bump under crest
- Fibular autograft: bump under ipsilateral hip, thigh tourniquet

Approach

Incision (Fig. 4-2)
- Historically, left-sided approach is preferred for the lower cervical spine due to more predictable course of the recurrent laryngeal nerve. However, the side of approach is often chosen contralateral to the decompression (if one side is worse than the other) to ease deep access and visualization.
- Revision cases: important to note function of recurrent laryngeal nerves
  - Approach from the same side as prior surgery, laryngoscopy optional
  - Approach from the contralateral side, direct laryngoscopy and vocal cord visualization should be performed to rule out unilateral (potentially asymptomatic) vocal cord paralysis preoperatively.
  - If laryngoscopy reveals normal vocal cord motion—contralateral approach allows dissection through native tissue and likely less risk of trachea, esophagus, and neurovascular injury
  - If laryngoscopy reveals abnormal vocal cord motion—approach through previous surgical incision to avoid risk of bilateral nerve injuries
- Transverse incision allows exposure for up to four-level vertebrectomy and provides a significantly better cosmetic result
- Longitudinal incision just anterior to the sternocleidomastoid (SCM) is rarely needed, but does allow a more extensile exposure if required, at the cost of a significantly worse cosmetic result
- Anatomic landmarks for incision: (see Table 4-1)
  - Use preoperative imaging to confirm correlation of landmarks and levels

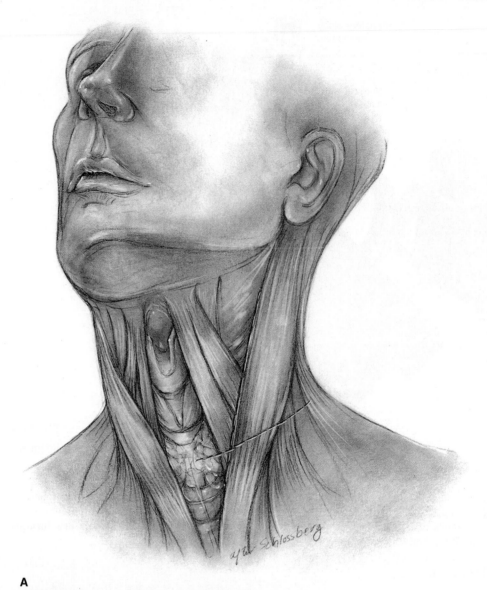

A

FIGURE 4-2

A: Transverse skin incision used for anterior cervical exposure for cervical vertebrectomy. The *dotted line* shows the midline of the cervical spine. **B:** A second photo of the transverse cervical incision, beginning 1 cm right of midline and extending over to the sternocleidomastoid musculature.

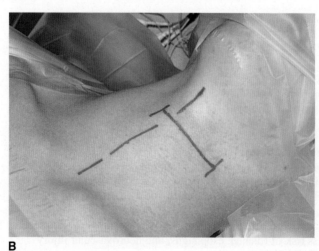

B

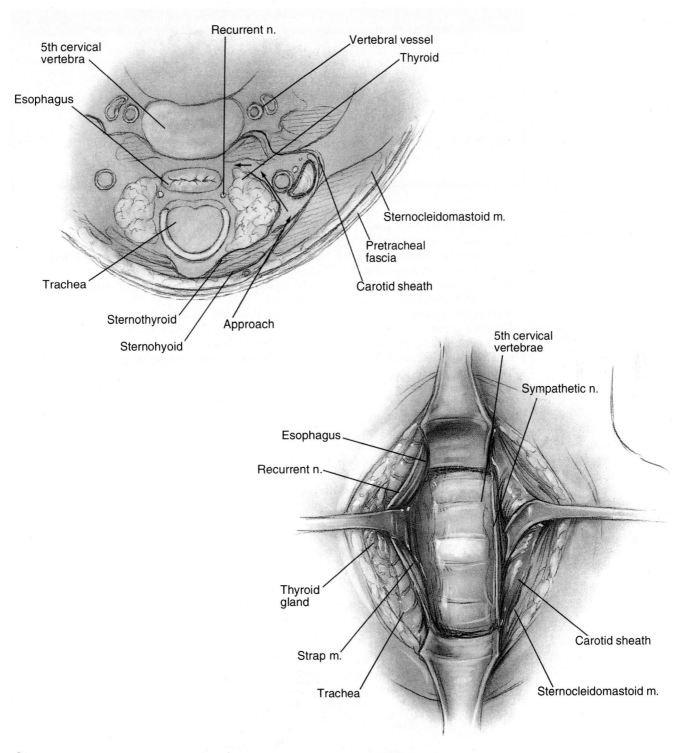

C

FIGURE 4-2 (*Continued*)

C, Top: Transverse view of the cervical spine through the fifth cervical vertebra. The *arrows* denote the anterior approach through the platysma, medial to the carotid sheath and lateral to the trachea, esophagus, and thyroid. **C, Bottom:** The view shows the complete exposure of the cervical spine with the retractors underneath the longus colli musculature.

TABLE 4-1	Superficial Anatomic Landmarks of the Cervical Spine
C-Spine Level	**Anatomic Landmark**
C3–C4	Hyoid bone; two finger breadths below mandible
C4–C5	Thyroid cartilage
C5–C6	Cricoid cartilage
C6	Carotid tubercle
C6–C7	Two finger breadths above the sternal notch

Dissection (Figs. 4-3 and 4-4)

Platysma can be incised horizontally or vertically

> We incise horizontally along the length of the wound, *after bluntly dissecting it from deep structures*, without preplatysmal dissection, which improves wound closure.

Underlying superficial cervical fascia can be separated off of the deeper SCM and anterior jugular vein with Metzenbaum scissors, usually bluntly

> Vein can be ligated with suture if necessary, but is usually retracted

> Cranial and caudal subplatysmal release of anterior cervical fascia is key to a wide exposure

SCM is retracted laterally, and the omohyoid is often seen traversing the field

Carotid sheath is palpated with index finger (contents = carotid artery, internal jugular vein, and vagus nerve)

Interval directly medial to SCM/carotid sheath is developed bluntly, and a Cloward or Richardson retractor is used to retract the trachea, esophagus, thyroid, and other anterior neck structures medially.

> Digastric and stylohyoid muscles can impede exposure of upper cervical spine; omohyoid can impede visualization of middle/lower cervical spine

> These muscles can usually be retracted, but can be divided if necessary

Crossing veins (superior and middle thyroid) and small nerves (deep ansa cervicalis) are retracted as necessary.

Pretracheal fascia split bluntly with Kittner dissector, allowing visualization of anterior surface of the cervical spine

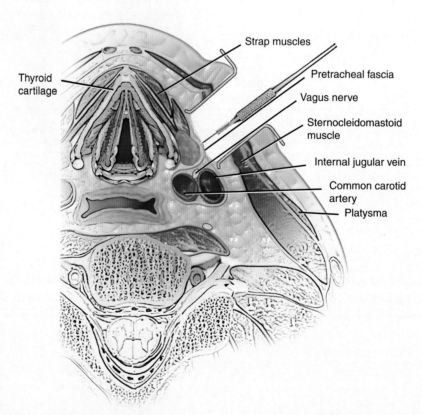

Strap muscles

Pretracheal fascia

Vagus nerve

Sternocleidomastoid muscle

Internal jugular vein

Common carotid artery

Platysma

Thyroid cartilage

FIGURE 4-3

Axial neck drawing with dissection plane and drawing of surgical dissection from surgeon's viewpoint.

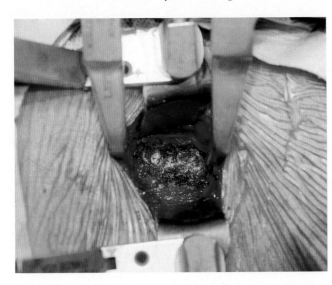

FIGURE 4-4

Photo of dissection with retractors in place.

Prevertebral fascia can be dissected off the center of the vertebral bodies bluntly with a Kittner or sharply with scissors or electrocautery revealing the longus colli muscles, anterior longitudinal ligament (ALL), and anterior surface of the vertebral bodies

KEY—Obtain a lateral fluoroscopic image with a hemostat clamped on the ALL directly overlying a disc space or with a spinal needle within the disc to confirm level

Carefully dissect the longus colli muscles to the lateral border of the vertebral bodies with electrocautery or a Freer dissector to allow full exposure of the uncovertebral joints during decompression

Vertebral arteries are usually lateral and deep to this dissection

Penfield elevator can be used to palpate the transverse processes and provide an estimation of the depth and width of the vertebral body

Dissection should proceed superficial to the transverse process

Retractor Placement

Wide, smooth-edged, or small-toothed medial/lateral retractors should be placed first and must be below the longus colli muscles to avoid damage to the overlying sympathetic chain

Sharp-edged long-toothed retractors should be used with care as they can damage the esophagus medially and the carotid sheath laterally

Narrow retractors can slip between the transverse processes and damage the vertebral artery

Place Caspar distraction posts (14 mm length) into the vertebral bodies above and below the corpectomy level(s) to provide local retraction.

Distractor pins can be placed in a diverging alignment to reduce kyphotic deformity if present

Cephalad/caudad retractors should be avoided, as they increase the risk of postoperative dysphagia; the distractor posts are often enough to hold cranial and caudal tissues

If exposure is inadequate, consider more aggressive fascial release

Confirm adequate exposure, should be able to visualize lateral border of all vertebral bodies to be resected uncovertebral joints and intervertebral discs at every level of resection.

NOTE: If wanting to dissect more laterally (under longus colli) to confirm boundaries of the vertebral body, it is safe to perform this at vertebral body level where there is bony protection of the vertebral artery, rather than at disc level where the vertebral artery is exposed (Fig. 4-5).

Decompression/Vertebrectomy (Figs. 4-5 and 4-6)

Review the course of the vertebral arteries (again)

Begin with discectomy at the cranial and caudal extent of the planned resection

Complete discectomies should all be performed prior to vertebrectomy—this allows for knowledge of depth and identification of the uncovertebral joints that mark the lateral boundaries of the planned corpectomy

Remove posterior osteophytes to clearly visualize the uncovertebral joints bilaterally at every involved level

Confirm adequacy of foraminotomies by passing a nerve hook just anterior to the exiting nerve root through the foramen

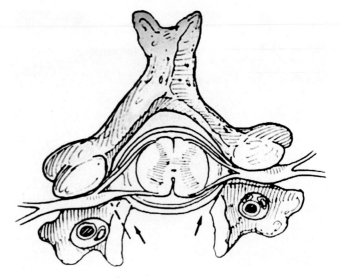

FIGURE 4-5

Axial image of planned bone resection. (Reprinted from Sherk HH. *The cervical spine: An atlas of cervical procedures.* Philadelphia, PA: JB Lippincott, 1993. Illustrator: Bernie Kida, with permission.)

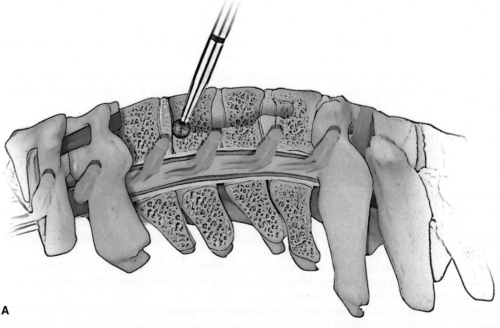

A

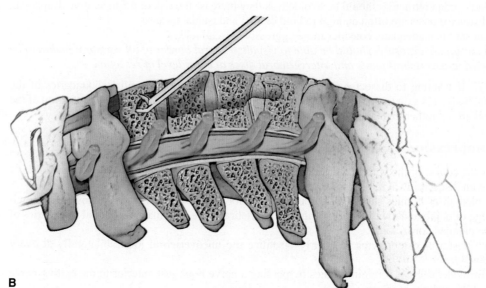

FIGURE 4-6

A: Sagittal image with burr at corpectomy level. **B:** Sagittal image with forward angle curette/pituitary rongeur.

B

Mark planned resection with electrocautery or high-speed burr
    Use uncovertebral joints to center resection
Debulk ventral vertebral bodies with rongeur
Resect vertebral bodies with high-speed burr using uncovertebral joints at the cranial and caudal disc spaces to determine width of resection
    Width should be between 15 and 18 mm to accommodate graft
    Thrombin-soaked collagen power or sponges can be used to control bleeding from bone surface
    Remove the posterior cortical bone of vertebral body with small anterior-angled curette, high-speed burr, or 1- or 2-mm Kerrison rongeur
    Leave a thin shell of the posterior wall attached to the posterior longitudinal ligament to avoid dural tear in patients with OPLL

NOTE: In OPLL, because the posterior longitudinal ligament cannot always be dissected off of the underlying dura, a small bone island over dura can be left behind; it will float up as decompression is completed.

This dissection can be difficult, and a skin hook can be used to pull the posterior longitudinal ligament away from the cord, which is released with a fine curette. A modified valvulotome can be used for this dissection (modified by a change in handle). This has a small ball tip for dissecting and a sharp cutting blade behind the ball that can be used by pulling back on the instrument.

Graft Preparation (Figs. 4-7 and 4-8)

Docking sites for the graft are created with a high speed burr—flatten the endplates to smooth punctate-bleeding cortical surfaces (remove all cartilage).
    NOTE: Leave rim of cortical bone to provide stability to graft
    NOTE: Remove anterior osteophyte at the superior endplate of the caudal vertebral body to avoid placing graft too anterior
Measure the bone defect with surgical calipers, a ruler, or an 18-gauge wire
    Measure distance between endplates, as well as width and AP depth of defect
Obtain donor graft (fibula, iliac crest, allograft) at least 5 mm longer than measured defect.
    Iliac crest: after safe dissection to the crest, an oscillating saw is used to resect a tricortical graft (larger than defect in length and width)
        Iliac crest curvature can make it difficult to use when more than two vertebral bodies are removed
        Anterior cortex of Iliac crest graft is used to recreate the posterior vertebral body wall
    Fibula: after safe dissection, an oscillating saw is used to resect a section of fibula (longer than defect)
    Trim to final dimensions with saw, high-speed burr, or small rongeur
Graft is held with Kocher clamp and placed with the assistance of up to 30 to 40 pounds of cervical traction and gentle tapping with a bone tamp.
Traction is released, and the graft is checked to ensure stability
    Kocher clamp can be used to gently pull on graft to verify fixation
AP and lateral fluoroscopic views to ensure proper graft placement

Plating (Figs. 4-9 and 4-10)

Anterior cervical plates for single or two-level vertebrectomies
Anterior plating for three or more level vertebrectomies is controversial because the forces from the longer lever arm may dislodge the plate and graft, causing more complications than graft dislodgement alone
Identify midline using anatomic landmarks to place the plate directly in midline (use fluoroscopy if needed)
Review preoperative imaging to measure the room available for screws in both the cranial and caudal vertebral bodies. Set the stop guide on the drill to the maximum screw length (usually 14 to 16 mm).
Choose the shortest plate that will span vertebrectomy to minimize risk of damaging adjacent levels during plating
Remove anterior osteophytes with rongeur or high-speed burr to ensure that plate sits flush against vertebral body
Hold plate in midline with a holding pin as the first screw is placed at the cranial and then caudal end (without final tightening of these screws)
Place the remaining screws and tighten all screws to "2-finger" tightness, so as to avoid stripping
Confirm the screw locking mechanism of the implant chosen
Fluoroscopy: AP and lateral views confirm position and alignment

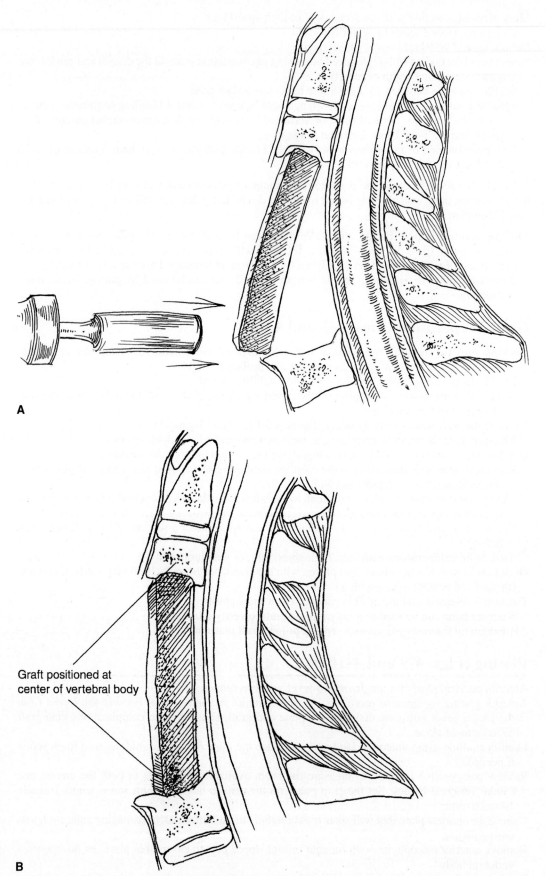

FIGURE 4-7

Sagittal drawing of graft positioning following multilevel corpectomy. **A:** Graft positioned cranially and tamp positioned to fit caudally. **B:** Graft in correct position at both ends.

Graft positioned at center of vertebral body

A

B

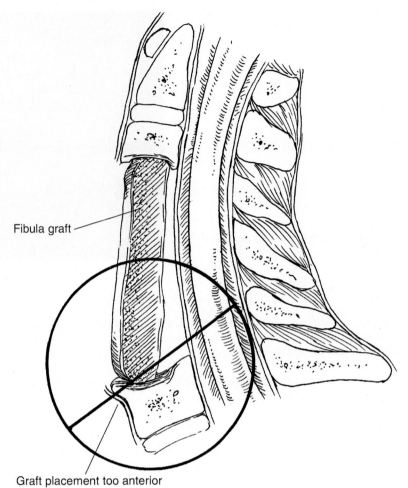

Fibula graft

Graft placement too anterior
at osteophyte

FIGURE 4-8
Anterior placement
of strut graft due to
incomplete removal of
osteophyte.

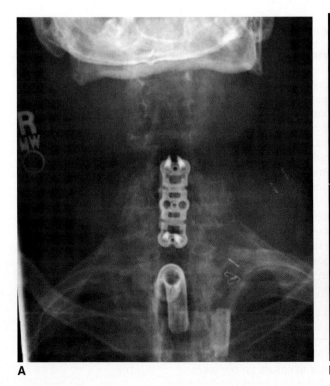

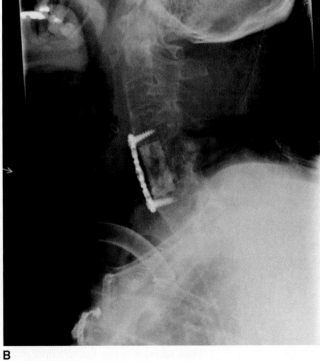

A

B

FIGURE 4-9
A,B: AP and lat XR of well-placed plate placed correctly.

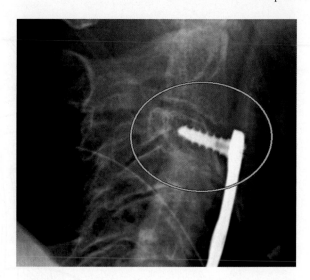

FIGURE 4-10
Anterior osteophyte limiting screw purchase.

Closure

Ensure completely dry wound at closure. Use bipolar electrocautery along the longus colli muscles.
    If not completely dry, place a suction drain.
Platysma and subcutaneous tissue can be closed together with interrupted stitches of 3-0 dissolvable
    suture
Skin is closed with a running subcuticular stitch, using 3-0 or 4-0 dissolvable suture and Steri-Strips,
    or with topical skin adhesive

Special Notes

Anterior Cervical Plate Fixation   The design of anterior cervical spine plates has evolved
from standard nonlocked plates to rigid plates with locking screws to variable-angle screws to
dynamic plating with either slotted plates to allow for compression through translation of the screws
in the plate or plates that translate by internal mechanism. Dynamic fixation may allow more load
sharing through the graft to decrease the risk of hardware failure and increase fusion rates.

Autograft versus Allograft versus Cages versus Cementation

Although it does carry donor site morbidity, autologous iliac crest bone grafting is a valid option for
one- or two-level vertebrectomies. With larger defects, fibular auto- or allograft provides appropriate
graft dimensions with minimal fashioning of the graft. The increased healing potential of autograft
is often overshadowed by the donor site morbidity and the fact that posterior stabilization in these
large defects minimizes any effect of bone graft choice on final functional outcome.

Several different types of cages have recently been introduced for reconstruction after anterior
cervical vertebrectomy with the proposed benefit of immediate anterior column stability without
donor graft site morbidity. The most commonly used are titanium mesh cages, ceramic cages, PEEK
cages, and carbon-fiber reinforced polymer cages. Although well-designed prospective studies are
lacking, all appear to have excellent fusion rates with acceptable subsidence and similar short-term
outcomes (4).

PMMA cement constructs with or without Steinmann pins or screws for additional fixation
(not FDA approved for this use) can be employed successfully for anterior column reconstruction in patients with metastatic cervical spine disease to provide immediate stability without donor
site morbidity. PMMA cementation does not allow for bony healing and is thus best suited for
patients with life expectancies less than 6 months (7). (Sayama, Schmidt, Bison Cervical Spine
Metastases: tech)

PEARLS AND PITFALLS

Review location of vertebral arteries on MRI preoperatively
Mark incision under fluoroscopic guidance to ensure proper level
Can use transverse incisions for up to at least four-level vertebrectomy
Intraoperative traction is optional for many cases but is particularly important in patients with
    myelopathy

Preoperative direct laryngoscopy and assessment of vocal cord function is necessary in revision cases when approaching the anterior cervical spine from the contralateral side of original approach

Horizontal incision through the platysma and avoidance of extensive dissection between the platysma and the skin allows the platysma and skin to be closed in one level and improves strength of skin closure and cosmesis

Obtain a lateral fluoroscopic image with a hemostat clamped on the ALL directly overlying a disc space or with a spinal needle within the disc to confirm level

Cephalad/caudad retractors may increase post-op dysphagia, and the distractor posts are often enough to hold cranial and caudal tissues

If wanting to dissect more laterally (under longus colli) to confirm boundaries of the vertebral body, it is safe to perform this at vertebral body level where there is bony protection of the vertebral artery, rather than at disc level where the vertebral artery is exposed

We can't always dissect bone off of the dura in OPLL, so frequently we will leave a small bone island over dura that can float up as decompression is completed

Graft docking site preparation—flatten the endplates to smooth punctate-bleeding cortical surfaces (remove all fibrocartilage). Creating concave docking sites to improve graft stability carries a risk of graft subsidence since the cortical bone has been thinned and weakened.

Use anatomic landmarks and fluoroscopy to ensure central placement of anterior plate without encroachment upon the adjacent level intervertebral discs.

POSTOPERATIVE MANAGEMENT

At the conclusion of the surgery, patients can be fit with a semirigid cervical orthosis for 6 to 10 weeks depending on perceived stability of construct during surgery. Patients should be encouraged to get out of bed and ambulate with PT on POD no. 0 or 1 and surgical drains are pulled on the first postoperative day. Postoperative pain control begins with preoperative education. Preoperative treatment with pregabalin and oxycontin may be considered. Postoperatively, pain treatment may include acetaminophen, IV, and oral narcotic medications (both short and long acting), as well as nerve modulating medication (gabapentin). The patient should begin on a mechanically soft diet as it is the least likely to cause an aspiration. Some patients will have swallowing discomfort for the first 2 to 4 days after surgery due to retraction on the esophagus intraoperatively. Any difficulties with swallowing should be evaluated by a speech and swallow exam before the patient takes further oral intake. An appropriate bowel regiment should be started in the immediate postoperative period to minimize the risk of developing an ileus.

Anterior cervical spine hematomas are rare but can progress quickly and cause airway obstruction. Symptomatic hematomas must be urgently addressed by opening the incision to decompress the anterior neck.

After discharge from the hospital, patients are routinely seen at 2 weeks, 6 weeks, 12 weeks, 6 months, and 1 year. Patients are encouraged to ambulate as often as possible from the time of discharge, with a limited lower extremity strengthening program beginning at 2 to 4 weeks. Overhead lifting, cervical spine twisting, and bending are discouraged until fusion is obtained.

COMPLICATIONS

The complications encountered after vertebrectomy and plating range from the relatively common and bothersome transient postoperative dysphagia to the rare and devastating cervical cord injury or dominant vertebral artery injury. Early complications can be organized based upon the area involved: neurologic, vascular, central neck structures (trachea and esophagus), and bone graft/hardware failures. Long-term adverse effects can also be seen in the form of decreased range of motion, symptomatic nonunions, and adjacent segment degeneration. Once again, adequate preoperative patient education regarding both the risks and benefits of surgery is critical to dealing with postoperative complications.

Trachea/Esophageal Trauma

Postoperative transient hoarseness and/ or dysphagia occurs in at least 5% to 10% of patients, and the incidence is likely higher for dysphagia. It nearly always resolves within 2 months (5). These symptoms are thought to be due to retraction on the esophagus, and/or trachea, intraoperatively and can be minimized by reducing time of retraction and ensuring that the retractors remain under the longus colli for the entire surgery. Some surgeons also will deflate the endotracheal cuff after retractors are placed and reinflate to reduce the incidence of hoarseness (1). Appropriate antibiotic treatment should be initiated after any recognized intraoperative tracheal or esophageal perforation to minimize the risk of infection. Such patients should be followed for clinical symptoms of a tracheal-esophageal fistula and managed by an ENT surgeon.

Neurologic Injuries

The most common neurologic complication after vertebrectomy and fusion is a C5 palsy, with a reported incidence of 0% to 17%, and nearly all patients improve over 2 to 3 months. The etiology, risk factors, and prognostic factors for this complication remain unknown. Potential causes include direct nerve root trauma, excessive traction of the nerve root caused by shifting of the cord after decompression, and ischemia caused by damage to the radicular arteries. Regardless, C5 radiculopathy occurs at a similar frequency after posterior or anterior cervical decompressive surgeries (2).

Intraoperative damage to the sympathetic chain can lead to Horner syndrome, which is diagnosed based on the clinical findings of unilateral ptosis (drooping eyelid), meiosis (constriction of pupil), and facial anhidrosis. This occurs if dissection is carried out lateral to the longus colli muscles. Supportive care is adequate for transient symptoms, and a neurology consult may be helpful for unrelenting cases.

- Cerebral spinal fluid leak from intraoperative dural injury is relatively rare and can usually be managed with a drain for 12 to 24 hours and a compressive dressing. A fibrin glue may be placed on the durotomy to seal the tear. Symptoms may be aided by maintaining an upright posture to decrease hydrostatic pressure in the cervical spine. Myelopathy and complete cord injury are thankfully very uncommon and can likely be minimized with spinal cord monitoring and meticulous surgical technique.

Vascular

The most feared vascular complication is the rare vertebral artery injury. Treatment options include local control with pressure and hemostatic agents versus direct repair or ligation. Close monitoring of blood pressure is critical to maintain cerebral perfusion. If a vertebral artery is suspected or identified, further dissection around the contralateral vertebral artery should be avoided (this may leave inadequate fixation that necessitates external or posterior stabilization). If local control has been obtained during surgery, the patient should nonetheless be evaluated by arteriography postoperatively to confirm repair or occlusion and lack of ongoing leak.

Graft/Hardware Related

Subsidence, migration, and frank dislodgement of the bone graft used for anterior column reconstruction can all lead to clinical symptoms and revision surgery. Similarly, failure of the anterior plate or screws can lead to compression of any of the anterior neck structures and often requires further surgical intervention. The reported incidence of graft dislodgement and hardware failure are each approximately 5% (8).

Long-Term Issues

Patients can expect to lose approximately 10 to 20 degrees of motion in all planes with each vertebral body removed. Reported nonunion rates vary between 0% and 28%, with an average of approximately 8% (8).

RESULTS

Long-term data have shown that anterior vertebrectomy and plating halts progressive myelopathy and results in clinically significant improvements in functional outcome scores (JOA score) (3).

A recent systematic review of ACDF versus vertebrectomy and fusion for multilevel cervical spondylosis found that vertebrectomy resulted in increased blood loss and an increased rate of graft dislodgement but also increased fusion rates for both 2 and 3 disc level surgeries. They also found that clinical outcome scores were greater in the vertebrectomy group in three studies, similar between ACDF and vertebrectomy in six studies, and no studies found ACDF clinical results superior to vertebrectomy (8). Two-level ACDF and single-level vertebrectomy and fusion have comparable results in terms of infection rates, dysphagia, sagittal alignment, cervical lordosis, graft subsidence, and adjacent-level radiographic deterioration (6,8).

RECOMMENDED READING

1. Apfelbaum RI, Kriskovich MD, Haller JR: On the incidence, cause, and prevention of recurrent laryngeal nerve palsies during anterior cervical spine surgery. *Spine* 25(22): 2906–2912, 2000.
2. Gandhoke G, Wu J-C, Rowland NC, et al.: Anterior corpectomy versus posterior laminoplasty: is the risk of postoperative C-5 palsy different. *Neurosurg Focus* 31(4): E12, 2011.
3. Gao R, Yang L, Chen H, et al.: Long term results of anterior corpectomy and fusion for cervical spondylotic myelopathy. *PloS one* 7(4): e34811, 2012.
4. Kabir SM, Alabi J, Rezajooi K, et al.: Anterior cervical corpectomy: review and comparison of results using titanium mesh cages and carbon fibre reinforced polymer cages. *Br J Neurosurg* 24(5): 542–546, 2010.
5. Lin, Zhou, Wang, et al.: A comparison of anterior cervical discectomy and corpectomy in patients with multilevel cervical spondylotic myelopathy. *Eur Spine J* 21(3): 474–481, 2012.
6. Park Y, Maeda T, Cho W, et al.: Comparison of anterior cervical fusion after two-level discectomy or single-level corpectomy: sagittal alignment, cervical lordosis, graft collapse, and adjacent-level ossification. *Spine J* 10(3): 193–199, 2010.
7. Sayama C, Schmidt M, Bisson E: Cervical spine metastasis: techniques for anterior reconstruction and stabilization. *Neurosurg Rev* 35(4): 463–474, 2012.
8. Sheng-Dan J, Lei-Sheng J, Lig-Yang D: Anterior cervical discectomy and fusion versus anterior corpectomy and fusion for multilevel cervical spondylosis: a systematic review. *Arch Orthop Trauma Surg* 132: 155–161, 2012.
9. Vaccaro A, Falatyn S, Scuderi GJ: *Early failure of long segment anterior cervical plate fixation. J Spinal Disord* 11(5): 410–415, 1998.

5 Cervical Osteotomy

Justin W. Miller and Rick C. Sasso

Techniques for spinal osteotomy have evolved over the past 75 years, and although basic principles remain the same, certain technical advances have occurred. Smith-Petersen et al. (7) were among the first to describe such techniques with their series of posterior lumbar osteotomies in 1945. LaChapelle (2) followed soon thereafter with his description of staged anterior and posterior lumbar osteotomies in 1946. Mason et al. (3) described his osteotomy of the cervical spine in 1953.

In 1972, Simmons (6) popularized the idea that cervical osteotomy could be performed in ankylosing spondylitis (AS) patients under local anesthesia with continuous neurologic monitoring. Urist (8) is credited with first describing this awake-sitting technique under local anesthesia in 1958. Urist also recommended that the osteotomy occur at the C7–T1 junction if possible. There are several benefits of performing the osteotomy at the cervicothoracic junction: (a) the spinal canal is relatively wide with more space available for the neural elements, (b) damage to the cord and/or nerve roots at this level would be less catastrophic than if in the midcervical region, and (c) the risk of injuring the vertebral artery is less, as the artery typically passes anterior to the transverse processes in this region.

Simmons (6) advocated a posterior wedge-shaped osteotomy to perform the correction. Removal of the lamina and spinous processes from C6 to T1 is done. Facetectomies are performed bilaterally to widely expose the C8 nerve roots. The head is extended in order to perform an osteoclasis of the anterior and middle columns of the cervical spine with the instantaneous axis of rotation at the base of the C7 pedicle. This causes lengthening of the anterior spine while the posterior elements are shortened. No instrumentation was used, and a halo was applied until fusion occurred. This technique was associated with a 4% mortality and 2% incidence of nerve root lesions.

Bohlman (1) expanded on Simmons' cervical osteotomy technique with the addition of instrumentation to stabilize the cervical spine after the osteotomies were performed. Bohlman utilized a small Luque rectangle with Drummond wires and buttons supplemented by autograft. Patients, however, were still immobilized postoperatively in halo vests. Like Simmons and Urist, Bohlman preferred to perform his osteotomy at the C7–T1 junction.

In order to limit the possibility of sagittal translation during the Simmons osteotomy technique, Mehdian and Arun (4) devised a more controlled method of reduction at the osteotomy site. The Mehdian method involves the use of a posterior cervicothoracic screw-rod system that is implanted prior to completion of the osteotomy. Provisional, malleable rods are temporarily inserted. These rods allow the thoracic pedicle screws to slide along the rod as the reduction is performed without allowing translation. This allows for a more controlled reduction maneuver before the definitive titanium rods are placed.

INDICATIONS/CONTRAINDICATIONS

The primary indication for cervical osteotomy is the correction of a fixed cervical kyphotic deformity. This can occur in patients with AS, previous trauma, or prior surgery. This deformity may result in difficulty with activities of daily living, respiratory compromise, difficulty eating, loss of horizontal gaze, and/or disabling pain. Cervical osteotomy is contraindicated when the major deformity is in the thoracolumbar spine, when a flexion contracture of the hip is present, or if the cervical kyphosis is flexible. Other general contraindications include significant medical comorbidities that would prohibit normal recovery and rehabilitation.

PREOPERATIVE PREPARATION

Patient Evaluation

Medical comorbidities should be noted, evaluated, and optimized. Special attention should ensure that the cardiopulmonary status of the patient is satisfactory to undergo a spinal reconstructive procedure. Patients with AS, for instance, often have significantly restricted chest expansion due to ankylosed costovertebral joints. The surgeon should be aware of such issues.

Routine preoperative lab work should exclude anemia and coagulopathy. We recommend a lengthy discussion with the patient regarding the potential risks and benefits of surgery. Major surgical risks of cervical osteotomy include dysphagia, infection, malunion, nonunion, neurologic injury, vertebral artery injury, and death.

Preoperative Radiographic Evaluation

Cervical kyphotic deformities can occur at any age and may be associated with thoracic and/or lumbar deformities. It is important, therefore, to look at global sagittal and coronal balance (with full-length PA and lateral 36-inch scoliosis x-rays) in these patients to ensure that the planned correction does not cause decompensation in overall spinal balance (Fig. 5-1). You must assess cervical, thoracic, and lumbar sagittal alignment individually as well as globally and define the site of maximal deformity. The degree of correction to be obtained depends on the angle of the cervical deformity and the chin-brow to vertical angle. Meticulously plan the procedure on printed or digital x-ray including the size of the osteotomy and hardware position. Determination of osteotomy size/angle can be done via radiographic tracing and film cutout or simple mathematical calculation (5). Planning is crucial to ensure you do not overcorrect the deformity. In addition, we recommend preoperative radiographic evaluation with computed tomography (CT), and magnetic resonance imaging (MRI). Sagittal and coronal reconstructions are helpful to better visualize the deformity. The CT scan is useful to measure the dimensions of the vertebral bodies, the cervical pedicles, and the cervical lateral masses. This information is crucial for selection of the appropriate implants and accurate planning. The MRI is useful to evaluate not only spinal cord and nerve root compression but also size and position of the vertebral arteries.

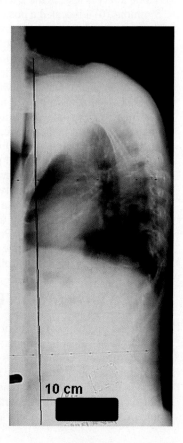

FIGURE 5-1

Lateral standing radiograph demonstrating significant sagittal imbalance with the C7 plumb line approximately 10 cm anterior to the sacral promontory.

TECHNIQUE

Anesthetic Considerations

Intubation of a patient with a significant cervical deformity can be challenging. A real potential exists for spinal cord injury during intubation, as well as throughout the case due to hemodynamic changes or direct cord injury. Consequently, modern anesthetic techniques involve monitoring the cardiovascular and neurologic status of the patient. To this end, arterial line placement and motor evoked (MEP) and somatosensory evoked potentials (SSEP) are recommended to monitor blood pressure and spinal cord integrity respectively throughout the case. Subclavian central line placement for monitoring the central venous pressure can also be done if deemed necessary. We caution, with regard to neuromonitoring, that SSEPs are not always accurate and there have been cases where changes in evoked potentials have not been accompanied by changes in neurologic status (i.e., false positives). There have also been cases where a neurologic injury occurred without accompanying changes in the evoked potentials (i.e., false negatives).

One relatively safe method of intubation is awake, nasotracheal, fiberoptic intubation. Performing the intubation awake is important because the patient's neurologic status can be continuously assessed. The abnormal fixed chin-brow vertical angle does not allow for the patient's head to be extended, and fiberoptic intubation is necessary to visualize the vocal cords and ensure appropriate placement of the endotracheal tube. Orotracheal intubation with a chin-on-chest deformity is difficult at best due to restricted access to the oral cavity. Nasotracheal intubation is easier and can proceed after the nasal cavity has been anesthetized.

The choice of anesthetic agents is critical when evoked potentials are utilized. Paralytics and nitrous oxide are not used in these cases as they blunt the MEPs and SSEPs respectively. Total IV anesthesia is ideal in the setting of neuromonitoring.

It is important to obtain pre– and post–general anesthesia baseline readings of the evoked potentials. Since changes in the anesthetic regimen can cause changes in the evoked potentials, we do not recommend changing the drugs or dosages throughout the case.

Ensuring adequate spinal cord perfusion throughout the case is crucial. The patient's mean arterial pressure (MAP) prior to intubation is assessed, and this MAP is maintained throughout the case (even in the face of blood loss). We do not hesitate to use transfusions and/or pressors as needed throughout the case to maintain the MAP.

Osteotomy Considerations

Numerous osteotomy techniques have been described as previously mentioned. All include some variation of opening versus closing wedge osteotomy. We will describe two cervical techniques felt to be the most efficacious and biomechanically sound depending on where the apex of the deformity occurs. The majority of deformities involving the cervical region are most severe at the cervicothoracic junction, which is also an ideal place for the osteotomy due to the reasons discussed earlier. Deformities, however, may be within the actual cervical region and necessitate osteotomy above the cervicothoracic junction.

CERVICOTHORACIC PEDICLE SUBTRACTION OSTEOTOMY

Stage I—Positioning

After induction of anesthesia, a Foley catheter, sequential compression stockings, and pneumatic compression devices are applied. Baseline readings of SSEPs and MEPs are obtained before positioning the patient. The preoperative x-ray with the operative plan is hung in the operating room for all physicians and assistants to reference.

The patient is placed in Mayfield pins while in the supine position. The Jackson table is set up such that the foot of the bed is placed at the lowest rungs and the head of the bed at the highest rungs. The patient is then transferred to the prone position on the Jackson table. Due to the significant kyphotic deformity, positioning can be a challenging task. In order to raise the head into the operative field, blankets can be used to elevate the chest. A second option involves removing the hip pads on the table and using the leg sling only provided the patient's body habitus allows the pelvic region to pass between the bars of the table. Arms are secured at the patient's side with a circumferential sheet and towel clips. The head is secured to the table by attaching to the Mayfield head holder. The patient's buttocks should be taped to the table to prevent distal migration of the patient on the bed. The shoulders are taped to aid with imaging. The table is placed in reverse Trendelenburg to also aid with elevation of the head into the operative field.

It is important that the surgeon pay close attention to the plane of the patient's body in relation to the floor. The chin-brow vertical angle should be noted, and this angle should be corrected, allowing the face to be parallel to the plane of the body. It is better to slightly undercorrect the deformity than to overcorrect. After positioning is complete, repeat SSEPs and MEPs are performed to ensure integrity of the spinal cord.

The posterior cervicothoracic region is prepped and draped in the normal sterile fashion. A permanent surgical marker is used to outline the incision prior to draping. It is best to drape wide from the occiput down to the midthoracic region.

Stage II—Exposure and Instrumentation

A standard posterior cervical exposure is performed. The lateral masses in the cervical region are fully visualized as are the transverse processes in the thoracic region. Care is taken at both the proximal and distal extent of the fusion area to protect the facets and posterior ligamentous complex in hopes of avoiding iatrogenic adjacent level problems (Fig. 5-2).

Lateral mass screws are inserted in the cervical region via the Magerl technique. The starting point is in the middle of the lateral mass, and the trajectory aimed at the upper and outer quadrant of the lateral mass. We typically use 14-mm screws that are placed unicortically.

Upper thoracic pedicle screws are placed via standard anatomic landmarks. The craniocaudal entry point is at the junction of the upper and middle third of the transverse process, and this point is usually approximately 3 mm below the facet joint itself. The mediolateral entry point is at the center of the facet joint. In addition, a laminoforaminotomy may be performed to allow the surgeon to visualize and palpate the medial border of the pedicle. Use of image guidance can also assist with placement of the thoracic screws. Use a high-speed drill to burr the posterior cortex at pedicle screw entry points. Typically, a bleeding area of bone (this is the cancellous bone within the pedicle) is exposed with this maneuver. We then utilize the awl and tap to enter the pedicle. These instruments usually pass down the pedicle with minimal force without perforating the pedicle walls. Pedicle screws are then placed.

Next we attach provisional rods to the lateral mass and thoracic pedicle screws. The provisional rods are hollow stainless steel tubes that are fairly easy to bend, thus allowing sagittal plane correction while preventing translation. These provisional rods are attached to the polyaxial screw heads with small lateral connectors. The lateral attachment of the provisional rods is necessary to allow for the upcoming posterior wedge osteotomy of the cervical facets. Locking caps are placed and tightened to secure the connectors to the polyaxial screw heads. Locking caps are also used to secure the connectors to the rods; however these are not tightened, allowing the connectors to translate along the rod during deformity correction (Fig. 5-3).

Stage III—Osteotomy

The osteotomy begins with a complete laminectomy of C7, removing the entire spinous process and lamina. The inferior half of the C6 lamina and superior half of the T1 lamina are removed. If needed, the caudal and cephalad aspects of the spinous processes of C6 and T1 respectively, can also be removed. The C7 lateral mass must be completely removed as well as the transverse process laterally. The inferior facets of C6 and the superior facets of T1 are also removed flush with the edge

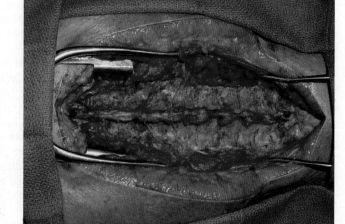

FIGURE 5-2

Complete exposure is performed of the lateral masses within the cervical region and out to the transverse processes within the upper thoracic region.

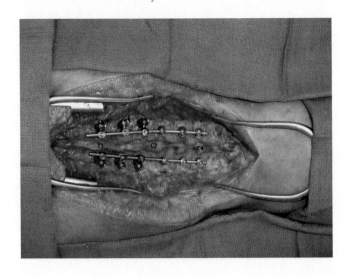

FIGURE 5-3

Instrumentation is placed above and below the C7 vertebra with a provisional rod. Note that off-set connectors are used in the thoracic spine from T1 to T3.

of the respective pedicle. It is crucial to remove any overhanging bone whether from residual facet overhang or lamina to prevent impingement of the neurologic structures during closure of the osteotomy. At this juncture, the spinal cord, C7, and C8 nerve roots should be fully visible and the C7 pedicle between the roots (Fig. 5-4). Hemostasis is maintained with Gelfoam thrombin and Floseal (Baxter Healthcare Corp.)

Decancellation of the C7 vertebral body is then begun. Several methods can be employed to perform the removal of bone from the vertebral body. The pedicle walls should be left intact if possible during this process to aid with protection of the neurologic structures. One method is use of a high-speed burr to thin the bone within the pedicle and subsequently remove the cancellous bone within the vertebral body. A second method is the use of successively larger taps, passing through the pedicles and into the vertebral body. Various forward and backward angle curettes also can assist with bone removal. Whether using the burr or taps, a wedge cavity is created via access through both pedicles such that only a cortical shell of bone remains. It is imperative that a uniform area of bone be resected to allow a symmetric closure of the osteotomy. A Penfield elevator is then used to expose the lateral walls of the vertebral body and a V-shaped area of bone is resected (Fig. 5-5). The resection is carried to the anterior cortex of the body. This is done with a narrow Leksell rongeur. The final area of bone to be removed is the posterior cortex and any remaining aspect of the C7 pedicle wall. This is done with a backward angle curette and should occur with relative ease if decancellation was done properly. The posterior cortex is carefully pushed downward into the wedge cavity, taking care not to retract the cord.

Stage IV—Correction of the Deformity

Once the osteotomy is complete, an unscrubbed assistant loosens the Mayfield attachment and gently elevates the patient's head. The surgeon helps to guide the head and closure of the osteotomy under direct visualization. Within the wound, close attention is paid to the exiting C7 and C8 nerve

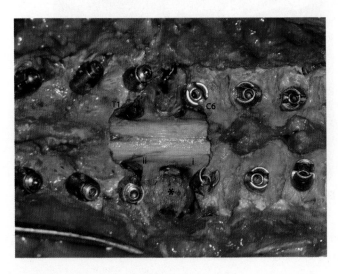

FIGURE 5-4

Complete removal of the C7 posterior elements has been performed. The caudal aspect of C6 has been removed as well as the inferior facets of C6 bilaterally. The cephalad aspect of T1 has been removed as well as the superior facets of T1 bilaterally. (Note the provisional rods have been removed for visualization purposes.) *, C7 pedicle; *i*, C7 nerve root; *ii*, C8 nerve root.

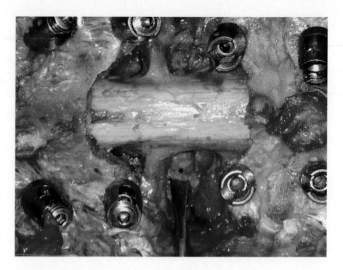

FIGURE 5-5

Note the Penfield 4 retractor lateral to the *decancellated C7 pedicle wall.

roots as well as the spinal cord and buckling dura (Fig. 5-6). If there is any impingement evident during closure of the osteotomy, or neuromonitoring signals change, the osteotomy should be gently reversed and the offending agent (i.e., bone) should be resected. The lamina may need to be undercut or further facet resection may be necessary. After the osteotomy is closed the provisional rods should be locked in place and the Mayfield attachment secured to the table again. Assessment of the chin-brow to vertical angle should be done at this time to assure that adequate correction has occurred. It is important not to overcorrect the deformity. The overall alignment is assessed via fluoroscopy imaging as well as gross examination of the patient's head in relation to the torso. We then proceed to replace the provisional rods with the appropriate length permanent titanium rods. The final set screws are secured and finally tightened with the torque wrench.

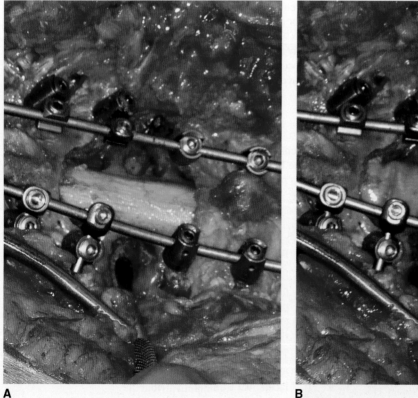
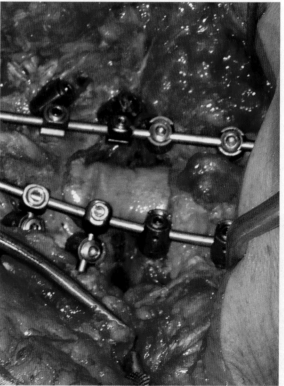

A   **B**

FIGURE 5-6

A,B: Note the Penfield 4 retractor within the osteotomy defect and the change in rod length and buckling of the dura following closure. The Penfield 4 retractor is no longer able to fit within the defect following closure of the osteotomy.

Stage V—Bone Grafting and Wound Closure

The wound should be copiously irrigated with normal saline. Decortication is performed at each facet joint and across each lamina within the fusion region using the high-speed burr. Local autograft is then placed along the decorticated regions. If additional graft is needed, iliac crest bone can be harvested. The wound is then closed in a layered fashion. A meticulous layered closure should be done to ensure proper healing occurs. It is especially critical that the fascial layer be reapproximated, as this layer tends to retract throughout the case, and if not careful can be missed. Poor wound closure can result in numerous complications including infection, fascial and/or wound dehiscence, hematoma, and poor cosmesis.

MIDCERVICAL EXTENSION OSTEOTOMY

Stage I—Anterior Release and Osteotomy

After induction of anesthesia, a Foley catheter, sequential compression stockings, and pneumatic compression devices are applied. Baseline readings of SSEPs and MEPs are obtained before positioning the patient. The preoperative x-ray with the operative plan is hung in the operating room for all physicians and assistants to reference.

The patient is positioned supine on the operating table with the head on a foam headrest, elevated with blankets and pillows to adjust for the kyphotic deformity. If there is a significant submandibular pannus, the soft tissue is retracted with wide tape to allow for greater access to the anterior cervical region. The shoulders are pulled caudally with tape. Rarely, the chin-on-chest deformity is so severe that the surgeon cannot access the anterior neck, and the procedure is abandoned. Patients with such severe kyphotic angulation may benefit from a trial of cervical traction.

We prefer to perform the anterior cervical approach through a transverse right side incision when above C7/T1. For illustrative purposes, we discuss the treatment of a C5/C6 kyphotic deformity for the remainder of this chapter.

After the standard Smith-Robinson anterior cervical exposure is performed, we place distraction pins into the bodies of C5 and C6 and then obtain a localizing x-ray to confirm the level. The pins are placed perpendicular to the longitudinal axis of the vertebral bodies in order to help with orientation during the anterior resection. It is sometimes difficult to confirm levels in patients with AS because the disc spaces are fused. In these patients, the surgeon may confirm levels by counting the spinous processes, looking for the angulation in the cervical spine, or by assessing the location of the deformity in relation to the hyoid bone.

Following localization of the appropriate level, a generous discectomy is performed. If the disc space is completely fused, then a power drill may be used. The posterior endplates of C5 and C6 and all posterior vertebral osteophytes are removed. The posterior aspect of the disc space is "trumpeted" by undercutting the posterior body walls of C5 and C6.

After the generous wedge is created at C5/6, a left C6 pediculectomy is performed. The left C6 pedicle is accessible from a right-sided anterior cervical approach because the surgeon is looking across midline and can visualize the contralateral pedicle. The ipsilateral pedicle is difficult to visualize from the anterior approach, and the right pediculectomy will need to be completed during the posterior stage of the operation.

Subsequent to the pediculectomy, bilateral C6 foramen transversaria are exposed. The longus colli muscles are reflected at the cephalad aspect of the C6 body bilaterally, out to the edge of the foramen. The anterior portions of the foramen are then removed (Fig. 5-7). This is done to prevent

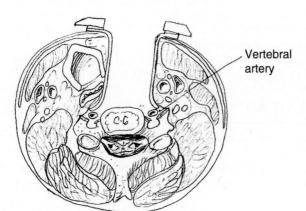

Vertebral artery

FIGURE 5-7

Note removal of the anterior portions of the foramen transversaria.

kinking of the vertebral arteries during the upcoming reduction maneuver. At the completion of the first stage, close the anterior cervical incision with staples only, and apply a sterile dressing. We anticipate coming back to the anterior approach in stage VI, so a typical layered closure is delayed.

Stage II—Posterior Exposure and Instrumentation

The patient is placed in Mayfield pins while in the supine position. We attempt to place a rigid cervical collar (occasionally, this is not possible due to the chin-on-chest position), and then carefully flip the patient prone onto another operating table. The prone setup is exactly as described previously for the pedicle subtraction osteotomy (PSO).

The exposure of the posterior elements and insertion of hardware is virtually identical to that described previously for the PSO, with the exception of vertebral levels. Anchors are placed three levels above and three levels below the deformity. Consequently, for a C5–C6 deformity, we place lateral mass screws at C3–C5 and pedicle screws at C7–T2.

Stage III—Osteotomy

The osteotomy begins with removal of the inferior half of the C5 spinous process and lamina (if this bone is not removed, it will impinge on the posterior dura when the correction is performed). The inferior articular process of C5 is removed below the C5 lateral mass screw. All of the posterior elements of C6 are removed including the spinous process, lamina, superior articular process, inferior articular process, and the residual C6 pedicles (the portion of the C6 pedicles that was not removed during the anterior approach). Use of a high-speed burr, fine curettes, and rongeurs allows efficient removal of bone. The exiting C6 and C7 nerve roots are completely exposed when the resection is complete. Removal of the posterior portion of the foramen transverium completes the bilateral foramen transversectomies at C6. This step is necessary to prevent kinking of the vertebral artery during correction. There is often abundant venous bleeding from the periarterial venous plexus, and this can be controlled with thrombin-soaked Gelfoam and/or Floseal (Baxter Healthcare Corp.). Finally, the cephalad half of the spinous process and lamina, and the superior articular facet of C7 are removed (also to prevent impingement of the posterior dura during correction). Prior to correction, the exposure and bone resection should look very similar to that described in the PSO section and seen in Figures 5-4 to 5-6.

Stage IV—Correction of Deformity

The deformity is corrected in the same manner as described previously for the PSO.

Stage V—Bone Grafting and Closure

The fusion area is prepared and wound closed in the same manner as described previously for the PSO.

Stage VI—Anterior Instrumentation

The patient is positioned supine again onto a separate operating table. After repositioning, evoked potentials are assessed. The head is placed on a foam cushion and the Mayfield attachment removed. The prior anterior incision is prepped and the skin staples removed.

The anterior exposure is redeveloped. The distraction pins are placed again into the vertebral bodies of C5 and C6, and mild distraction is applied. A tricortical iliac crest autograft is measured, cut to size, and inserted into the now parallel interbody space at C5–C6. The distraction pins are removed, and an appropriate-size anterior cervical plate is applied (Fig. 5-8).

The platysma is then reapproximated, and the anterior skin incision is closed with a subcuticular suture. A rigid collar is applied.

POSTOPERATIVE MANAGEMENT

The patient remains intubated and is taken to the recovery room. Postoperatively, the patient is allowed to temporarily emerge from the anesthetic in order to perform a neurologic exam. The patient is extubated after the anesthesiologist assesses airway edema with a leak test. Progressive ambulation is initiated immediately, and the cervical hard collar is kept in place for 6 weeks.

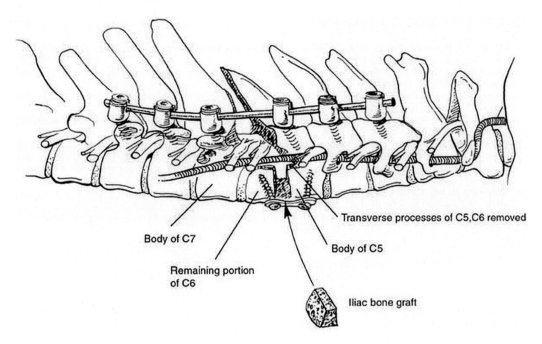

Transverse processes of C5,C6 removed

Body of C7

Body of C5

Remaining portion
of C6

Iliac bone graft

FIGURE 5-8
Final construct with
kyphotic reduction.

CONCLUSION

Patients with chin-on-chest deformity pose an anesthetic and surgical challenge. Modern anesthetic and surgical techniques allow for a relatively safe correction of this deformity (Fig. 5-9). Provisional rods allow for controlled reduction of the deformity after the osteotomy has been performed. Our techniques are not the only methods of achieving reduction of this deformity; however we have used them with success on a number of cases. The potential complications of this procedure include all of those relevant to cervical spine surgery including dysphagia, infection, radiculopathy, pseudarthrosis, loss of sagittal correction, spinal cord injury, and anesthetic risks.

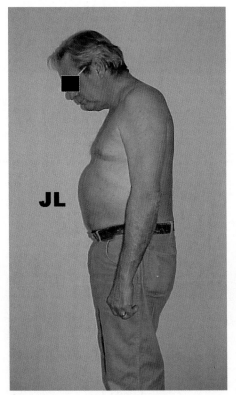

JL

A

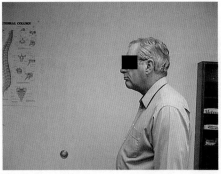

B

FIGURE 5-9
A: Preoperative.
B: Postoperative.

RECOMMENDED READING

1. Belanger TA, Milam RA, Roh JS, et al.: Cervicothoracic extension osteotomy for chin-on-chest deformity in ankylosing spondylitis. *J Bone Joint Surg Am* 87: 1732–1738, 2005.
2. LaChapelle EH: Osteotomy of the lumbar spine for correction of kyphosis in a case of ankylosing spondylitis. *J Bone Joint Surg Am* 28: 851–858, 1946.
3. Mason C, Cozen L, Adelstein L: Surgical correction of flexion deformity of the cervical spine. *Calif Med* 79: 244–246, 1953.
4. Mehdian S, Arun R: A safe controlled instrumented reduction technique for cervical osteotomy in ankylosing spondylitis. *Spine* 36: 715–720, 2011.
5. Ondra SL, Marzouk S, Koski T, et al.: Mathematical calculation of pedicle subtraction osteotomy size to allow precision correction of fixed sagittal deformity. *Spine* 31: E973–E979, 2006.
6. Simmons EH: The surgical correction of flexion deformity of the cervical spine in ankylosing spondylitis. *Clin Orthop* 86: 132–143, 1972.
7. Smith-Petersen MN, Larson CB, Aufranc OE: Osteotomy of the spine for correction of flexion deformity in rheumatoid arthritis. *J Bone Joint Surg Am* 27: 1–11, 1945.
8. Urist MR: Osteotomy of the cervical spine: report of a case of ankylosing spondylitis. *J Bone Joint Surg Am* 40: 833–843, 1958.

6 Anterior Odontoid Fixation

Ronald I. Apfelbaum and Rick C. Sasso

INDICATIONS

Direct anterior odontoid screw fixation is indicated in patients with acute type II and high type III (with a shallow base) odontoid fractures (Fig. 6-1). The rationale for direct anterior fixation is the achievement of immediate fixation in anatomical alignment, stabilizing the atlantoaxial complex while providing the best environment for fracture healing. The construct preserves C1–C2 rotation while providing rigid internal fixation and avoids restrictive bracing and the complications associated with bone grafting techniques. It has a higher success rate than and reduces the morbidity associated with prolonged halo immobilization, which had been used preferentially in the past. Direct anterior osteosynthesis of the odontoid fracture with anterior odontoid screw fixation is often the preferred alternative to atlantoaxial arthrodesis for management of odontoid fractures. This technique has been shown to achieve a high healing rate, similar to that of posterior atlantoaxial arthrodesis (88% to 100%), with a similarly low complication rate (1,4,9,27,30,31), and has the advantage over posterior methods of achieving this without intentionally sacrificing atlantoaxial motion (2,27,30).

Polytrauma patients, in whom immediate mobilization has proved beneficial, are also good candidates for anterior odontoid screw fixation as they often are not candidates for halo-vest stabilization. Direct osteosynthesis also can be used in patients who refuse halo treatment and in those in whom fracture reduction can be obtained but not maintained in this apparatus.

CONTRAINDICATIONS

Caution should be used in osteopenic patients; many patients with odontoid fractures are elderly and will have decreased bone mineralization. There is less reason to be concerned about the bone density of the cancellous interior of the odontoid and the C2 body because healing occurs primarily across the cortical bone at the junction of these two. Therefore, if the cortical shell of C2 and the odontoid are reasonably well ossified and there is good apical bone at the tip of the odontoid, screw fixation maybe considered. The lag screw needs to have good purchase in the strongest region of the odontoid—the dense apical cortex—and have a good buttress at the strong anterior inferior aspect of the C2 body to be effective (Fig. 6-2).

A fixed kyphotic angulation of the neck or a barrel chest with a short neck may preclude obtaining the low trajectory needed to place a screw from the inferior edge of C2 to the odontoid apex. This can be checked before surgery using lateral fluoroscopy when the patient is optimally positioned. If the trajectory is not adequate, we will not proceed with direct odontoid screw fixation but rather reposition the patient and perform a C1–C2 instrumented fusion. Compromising the trajectory and accepting an entry site for the screw on the anterior face of C2 rather than the inferior one is not recommended.

Anatomic reduction of the odontoid fracture is imperative before the fixation screw is placed across the fracture. Inability to achieve reduction prior to commencing surgery was therefore previously considered to be an absolute contraindication to the procedure; however, intraoperative reduction and perfection of the alignment of the odontoid to the body of C2 can be obtained using the techniques and instrument system described in this chapter, so this is no longer a contraindication. An absolute contraindication to anterior screw fixation is (the relatively rare) concomitant transverse atlantal ligament (TAL) disruption since, in such a case, fixation of the odontoid alone will not stabilize the C1–C2 complex.

75

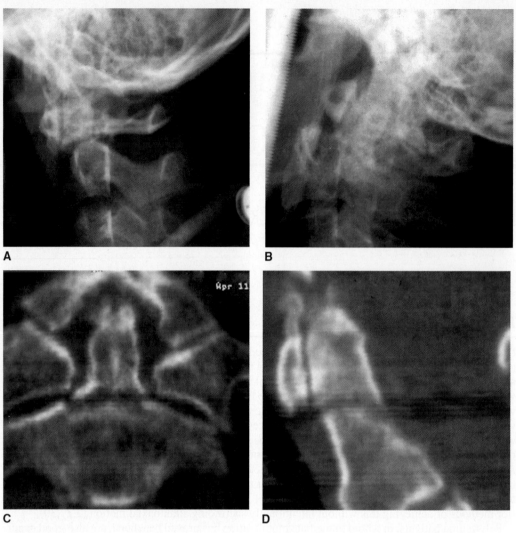

FIGURE 6-1
Type II odontoid fractures: with odontoid anterolisthesed **(A)** and retrolisthesed **(B)**. High Type III odontoid fracture **(C, D)**. (Copyright Dr. Ronald I. Apfelbaum).

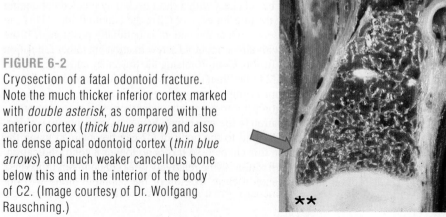

FIGURE 6-2
Cryosection of a fatal odontoid fracture. Note the much thicker inferior cortex marked with *double asterisk,* as compared with the anterior cortex (*thick blue arrow*) and also the dense apical odontoid cortex (*thin blue arrows*) and much weaker cancellous bone below this and in the interior of the body of C2. (Image courtesy of Dr. Wolfgang Rauschning.)

Chronic fracture nonunions over 6 months old and oblique fractures in an anteroinferior-to-posterosuperior plane that could cause the odontoid fragment to shear anteriorly at the fracture site during lag compression are relative contraindications. The success rate of direct screw fixation for fractures over 6 months of age (25%) has been substantially lower than in those treated earlier. Patients with fractures treated within the first 6 months, such as those treated after failure of a trial of halo immobilization, did as well as those with fresh fractures (4). This is similar to the experience in treating patients with nonunions of anterior cervical interbody fusions with posterior rigid fixation. Once the motion is eliminated, a high percentage of patients with anterior nonunions go on to achieve solid fusion. In regard to oblique fractures, if the overall bone quality is adequate, fixing them in a slight retrolisthesed position in anticipation of the translation of C1 anteriorly on C2 can result in the final alignment being anatomic. In such a case, we would also use a hard collar for 6 weeks to restrict neck flexion. Others also have reported good success with shallower anterior oblique fractures (11).

PREOPERATIVE PREPARATION

Examination and Evaluation/Pathology

Odontoid fractures are relatively common upper cervical spine injuries, constituting nearly 60% of all fractures of the axis and 10% to 18% of all cervical spine fractures (6,24,30). Proportionally greater space is available for the spinal cord in the upper cervical spine than in the lower cervical spine. Therefore, the incidence of neurologic involvement in upper cervical spine injury is relatively low (18% to 26%) (12,38). Furthermore, when significant cord damage does occur in the upper cervical spine, patients frequently do not survive because of respiratory arrest. Modern immobilization and transportation techniques have reduced the incidence of secondary injuries at this level and resulted in more survivors with injuries that previously might have been fatal.

Although odontoid fractures occur in all age groups, the bimodal distribution observed in the past is changing. In younger patients, who represent the first peak incidence, these fractures are usually secondary to high-energy trauma; motor vehicle accidents are responsible for the majority of the odontoid injuries (6,13). Often, the injured patient was a nonrestrained passenger in the front seat whose neck was violently hyperextended when his or her head or face struck the windshield. Concomitant spinal injuries are present in up to 34% of patients; 85% of these associated injuries occur in the cervical spine, most commonly the atlas (12,23,38). These injuries have become much less frequent with the increased use of seat belts and the proliferation of passive restraints such as airbags. The second peak in the incidence of odontoid fractures occurs among the elderly (30). In fact, odontoid fractures are the most common cervical spine fracture in patients older than 70 years (34,35,37). These fractures, unlike those in the younger patients, tend to result from low-energy injuries, such as falls from a standing height. The mechanism of injury is often hyperextension that results in posterior displacement of the odontoid. Associated spinal trauma is much less common in elderly patients (7,12). With increased longevity, these injuries are being seen more frequently and make up the clear majority of odontoid fractures.

Preoperative Radiographic Evaluation

Which imaging studies should be obtained for a comprehensive, diagnostic approach in evaluating suspected upper cervical spine injuries remains a topic of controversy, particularly in the presence of polytrauma or for obtunded patients. The standard, initial cervical spine radiographic series in trauma patients includes a cross-table lateral view, an anteroposterior (AP) view, and an open-mouth view. The value of the AP view has been questioned because it provides little additional information (18). Although this three-view screening series can detect 65% to 95% of axis injuries (30), the C2 vertebra is often obscured by overlying bony maxillary, mandibular, and dental structures; therefore, C2 fractures may be missed. Thin-section computed tomography (CT) is the best study for evaluating C2 bony fractures (8). Sagittal reconstruction of CT images is important because axial images may not show a transverse odontoid fracture. These views can also provide valuable information about the cortical bone density, the status of the subaxial spine, and the presence of anterior osteophytes that may factor into the decision regarding choice of approach.

Although CT is excellent in demonstrating bony injuries, soft tissue and significant ligamentous injuries may not be apparent. Therefore, dynamic flexion/extension lateral fluoroscopic evaluation has been advocated for polytrauma patients to identify occult ligamentous instabilities and confirm that the cervical spine is uninjured (25). Magnetic resonance imaging (MRI) also is helpful in assessing the spinal cord in patients with and without neurologic deficits and gives important information about the subaxial spine. It also is becoming increasingly important in evaluating the status of ligamentous structures such as the TAL.

The assessment of TAL integrity in patients with odontoid fractures is an important consideration in selecting appropriate treatment options (15). Anterior odontoid screw fixation will not provide C1–C2 stability if the TAL is not competent. TAL disruption has been reported to occur in 10% of patients with odontoid fractures (22); however, in our experience, we have rarely noted instability when evaluating TAL integrity by flexing the patient's neck under fluoroscopy after odontoid fixation. This brings into question the accuracy of the MRI criteria. Nevertheless, the combination of MRI, CT, and plain radiographs is important for evaluating unstable C2 fractures and planning a rational treatment course. When a C2 fracture is identified, it is necessary to also evaluate the subaxial spine carefully because 16% of patients have a noncontiguous fracture (39).

TECHNIQUE

Positioning

Before beginning the operation, the surgeon must ensure that reduction of the odontoid to a more anatomic position is possible. Some prefer to do this by simple traction or manipulation while the patient is awake, with lateral fluoroscopic imaging. Typically, we will place the patient on the operating table with a folded blanket or other suitable padding under the shoulders and a similar padding under the head to keep the neck in a neutral position (Fig. 6-3). If the patient's odontoid in this position is anterolisthesed, we extend the patient's neck while observing the alignment under fluoroscopy and gradually remove the head pads. This may reduce the anterolisthesis of C1 and the odontoid process relative to C2 while also optimizing the patient's head position for both intubation and screw placement. If the patient's odontoid is retrolisthesed, the degree of mobility can be assessed under fluoroscopy when the neck is slightly flexed. These preliminary maneuvers help ascertain that reduction will be possible intraoperatively. Intubation should be done without moving the patient's neck in the direction that increases the subluxation. This may require fiberoptic intubation techniques.

To achieve a proper screw trajectory and clear the anterior chest with the instrumentation, it is usually necessary to extend the patient's neck; however, unless this position results in optimal reduction and alignment, this is best done once the screw guidance tubes are in place as is described below. In essence, we will accept the best aligned position to begin the approach but prepare the setup to allow us to modify the patient's head position once the C1–C2 relationship is perfected intraoperatively. Therefore, "perfect" preoperative reduction is *not* required to proceed.

Once the patient is intubated, a radiolucent mouth gag is placed to allow for transoral imaging. A wine bottle cork notched for the patient's teeth or gums is excellent for this. We then use halter

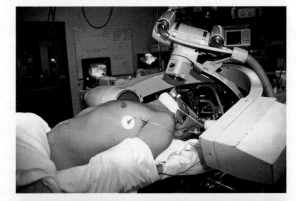

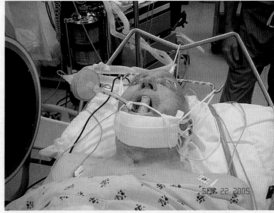

FIGURE 6-3

Patient positioning. Note padding under the patient's shoulders (**top**), radiolucent mouth gags, halter traction to allow head repositioning if needed during surgery, and biplanar fluoroscopes. (Copyright Dr. Ronald I. Apfelbaum.)

traction, with the patient's head resting on a foam donut rather than any type of pin fixation so further intraoperative position changes can be made. If C1 and the odontoid are in an anterolisthesed position, we can optimize the alignment as achieved in the preanesthetic evaluation described above, slowly removing any additional padding, other than the donut, and then dropping the head of the table if necessary under fluoroscopic control to maximize the reduction (Fig. 6-3, top). If C1 and the odontoid are in a retrolisthesed position, rotating the patient's head about a transverse axis approximately through the ear canals by placing one hand under the chin and the other on the occiput may reduce this completely or partially (Fig. 6-4). This occurs because the center of rotation is above the odontoid, so this motion brings the odontoid anteriorly. These maneuvers may result in full or partial reduction. Biplanar fluoroscopy using two C-arms is used not only for the initial reduction but also for tracking the progress of the operation and screw placement. Excellent visualization of the odontoid in both planes is mandatory. The recent application of fluoroscopic-derived CT imaging and stereotactic guidance systems allows for the use of this modality to substitute for the AP images once the reduction is obtained. Because the scan will only be accurate if no further motion has occurred, it must be used with caution and not relied upon until the final position is obtained.

Before the incision is made, the trajectory of the drill is ensured by placing a Steinmann pin or other long straight tool along the lateral aspect of the patient's neck while observing the lateral fluoroscopic image. If the surgeon's hand does not clear the chest, repositioning may be required. As noted above, this may be difficult in a large barrel-chested patient, one with a short neck, or a patient with a fixed kyphotic deformity in the subaxial spine. If an adequate approach path cannot be achieved, then the procedure should be converted to a C1–C2 posterior instrumented fusion.

Approach

A small 3- to 4-cm transverse skin incision is made at the C5–C6 level in the same manner as is done for an anterior cervical discectomy (3). The platysma muscle is then incised sharply but not undermined. The sternocleidomastoid muscle fascia is opened sharply, and this opening is carried cranially for several centimeters. Blunt dissection through the natural tissue planes medial to the carotid artery and lateral to the trachea and esophagus is then carried down to the anterior cervical spine at about the C5–C6 level. We then make an incision in the midline and elevate the longus colli muscles over about 1½ vertebral bodies. We use electrocautery for the midline incision but use a periosteal elevator to elevate the muscles to keep them intact. A modified Caspar retractor is placed with toothed blades fixed under the longus colli muscles to anchor it in place. This serves as a base for a special retractor used to keep open a tunnel to C2 in the midline (Fig. 6-5). Blunt dissection anterior to the longus colli muscles in the midline using a "peanut" or Kittner dissector held in an angled hemostatic clamp and swept side to side will quickly open the prevertebral space up to C1. An angulated retractor blade is placed to hold this plane open. It retracts the soft tissues including the esophagus and posterior oropharyngeal wall to keep them out of harm's way. It is mated to a special retractor that attaches to one side of the previously placed Caspar retractor to maintain the working tunnel up to C2 (17). In addition to creating a safe working tunnel up to C2 in the direction needed for the drilling and screw placement, approaching C2 in this manner rather than directly from the incision area avoids crossing structures such as the superior laryngeal nerve.

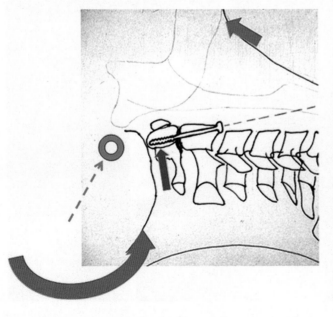

FIGURE 6-4
Maneuver to help realign a retrolisthesed odontoid: The patient's head is rotated in the sagittal plane by lifting up the chin and also rotating the occipital area as shown by the *red arrows*. This will rotate the head about a center of rotation indicated by the *green circle*, which is superior to the odontoid. The odontoid will therefore be translated anteriorly as a result (*blue arrow*), and the screw can then be placed to hold it in anatomic alignment. (Copyright Dr. Ronald I. Apfelbaum.)

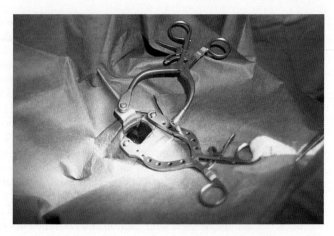

FIGURE 6-5
The retractor system creates a stable working tunnel and allows a midline approach through a small midcervical incision. Note that there is no inferior retractor blade that would interfere with the low trajectory needed to place the screw. (Copyright Dr. Ronald I. Apfelbaum.)

Screw Placement

The entry point for the fixation screw is on the anterior aspect of the inferior endplate of C2, *not on the anterior surface of C2*. To achieve this, we initially place a K-wire and optimize its position fluoroscopically (Fig. 6-6). If one screw is to be placed, we will insert it in the midline through the anterior annulus at C2–C3 and tap it into the bone. If two screws are to be placed, we will offset their entry points by about 3 mm from the midline. The K-wire is placed to create an entry point and to guide the placement of a guide tube system. *We do not drill with the K-wire*, as it is not rigid enough to maintain an accurate trajectory and any changes in the trajectory are hard to achieve because the K-wire will revert to the original hole.

Once the entry site is selected, we first remove a small amount of bone from the anterior surface of C3 inferior to the C2–C3 interspace to accommodate the guide tube system (5). To do this, a hollow 7-mm drill is placed over the K-wire and rotated by hand to create a shallow trough in C3 (not C2) up to the inferior edge of C2 without removing any bone from C2 (Fig. 6-7). We then place the guide tube system over the K-wire. The system has outer and inner components, the latter of which can be extended beyond the outer tube as needed. They are mated together, with the inner tube retracted, and placed over the K-wire until the spikes on the guide tube contact C3 (Fig. 6-8). The K-wire is cut off so only about an inch protrudes from the guide tube, and a plastic impactor sleeve is placed over the guide tube. Tapping on this with a mallet drives the spikes into C3 to secure the guide tube system.

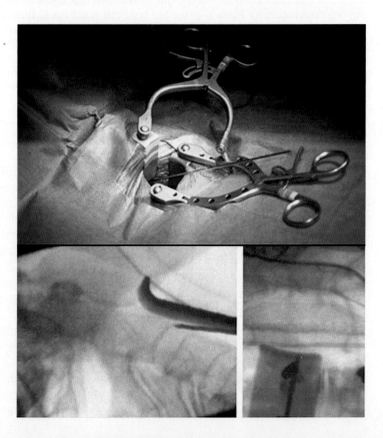

FIGURE 6-6
Placement of the K-wire to create a starter hole and align the guide tube system to the entry site for drilling on the anterior inferior aspect of C2, as seen on the lateral view (**lower left**). In this case, one screw was planned and therefore a midline entry site was chosen, as seen on the AP view (**lower right**). (Copyright Dr. Ronald I. Apfelbaum.)

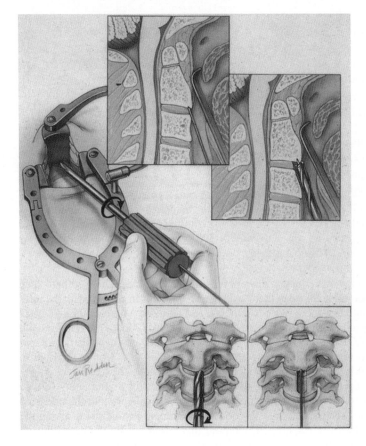

FIGURE 6-7
A shallow trough in the face of C3 is created with a hand drill to allow placement of the guide tube system to the inferior edge of C2. (Copyright Dr. Ronald I. Apfelbaum.)

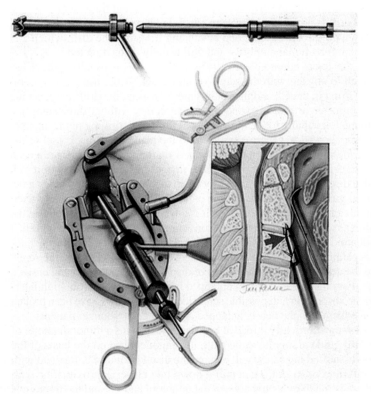

FIGURE 6-8
The outer and inner guide tubes are mated together and passed over the K-wire until the spikes on the outer guide tube can engage C3. After seating the spikes with the impactor, the inner guide tube is extended to the bottom of C2 (*blue arrow*). This provides a secure pathway to the selected entry hole and allows adjustment of the drilling trajectory as the drill is advanced. It also allows realigning C2 into an optimal relationship with the odontoid process (see Fig. 6-9). (Copyright Dr. Ronald I. Apfelbaum.)

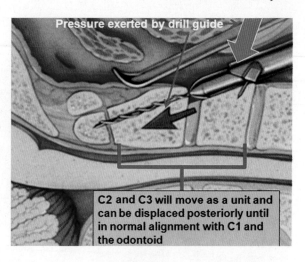

FIGURE 6-9
In the case of a retrolisthesed odontoid, the guide tube can be used to correct the alignment. Upward pressure is maintained at all times to keep the fixation pins engaged in C3 (*blue arrow*), and then C3 and C2 are displaced posteriorly by simultaneous posterior pressure on the drill guide (*red arrow*). When in optimal alignment, the drill is advanced across the fracture and into the apical odontoid cortex. (Copyright Dr. Ronald I. Apfelbaum.)

Once in place, the surgeon should maintain constant upward pressure on the guide tube system to keep the spikes engaged in C3. The inner guide tube can then be advanced until it is in contact with the inferior edge of C2 at the entry site, and then the K-wire is removed and replaced with a calibrated drill.

The guide tube is used not only to accurately direct the drill to the apical cortex of the odontoid but also to optimize the alignment of C2 and the odontoid. While keeping upward (cephalad) pressure on the guide tube at all times to maintain the engagement of the spikes in C3, it is possible to displace C3 and C2 posteriorly under a retrolisthesed odontoid (Fig. 6-9) or to lift C2–C3 anteriorly to realign with an anteriorly displaced odontoid. Unless we need to correct the alignment to initiate the drilling, we find it easiest to start drilling first, aiming for where the apical cortex of the odontoid will be in the reduced position and then perfect the C2–odontoid alignment just before crossing the fracture. If, however, the patient has a retrolisthesed odontoid that could not be realigned during the initial positioning, we would start the surgery with the head in a neutral position and proceed until the guide tube was anchored. Then C3 and C2 can be displaced posteriorly under the odontoid (Fig. 6-10). The anesthesiologist then slowly removes the extra padding under the patient's head; when the head is lowered, the patient's neck is extended while the alignment is maintained with the guide system. This can give the needed chest clearance to proceed. We would not try this unless we were convinced we could achieve the position by initial maneuvers such as displacing C2 posteriorly by direct posterior pharyngeal wall pressure once the patient was anesthetized.

The drilling is accomplished by advancing the drill slowly and using frequent fluoroscopic views. If any changes are needed as the drill is advanced, these can easily be done by backing up the drill slightly, correcting the trajectory with the drill guide, and advancing it again. The drill, which is 3 mm in outer diameter, has excellent directional authority and will usually go as directed.

It is important to drill through the apical odontoid cortex (Fig. 6-10C). This is usually quite dense and, if not drilled, may be difficult to engage with the screw or may crack. If the drilling is accomplished in the correct trajectory starting in the C2 endplate at its anterior aspect, the drill can penetrate from several millimeters to a centimeter or more beyond the apical cortex without threatening the thecal sac. Since the drill is coming tangentially to the dura and is in front of it, drilling in this manner is safe as long as the drill tip is not allowed to progress posterior to the plane of the back wall of the C2 body. Before removing the drill, note its depth on the calibrated shaft and take an image in each plane and store it on the second screen of the fluoroscopes. These images make it very easy to match the alignment that was obtained and achieve the same trajectory when tapping the hole and placing the screw. The drill and the inner drill guide are removed, but the outer drill guide is kept securely fixed in C3. A tap is then used to cut threads in the drilled hole. As it is advanced, it is easy to replicate the trajectory achieved with the drilling, making minor alignment corrections with the guide tube if needed to follow the same path in the odontoid (Fig. 6-11). In fact, the drill hole can usually be seen on the fluoroscopic images. The tap also is calibrated so the depth can be checked if needed. Tapping the screw hole allows the screw to engage the dense apical cortex instead of displacing the odontoid and ensures an optimal screw bone interface. Forcing a screw into an untapped bone hole can result in high interface pressures and subsequent bone absorption and possible screw loosening. Screws have been broken when attempts were made to force them into the dense, untapped apical bone of younger patients.

The tap is then removed, and a 4-mm cortically threaded lag screw, which has a minor diameter of 2.9 mm, is placed through the drill guide along the same path, its length chosen on the basis of the depth measurements. This smooth-shafted lag screw will engage the distal odontoid cortex and with its head buttressed against the inferior cortex of C2 can pull it down into closer approximation with the body of C2 (Fig. 6-11). If there is much of a gap between the odontoid and C2 and the fracture is

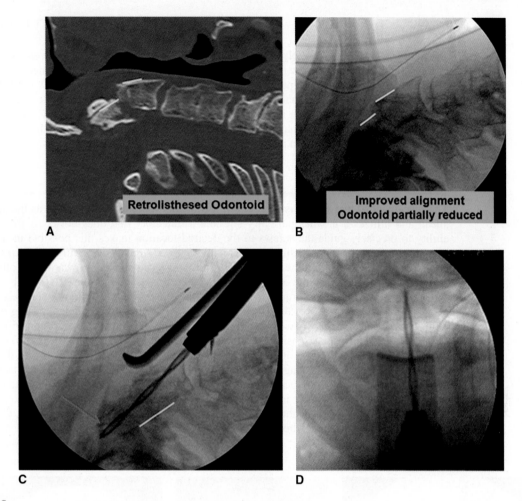

FIGURE 6-10
The alignment of this difficult retrolisthesed odontoid in an 80-year-old man **(A)** was improved **(B)** by the head-tipping maneuver (note less offset of the *yellow lines*), and we were then able also to further extend his neck (cf. **B** and **A**). This allowed us to proceed with drilling and achieve complete realignment (as indicated by the *yellow line*) **(C)** before crossing the fracture line. The final drill position **(C)** is through the apical cortex of the odontoid (*red arrow*). The AP view **(D)** just before penetrating the tip of the odontoid shows that we chose a paramedian position for the screw to accommodate a second screw. (Copyright Dr. Ronald I. Apfelbaum.)

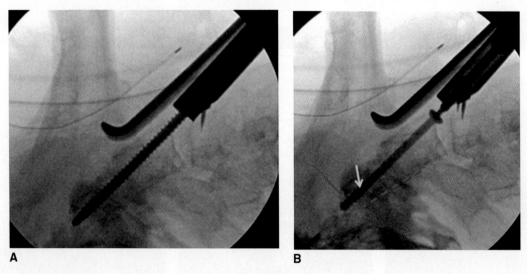

FIGURE 6-11
A: The pilot hole is tapped over its full length. **B:** The lag screw with threads extending only distally past the *short yellow arrow* is then placed. This lags (draws) the odontoid to the body of C2. Note also the apical penetration of the screw (*red arrow*). The head of the screw is against the inferior surface of C2, not its anterior surface, and the alignment is anatomic (*dashed red line*). (Copyright Dr. Ronald I. Apfelbaum.)

recent, the lag effect will usually close this substantially. It is important to fully engage the odontoid cortex, so we strive for a screw length that will allow the tip of the screw to penetrate a 0.5 to 1 mm through the apical cortex. Deeper penetration is acceptable as long as the screw tip does not extend posteriorly into the spinal canal. Because the drill hole is tapped, the screw can be removed and replaced if needed to optimize its length without damaging the bone pathway. This type of screw with a larger minor diameter has proven to be much stronger in resisting bending, and since it has been adopted we have not seen any screw breakage.

PEARLS

The placement of two screws is usually not technically more difficult as long as the surgeon plans ahead and utilizes a paramedian entry site and a trajectory that does not cross the midline. The ability to precisely guide the screws to the desired location makes this possible in most patients. The second screw is placed using the identical series of steps and an entry site into C2 that is on the opposite side of the midline (Fig. 6-12). The screws can converge toward each other to remain within the cortical shell of the odontoid. If the odontoid has a larger diameter in the AP plane, the screws can be placed so one comes to lie behind the other within the odontoid process. Only rarely is it not anatomically possible to place a second screw. While biomechanical testing has shown no biomechanical advantage of two screws in comparison with one-screw fixation in regard to sta-bilization of flexion and extension or resistance to screw fracture (16,26,27,33,36), this is not the complete picture. Two screws offer resistance to rotation of the odontoid relative to the body of C2 that is not achieved with one lag screw. This has not been addressed in studies such as that of Sasso et al. (36). Mechanically produced type II odontoid fractures were stabilized with either one or two 3.5-mm screws. Stability after internal fixation was 50% that of the unfractured odontoid. The use of two screws did not significantly enhance the stability in testing against re-failure. Graziano et al. (21) also found no difference between one and two screws in bending and torsional stiffness of the

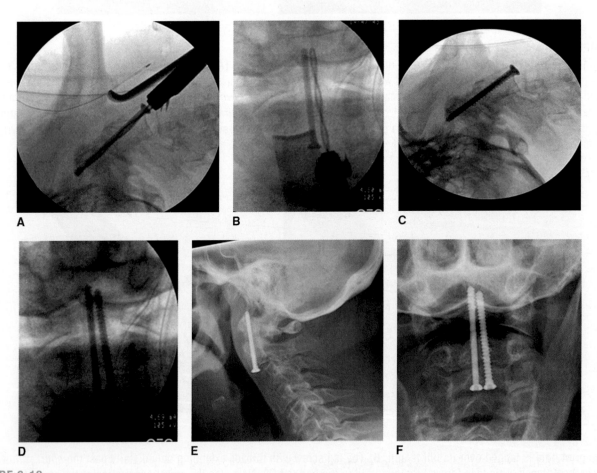

FIGURE 6-12
A,B: Drilling for the second screw. **C,D:** Final construct in the operating room. **E,F:** Two-month follow-up films. The second screw can be either a lag screw or a threaded screw because no further lag action is expected. (Copyright Dr. Ronald I. Apfelbaum.)

instrumented odontoid; however, the ability of one screw to limit rotation between the odontoid and C2 was not evaluated and is probably critical in achieving a solid fusion.

In younger patients with fresh fractures in whom the fracture line is often irregular, the lag effect alone may pull the irregular surfaces together and prevent rotation, but in fractures treated a few weeks or longer after their onset, such as after failure of a 3-month trial of halo immobilization, the single screw may not be adequate. This has not been adequately studied until recently when Dailey et al. (14) evaluated the results of odontoid screw fixation in elderly patients over the age of 70 years and found the difference between one and two screws to be highly significant. Fusion was achieved in only 56% of patients with one screw versus 96% when two screws were used. This likely is due to the weaker bone structure in older patients who may sustain smoother fracture surfaces. These may also not be able to be lagged as tightly, allowing rotation to persist when only one screw is used, thereby reducing the success rate. *In these older patients, we believe that two screws should always be placed unless anatomically prohibited.* In younger patients, we see no downside to using two screws when possible as it may be helpful in some, but we recognize it is not essential.

In some cases, especially in osteopenic patients, it can be difficult to positively identify the odontoid, and particularly its apex, on the lateral fluoroscopic images. In such situations, careful study of the CT sagittal reconstructions referencing the shape and height of the odontoid in relation to other better-seen landmarks, such as the top of the anterior arch of C1, can help define the actual borders of the odontoid on the fluoroscopic image.

PITFALLS

Odontoid screw fixation has been considered to be a technically demanding procedure; however, the refinement of the instrumentation, as described here, and improved imaging have made it less so. The procedure requires thorough preoperative planning and adequate surgical training. Determining the correct entry point, at the anterior margin of the inferior endplate, is critical. If entry is started more cephalad on the anterior surface of C2, the angle of inclination for fracture fixation often cannot be achieved, and the purchase is weaker, which may allow the screw to cut out of or migrate in C2 (Fig. 6-13). Poor odontoid purchase with subsequent screw back-out may also occur if the apical cortex of the odontoid tip is not fully engaged to ensure adequate purchase (Fig. 6-14). This is mandatory to achieve a lag effect between the fractured odontoid and the body of C2.

AP and lateral fluoroscopy are essential for constant monitoring during all stages of this procedure, and the procedure should not be attempted without adequate imaging equipment.

Clearly, choice of the proper screw length is also important for the screw to sit flush against the body of C2 proximally and not extend into the neural canal at its distal end. Failure to properly position the patient to achieve reduction and the needed trajectory to place the screws (both described in detail above) will make it difficult or impossible to achieve the desired result.

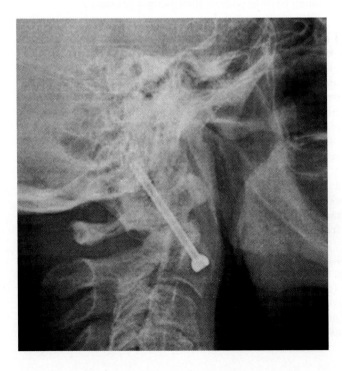

FIGURE 6-13
Poorly placed cannulated screw whose insertion was started on the anterior face of C2. The screw head has migrated into the body of C2, and the screw tip is within the neural canal, almost to the foramen magnum and in an uncertain relationship with the odontoid.

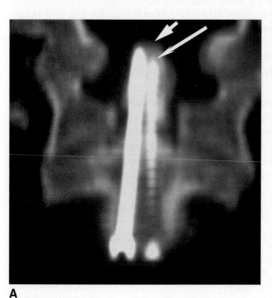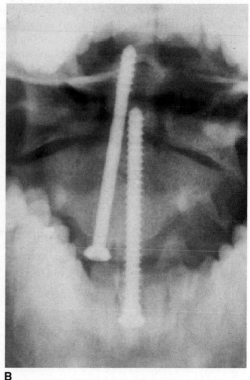

A   **B**

FIGURE 6-14
In another case, in an 18-year-old man, **A:** One screw went completely through the apical cortex (*short arrow*) while the other stopped a few millimeters short (*longer arrow*). That small difference was enough to prevent a firm grip and allow the second screw to back out within 6 weeks of the initial surgery. When revised with a longer screw, it held well. (Copyright Dr. Ronald I. Apfelbaum.)

The surgeon must realize that the whole procedure is performed using fluoroscopic guidance. It is not useful to try to retract the neck soft tissues any more than is necessary to create a working tunnel. The fixed retractors assure this. Hand retraction is difficult to limit and may result in excessive pharyngeal retraction and postoperative dysphagia. Trying to look up the tunnel to see C2 is not useful. All guidance must be obtained from the fluoroscopic images. No placement of the guide tubes and other tools to C2 and through the bone should be done without fluoroscopic guidance.

SPECIAL CONSIDERATIONS

Several options exist for treating odontoid fractures, which by definition are always unstable unless C1 is fused to C2. For many years, and especially before the development of this minimally invasive technique, halo immobilization was the preferred method. Despite the morbidity of prolonged immobilization, successful odontoid fusion can be achieved in approximately two-thirds of patients with halo immobilization. The risk of nonunion in patients over the age of 50 years with type II odontoid fractures, however, was 21-fold greater with immobilization in a case-controlled study (28), and studies have also shown that type II odontoid fractures with more than 6 mm of initial radiographic displacement have a very high incidence of nonunion despite immobilization in a halo for 3 months (6). For patients with these fractures, it is reasonable and preferable to consider direct fixation of the fracture or C1–C2 fusion. There are no studies looking at the maximum possible displacement in patients with odontoid fractures on flexion and extension images (for obvious reasons), so many patients with "nondisplaced fractures" also may have much greater offsets if the images had been taken at a different time.

If halo treatment is chosen but fails, then anterior odontoid screw stabilization is still an option for patients within 6 months of injury, and the outcomes have been equal to those in fresh fractures (4). Chronically nonunited fractures (over 18 months) have fared poorly, so for these established nonunions, the best surgical alternative is posterior C1–C2 arthrodesis, despite the accompanying loss of axial rotation. The morbidity and mortality of halo immobilization in the elderly is significantly higher than in younger patients, again suggesting that surgical fixation should be strongly considered (7).

The use of cannulated screws is controversial. In a prior version of this chapter, Dr. Sasso stated: "For three main reasons, I do not use this technique: First, it is very difficult to drive a K-wire exactly. It is much easier to make fine corrections to the trajectory of a 2.5-mm drill bit. It is imperative that the screw is perfectly placed in the odontoid fragment, and if the K-wire is not perfect, it is usually necessary to completely restart the drilling because the K-wire tends to follow the hole already made. Second, the K-wire may shear and break or may bind and drive into the spinal canal if the cannulated drill is not perfectly collinear. Finally, the bending and shear strength of the cannulated screw is less than a solid screw of the same diameter." Dr. Apfelbaum agrees and feels even more strongly about this technique. Having become aware of serious (but unreported in the literature) complications and fatalities from using a K-wire and cannulated screw technique, we feel even more strongly about this decision. These complications have resulted, in various instances, from not achieving the correct trajectory and/or from drilling or advancing the K-wire into the spinal canal, the spinal cord, and through the foramen magnum into the brain stem or vertebral artery. We are not aware of any such complications with properly placed solid screws.

If a partially threaded lag screw is used, concern has been raised that some circumstances such as a high fracture may not allow the threads to be completely contained in the dens fragment and that these threads crossing the fracture site would keep the fracture distracted. The currently used screws have only a 10-mm threaded portion, which will not cross the fracture site, but, even with longer threaded portion screws previously used, we saw no failure to lag or other ill effects because the central bone at the fracture site is structurally weak and does not hold the screw. For this reason, we have not found it necessary to overdrill the body fragment to obtain the lag effect as some have recommended.

Another concern has been raised that the anterior aspect of the C2–C3 disc space must be violated to obtain the proper entry point; however, this usually involves removing only a very small piece of the anterior annulus at the screw insertion site at the inferior endplate of C2. The nucleus should remain intact, as will the anterolateral annulus. No long-term ill effects at this level have been observed.

In elderly patients, osteopenia is a relative contraindication to anterior odontoid screw fixation. A perfectly placed screw, however, engages into the strongest bone at the tip of the dens (strengthened by the constant pull of the alar ligaments) and possesses a foundation in the very strong inferior endplate of C2. When good lag technique is implemented across the fracture, this construct may be quite stable even in osteoporotic patients. This strategy may be reasonable in the medically unstable geriatric population because the anesthetic morbidity is much less severe in the supine position than in the prone position required for a C1–C2 fusion. Also, surgical morbidity is much less severe with an anterior cervical approach than with a posterior approach, and the bone graft harvest site is eliminated.

POSTOPERATIVE MANAGEMENT

Progressive ambulation is initiated immediately after surgery. A hard cervical collar may be worn postoperatively when it is desirable to reduce a patient's motion or activity levels. In most of the older patients who are not very active it may be omitted or used for only a few days to weeks. If the patient is unstable on his or her feet and likely to fall again, it may be prudent to consider using a collar for a longer period of time, because, although the fixed fracture is stable, it is only 50% as strong as the intact odontoid (36). No correlation has been observed between collar usage and outcomes, so our preference is to not use them and to encourage gentle regular neck motion to preserve neck mobility as the fracture heals. We do advise against bouncing, jarring, or other strenuous activity and to delay return to work if such activities are required.

Mild dysphagia is common because of the retropharyngeal dissection and retraction. The latter can be minimized by using the self-retaining retractor system rather than handheld retractors. Most often the dysphagia will be mild and will resolve quickly, but occasionally it can be severe and require delayed feeding or the use of a feeding tube for a period of time. The incidence of dysphagia has been shown to be high in patients over the age of 70 years (14), so medical staff should monitor patients carefully, but if the patient is able, we will have the patient resume oral intake immediately after surgery and progress quickly from a soft to a normal diet.

Rehabilitation

Unless dysphagia is a problem or they have other limiting medical issues, patients can usually be discharged in a day or two after surgery. The patient is encouraged to be active immediately. In the elderly, who may be timid to be active, we recommend that they "get out of the house" and take a walk daily if the weather permits. Home exercise equipment if available can also be used. We also encourage gentle range-of-motion exercises, stretching, and strengthening the cervical spine to regain full function. Formal physical therapy can be used if the patient is not able to do this alone.

COMPLICATIONS

Complications of this procedure can be divided into approach-related ones and technical errors. The former group could involve injury to other structures in the neck, wound problems, and infections, but other than the dysphagia discussed above, these have rarely been observed or reported.

Technical problems include an inability to anatomically reduce the fracture, difficulty positioning the surgeon's hand for proper drill trajectory because of interference with the patient's chest, and poor visualization of the odontoid on fluoroscopy because of osteopenia. All of these can reduce the chance of a successful outcome; however, refinements in instrumentation and fluoroscopic devices have overcome many of these issues. With experience, we have learned that two screws are very important in older patients to get a successful fusion. We also learned years ago that using a larger-diameter, 3-mm solid screw virtually eliminated screw breakage. Finally, as noted, if a cannulated technique is used, the K-wire may shear, bind, and drive into the spinal canal, resulting in suboptimal screw placement at best and neurologic injury or death at worst.

A better understanding of methods to realign the spine preoperatively and intraoperatively and an understanding of the technique as described above can eliminate or minimize problems due to poor screw placement. Incorrect entry site selection, failure to engage the distal odontoid cortex, or using too long a screw to get the lag effect can all lead to a failed fusion and may require additional treatment.

With any biologic system, no treatment can be expected to be 100% effective; however, with careful preoperative and perioperative evaluation and careful attention to, and understanding of, the details of the procedure, anterior odontoid screw fixation has proven to be safe with a very high success rate and few serious complications.

RESULTS

Overall, studies reported in the literature have established this technique as an efficacious treatment of odontoid fractures (4,10,14,19,20,29,32). Complications and their incidences, reported in clinical series as results of direct anterior odontoid screw fixation, include screw malposition (2%), screw breakout (1.5%), and neurologic or vascular injury (less than 1%) (see comments above about nonreported serious complications). The procedure in several series has an aggregate fusion rate of 94.5% (9,31,32). If the fracture is morphologically appropriate and if the patient is not osteoporotic, then reliable fixation with minimal morbidity and quick return to function without a halo can be expected.

DISCLOSURES

The instrumentation described in this chapter was developed by Dr. Apfelbaum in conjunction with Aesculap, AG and is available from the manufacturer. The author has no ongoing financial interest in this product and receives no remuneration in any form related to either the instrumentation or screws.

RECOMMENDED READING

1. Aebi M, Etter C, Coscia M: Fractures of the odontoid process. Treatment with anterior screw fixation. *Spine (Phila Pa 1976)* 14(10): 1065–1070, 1989.
2. Apfelbaum R: Screw fixation of the upper cervical spine: indications and techniques. *Contemp Neurosurg* 16: 1–8, 1994.
3. Apfelbaum RI: Anterior approach for odontoid screw fixation. In: Zdeblick T, ed. *Anterior approaches in spine surgery.* St. Louis, MO: Quality Medical Publishing, 1999: 33–46.
4. Apfelbaum RI, Lonser RR, Veres R, et al.: Direct anterior screw fixation for recent and remote odontoid fractures. *J Neurosurg* 93(Suppl 2): 227–236, 2000.
5. Apfelbaum RI, Zileli M, Stillerman C: Upper cervical screw fixation techniques. In: Benzel E, ed. *Spine surgery: techniques, complication avoidance and management.* 3rd ed. Philadelphia, PA: Elsevier Saunders, 2012: 1373–1385.
6. Apuzzo ML, Heiden JS, Weiss MH, et al.: Acute fractures of the odontoid process. An analysis of 45 cases. *J Neurosurg* 48(1): 85–91, 1978.
7. Bednar DA, Parikh J, Hummel J: Management of type II odontoid process fractures in geriatric patients; a prospective study of sequential cohorts with attention to survivorship. *J Spinal Disord* 8(2): 166–169, 1995.
8. Blacksin MF, Lee HJ: Frequency and significance of fractures of the upper cervical spine detected by CT in patients with severe neck trauma. *AJR Am J Roentgenol* 165(5): 1201–1204, 1995.
9. Bohler J: Anterior stabilization for acute fractures and non-unions of the dens. *J Bone Joint Surg Am* 64(1): 18–27, 1982.
10. Borne GM, Bedou GL, Pinaudeau M, et al.: Odontoid process fracture osteosynthesis with a direct screw fixation technique in nine consecutive cases. *J Neurosurg* 68(2): 223–226, 1988.
11. Cho DC, Sung JK: Is all anterior oblique fracture orientation really a contraindication to anterior screw fixation of type II and rostral shallow type III odontoid fractures? *J Korean Neurosurg Soc* 49(6): 345–350, 2011.
12. Chutkan NB, King AG, Harris MB: Odontoid fractures: evaluation and management. *J Am Acad Orthop Surg* 5(4): 199–204, 1997.

13. Clark CR, White AA III: Fractures of the dens. A multicenter study. *J Bone Joint Surg Am* 67(9): 1340–1348, 1985.

14. Dailey AT, Hart D, Finn MA, et al.: Anterior fixation of odontoid fractures in an elderly population. *J Neurosurg Spine* 12(1): 1–8, 2010.

15. Dickman CA, Mamourian A, Sonntag VK, et al.: Magnetic resonance imaging of the transverse atlantal ligament for the evaluation of atlantoaxial instability. *J Neurosurg* 75(2): 221–227, 1991.

16. Doherty BJ, Heggeness MH: Quantitative anatomy of the second cervical vertebra. *Spine (Phila Pa 1976)* 20(5): 513–517, 1995.

17. Finn MA, Fassett D, Apfelbaum RI: Odontoid screw fixation. In: Vaccaro AR, Baron E, eds. *Operative techniques in spine surgery.* 2nd ed. Philadelphia, PA: Elsevier, 2012: 28–37.

18. Freemyer B, Knopp R, Piche J, et al.: Comparison of five-view and three-view cervical spine series in the evaluation of patients with cervical trauma. *Ann Emerg Med* 18(8): 818–821, 1989.

19. Fujii E, Kobayashi K, Hirabayashi K: Treatment in fractures of the odontoid process. *Spine (Phila Pa 1976)* 13(6): 604–609, 1988.

20. Geisler FH, Cheng C, Poka A, et al.: Anterior screw fixation of posteriorly displaced type II odontoid fractures. *Neurosurgery* 25(1): 30–37, 1989; discussion 37–38.

21. Graziano G, Jaggers C, Lee M, et al.: A comparative study of fixation techniques for type II fractures of the odontoid process. *Spine (Phila Pa 1976)* 18(16): 2383–2387, 1993.

22. Greene KA, Dickman CA, Marciano FF, et al.: Transverse atlantal ligament disruption associated with odontoid fractures. *Spine (Phila Pa 1976)* 19(20): 2307–2314, 1994.

23. Greene KA, Dickman CA, Marciano FF, et al.: Acute axis fractures. Analysis of management and outcome in 340 consecutive cases. *Spine (Phila Pa 1976)* 22(16): 1843–1852, 1997.

24. Hadley MN, Browner C, Sonntag VK: Axis fractures: a comprehensive review of management and treatment in 107 cases. *Neurosurgery* 17(2): 281–290, 1985.

25. Harris MB, Waguespack AM, Kronlage S: "Clearing" cervical spine injuries in polytrauma patients: is it really safe to remove the collar? *Orthopedics* 20(10): 903–907, 1997.

26. Heller JG, Alson MD, Schaffler MB, et al.: Quantitative internal dens morphology. *Spine (Phila Pa 1976)* 17(8): 861–866, 1992.

27. Jenkins JD, Coric D, Branch CL Jr: A clinical comparison of one- and two-screw odontoid fixation. *J Neurosurg* 89(3): 366–370, 1998.

28. Lennarson PJ, Mostafavi H, Traynelis VC, et al.: Management of type II dens fractures: a case-control study. *Spine (Phila Pa 1976)* 25(10): 1234–1237, 2000.

29. Lesoin F, Autricque A, Franz K, et al.: Transcervical approach and screw fixation for upper cervical spine pathology. *Surg Neurol* 27(5): 459–465, 1987.

30. Marchesi DG: Management of odontoid fractures. *Orthopedics* 20(10): 911–916, 1997.

31. Montesano PX, Anderson PA, Schlehr F, et al.: Odontoid fractures treated by anterior odontoid screw fixation. *Spine (Phila Pa 1976)* 16(Suppl 3): S33–S37, 1991.

32. Nakanishi T, Sasaki T, Tokita N, et al.: Internal fixation of the odontoid fracture. *Orthop Trans* 6: 176, 1982.

33. Nucci RC, Seigal S, Merola AA, et al.: Computed tomographic evaluation of the normal adult odontoid. Implications for internal fixation. *Spine (Phila Pa 1976)* 20(3): 264–270, 1995.

34. Pepin JW, Bourne RB, Hawkins RJ: Odontoid fractures, with special reference to the elderly patient. *Clin Orthop Relat Res* 193: 178–183, 1985.

35. Ryan MD, Taylor TK: Odontoid fractures. A rational approach to treatment. *J Bone Joint Surg Br* 64(4): 416–421, 1982.

36. Sasso R, Doherty BJ, Crawford MJ, et al.: Biomechanics of odontoid fracture fixation. Comparison of the one- and two-screw technique. *Spine (Phila Pa 1976)* 18(14): 1950–1953, 1993.

37. Seybold EA, Bayley JC: Functional outcome of surgically and conservatively managed dens fractures. *Spine (Phila Pa 1976)* 23(17): 1837–1845, 1998; discussion 1845–1846.

38. Southwick WO: Management of fractures of the dens (odontoid process). *J Bone Joint Surg Am* 62(3): 482–486, 1980.

39. Vaccaro AR, An HS, Lin S, et al.: Noncontiguous injuries of the spine. *J Spinal Disord* 5(3): 320–329, 1992.

7 Anterior Cervicothoracic Approach

C. Chambliss Harrod, Christian Klare, and Todd J. Albert

INDICATIONS/CONTRAINDICATIONS

The cervicothoracic junction anatomically and biomechanically is a complex region transitioning from the lordotic highly mobile cervical spine to the kyphotic, rigid thoracic spine (1). Anatomically, complex vascular, respiratory, alimentary viscera combined with local neurologic and osseous structures place a high demand on appropriate approach selection to obtain good outcomes (2). The spinal cord in this region is at its widest due to the cervical enlargement, while the bony canal volume is the smallest. Additionally, the upper thoracic cord is a watershed area with the anterior spinal blood supply transitioning from the vertebral and cervical arteries to the intercostals. Anterior- and posterior-based approaches both carry advantages and disadvantages. Careful analysis of disease etiology, extent, and surgical goals allows the correct approach to obtain surgical goals—namely, decompression, stabilization, and arthrodesis. Posterior-based approaches include direct posterior (laminectomy) and posterolateral approaches (transpedicular, transfacet, costotransversectomy, lateral extracavitary).

A number of anterior approaches to the cervicothoracic junction have been described including low cervical-supraclavicular (Smith-Robinson variant), transmanubrial-transclavicular, the modified anterior, the transsternal, and the high transthoracic (third rib resection) (3–12,14). Each of these techniques has its own unique advantages and disadvantages. Experience of the surgeon, cosurgeon availability, and familiarity with the approach and anatomy of the patient are of utmost importance when deciding on which approach to use. We discuss the transmanubrial-transclavicular approach, which offers extensive, simultaneous exposure of the lower cervical and upper thoracic vertebral bodies of the cervicothoracic junction.

Pathologic processes occurring at the cervicothoracic junction typically involve the vertebral bodies, making an anterior approach preferred. The most common indications for surgical intervention at the cervicothoracic junction include neoplasms (metastatic more common than primary), infections, and fractures (15–17). Metastatic lesions widely outnumber primary lesions in all regions of the spine. Lymphomas, myelomas as well as solid cancers such as lung, breast, prostate, renal, gastrointestinal, and thyroid lesions are common metastatic or systemic neoplasias. Primary lesions can be benign (hemangiomas, osteochondromas, osteoid osteomas, aneurysmal bone cysts, giant cell tumors), malignant (osteosarcomas, chondrosarcomas), or locally invasive chordomas less frequently. Perhaps, the most common spinal lesion to the cervicothoracic spine is a direct local invasion of a primary pulmonary mass (Pancoast tumor, historically tuberculomas) transpleural to the osseous spine or epidural space. Although these lesions may be approached posterolaterally in this region of the spine, sacrifice of unilateral or bilateral C8 and T1 nerve roots can be devastating and avoided by utilizing anterior resection and reconstructions (13). Also, mediastinal tumors such as neuroblastomas or ganglioneuromas can impinge on the spine or epidural space. Often, the natural progression of diseases at the cervicothoracic junction includes anterior collapse of the vertebral bodies with resultant kyphosis increasing the difficulty in obtaining adequate surgical exposure. Commonly, these procedures will need additional supplemental posterior stabilization.

PREOPERATIVE PREPARATION

Adequate preoperative planning entails two main factors: understanding the anatomy of the cervicothoracic junction and the thoracic inlet and adequately imaging/localizing the pathology. Cranially, the Smith-Robinson anteromedial approach to the lower cervical spine can be utilized with dissection proceeding through the platysma, between the strap muscles, trachea, esophagus, thyroid, and parathyroid glands medially and the sternocleidomastoid (SCM), carotid sheath (common carotid artery, internal jugular vein, and vagus nerve) laterally. Caudally, the first thoracic structures encountered are osseous and include the manubrium, sternum, medial third of the clavicle, and their articulations in addition to the insertions of the strap and SCM muscles. These structures protect the thymus, great vessels, thoracic duct, and pleural structures laterally. Notably, the brachiocephalic and subclavian veins right brachiocephalic artery and arch of the aorta, left subclavian artery, the carotid sheath, and recurrent laryngeal nerves (RLNs) will be encountered.

Imaging of this area is often difficult to assess with plain radiography though "winking eye" (pedicle erosions) can be seen while also being classified as osteolytic or osteoblastic. Swimmer's lateral, oblique, flexion-extension views can aid in visualizing the junction, neuroforamen, and destabilizing nature. However, computed tomography better assesses both fractures and the extent of osseous pathology. Most importantly, MRI best assesses the extent of spinal cord compression with or without intradural extension. Gadolinium administration with enhancement is particularly useful with neoplasms and infection associated with abscess formation. Vascularity of lesions is important to identify which patients might benefit from arteriography and embolization to avoid catastrophic blood loss. Lastly, careful attention to the lateral extension cervical spine radiographs and midsagittal CT or MRI images will allow identification of the most caudal vertebra or disc space to be accessed without splitting midline osseous structures. In thin, long-necked patients, T2 is possible via the standard anterior approach to the neck. Contrastingly, short-necked patients can make access even to C6–C7 difficult. The following technique relates to the anterior transmanubrial-transclavicular approach to the cervicothoracic junction.

PATIENT POSITIONING

The patient should be positioned supine on a regular radiolucent operating table with a rolled towel between the scapulae, allowing for slight extension of the neck. We use multimodality neuromonitoring employed with a combination of transcranial motor evoked potentials, somatosensory evoked potentials, and free-running EMGs to monitor the spinal cord throughout the procedure. After preintubation motor baseline potentials are obtained, intubation is performed along with appropriate hemodynamic access and monitoring via the anesthesia team. The table is then reversed 180 degrees from anesthesia to allow additional room for fluoroscopic imaging during the procedure. If intraoperative traction is used, Gardner-Wells skull tongs are placed after induction of anesthesia with baseline of 10-pound traction placed with aid of a Mayfield horseshoe head holder. We do not routinely use them for cases needing corpectomy at T1 or below. Care must be taken to pad bony prominences and ensure safety of peripheral nerves. The patient's arms should be tucked at his or her sides. We tape down the shoulders firmly to help with fluoroscopic evaluation of the cervicothoracic junction (or the most caudal cervical vertebrae). We also monitor the brachial plexus and check the signals after taping of the shoulders. We do clip any chest hair on male patients and then drape out our operative field from the lips to 3 cm below the xiphoid process caudally and laterally along the midaxillary lines crossing the acromioclavicular joints and then cranially to the SCM insertions at the mastoid processes. After scrubbing skin and prepping with ChloraPrep, a World Health Organization "time-out" is performed to verify the details of the procedure and equipment and review major intraoperative risks with the anesthesia, surgical, and nursing teams.

TECHNIQUE

Low Cervical Approach (Smith-Robinson)

We utilize an anterolateral oblique skin incision along the anterior border of the SCM muscle, extending to the sternal notch and continued along the anterior aspect of the sternum distal to the manubriosternal junction (Fig. 7-1). Supraplatysmal subcutaneous flaps are elevated (Fig. 7-2), and the platysma is split in line with the skin incision using Bovie electrocautery (Fig. 7-3). Subplatysmal flaps are then created with Metzenbaum scissors caudally to the sternal notch, sternoclavicular (SC) joint, and medial clavicle laterally. The external jugular veins may be sacrificed for increased exposure if necessary. Knowledge of the fascial layers of the neck is mandatory for safe dissection. The superficial cervical fascia (splits into superficial and deep layers enveloping the platysma),

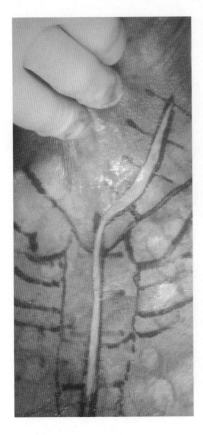

FIGURE 7-1

The field has been prepped and draped, and the combined oblique low cervical and midline transmanubrial incision has been made.

deep investing cervical fascia (splits anteriorly to envelop the SCM and posteriorly the trapezius muscles), pretracheal fascia (separates the trachea-laryngeal cartilage-esophagus medially from the carotid sheath laterally), and prevertebral fascia (between the longus colli muscles overlying the vertebrae and discs) compose the cervical fascia layers. The retropharyngeal space runs from the clivus into the mediastinum ventral to the prevertebral fascia. Careful dissection of the deep investing

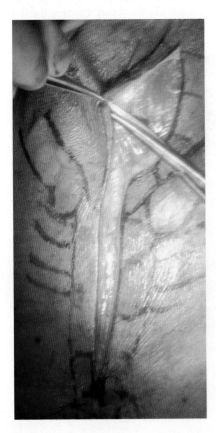

FIGURE 7-2

After incision, dissection is first performed cranially at the low cervical oblique Smith-Robinson approach. Metzenbaum scissors are being used to create supraplatysmal flaps to allow maximal wound mobility.

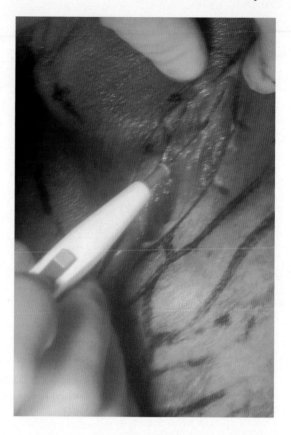

FIGURE 7-3

The platysma is split in line with the skin incision with the Bovie electrocautery. The superficial cervical fascia splits to encompass the platysma allowing supra- and subplatysmal dissection. We eventually repair this with absorbable 2-0 interrupted suture at the end of the procedure.

cervical fascia is performed medial to the SCM muscle, allowing for the mobilization and release of the omohyoid muscle (Fig. 7-4). This muscle does not typically need to be reapproximated or repaired unless operating on a vocalist.

Exposure and splitting of the pretracheal fascia allow for the careful dissection in an interval between the trachea and esophagus medially and the carotid sheath laterally (Fig. 7-5). The thoracic duct, located at the level of T1, is found lateral to the carotid sheath before entering the left

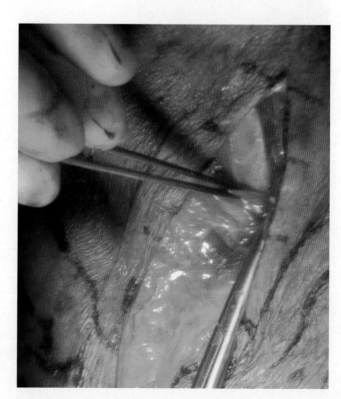

FIGURE 7-4

The strap muscles lie deep to the platysma medially, while the SCM lies laterally. The superficial strap muscles are the sternohyoid medially and the omohyoid laterally, which is being sacrificed here. We typically do not repair this muscle except in vocalists.

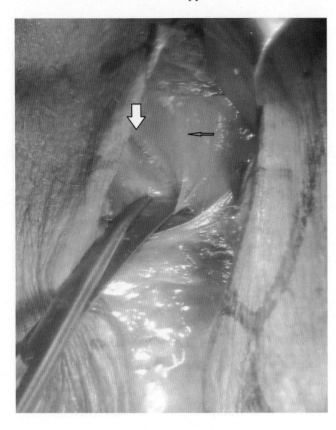

FIGURE 7-5

After splitting the middle fascial layer, the deep investing cervical fascia (*large white arrow*) of the neck (enclosing the SCM and trapezius muscles); the areolar plane between the laryngeal cartilage, thyroid gland, trachea, and esophagus medially; and the carotid sheath (common carotid artery seen at *small black arrow*) laterally after feeling for the pulse.

subclavian vein. The surgeon can minimize risk to the duct by staying medial to the carotid sheath. The RLN can be found in the tracheoesophageal groove on the left side after looping around the arch of the aorta caudally (nota bene, on the right side; the RLN enters more cranially and less predictably after looping around the subclavian vessels). The nerve can be safely retracted medially by keeping the retractor deep to the strap muscles, trachea, and esophagus. A Richardson or Cloward retractor is placed medially and an Army Navy retractor laterally. A Cloward or large Richardson retractor should be used because its broad, smooth face allows for an even distribution of pressure, minimizing risk of esophageal ischemia and perforation. The surgeon's assistant must keep the retractor deep to the esophagus and take care not to let the retractors slip superficially. Through superficial migration and/or repeated concussion with the retractor, they can cause a neuropraxia to the RLN. The surgeon then utilizes blunt finger dissection of the retropharyngeal space to expose the prevertebral fascia (Fig. 7-6) and continues this dissection retrosternally.

Thoracic Transmanubrial-Transclavicular (Medial Third) Osteotomy

Attention is then turned to the caudal thoracic extent of the approach. After incising the sternohyoid superficially and sternothyroid muscles deep to access the sternal notch, retrosternal finger dissection allows for displacement of the thymus, great vessels, and inferior thyroid arteries in order to protect these structures, while Bovie electrocautery is being used to expose the manubrium down to the angle sternomanubrial angle of Louis (Fig. 7-7). A sponge takes the place of the surgeon's finger and is placed retrosternally while the manubrium is split along the midline using a saw with footplate attached to protect the mediastinal structures (Fig. 7-8). The junction of the medial and middle third clavicular diaphysis is exposed subperiosteally with Bovie electrocautery dorsally and then a bone elevator to stay strictly subperiosteal to avoid injury to the left subclavian vein, which is closely apposed to the posteroinferior surface of the clavicle. After passing a sponge beneath the clavicle, a Gigli saw, sagittal saw, or osteotome may be used to split the clavicle (Fig. 7-9). With great care to ensure no medial internal mammary artery exists, a transverse manubrial osteotomy is then performed (Fig. 7-10), creating and allowing elevation of a manubrial window (Fig. 7-11).

After the retractors have been carefully placed, the left brachiocephalic vein and arch of the aorta are seen distally. Along with the esophagus and trachea, the right brachiocephalic artery and vein are retracted to the patient's right with handheld dynamic Cloward retractors or static retractor systems. Retracted to the left are the sternomanubrial bone fragment with attached SCM, carotid sheath, and subclavian veins. A malleable Deaver retractor with sponge is used in the inferior aspect

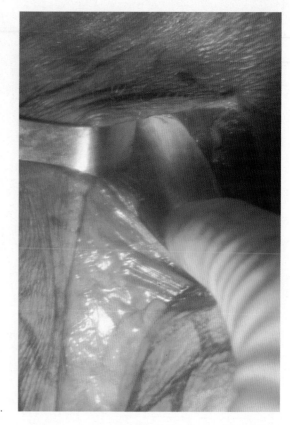

FIGURE 7-6

Blunt finger dissection best defines the plane to prevertebral fascia overlying the "humps" (discs) and "valleys" (vertebral bodies) lying between the longitudinal longus colli muscles.

of the operative field to gently retract the thymus, left brachiocephalic vein, and arch of the aorta (Fig. 7-12). With the retractors in place, caudal exposure of the prevertebral fascia can be performed down to T3. At this point, the exposure is adequate for the remainder of the indicated procedure. We will discuss corpectomy of T1 and T2 with placement of a cage followed by anterior stabilization with a plate.

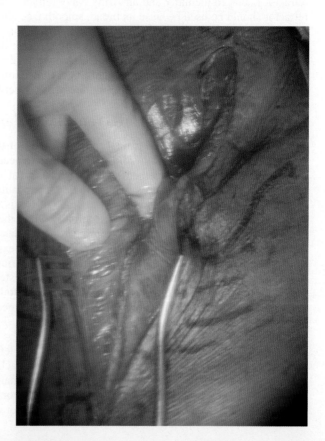

FIGURE 7-7

After incising the sternohyoid superficially and sternothyroid muscles to access the sternal notch (but preserving the SCM attachment to the medial clavicle and SC joint capsule), retrosternal finger dissection allows for displacement of the thymus, great vessels, and inferior thyroid arteries in order to protect these structures while Bovie electrocautery is being used to expose the manubrium down to the angle sternomanubrial angle of Louis.

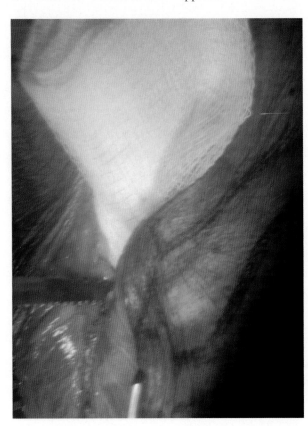

FIGURE 7-8

Midline manubrial osteotomy. A sponge takes the place of the surgeon's finger and is placed retrosternally while the manubrium is split along the midline using a saw with footplate attached to protect the mediastinal structures.

Decompression

Level confirmation of the appropriate vertebral levels is crucial and is accomplished with a lateral radiograph taken with a spinal needle bent 90 degrees twice inserted into a cervical disc space with counting down from the C2 body (Fig. 7-12). Once the proper levels are confirmed, annulotomy and initial disc removal with a combination of pituitary rongeurs, curettes, Kerrison, and a

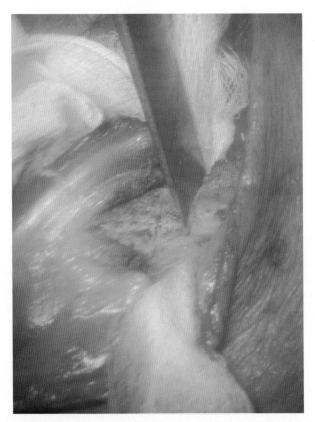

FIGURE 7-9

Medial clavicular exposure and osteotomy. After passing a sponge beneath the clavicle, a Gigli saw, sagittal saw, or osteotome may be used to split the clavicle.

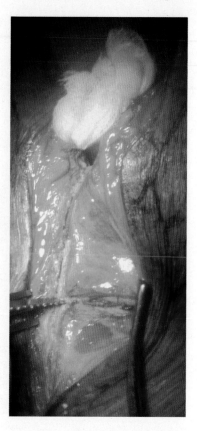

FIGURE 7-10

Transverse manubrial osteotomy. With great care to ensure no medial internal mammary artery exists, a transverse manubrial osteotomy is then performed, creating and allowing elevation of a manubrial window.

high-speed burr with a 3-mm matchstick or acorn-style tip are used to perform cranial and caudal discectomies back to the posterior osteophytes or the posterior longitudinal ligament (PLL). Caspar pins are placed into the vertebral bodies immediately cephalad and caudad to the level of planned corpectomy, in this case C7 and T3 (Fig. 7-13A and B). Distraction across the Caspar pins will aid in posterior discectomy. The midline is marked and a ruler used to measure the width of the planned corpectomies (Fig. 7-14A). Initial burr troughs laterally set the boundaries; then a large

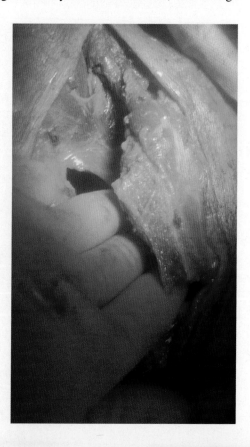

FIGURE 7-11

Resulting manubrial window. Note the intact SCM, SC capsule and joint, and medial clavicle.

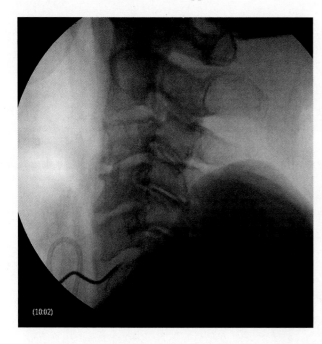

FIGURE 7-12

Level identification. Level confirmation of the appropriate vertebral levels is crucial and is accomplished with a lateral radiograph taken with a spinal needle bent 90 degrees twice inserted into a cervical disc space with counting down from the C2 body.

rongeur is used to remove the vertebral bodies down to the posterior vertebral wall (Fig. 7-14B). The corpectomy is then completed with a nerve hook elevating the PLL and posterior vertebral wall carefully, while a 2-mm Kerrison punch completes the bony and PLL resection along the entire defect from C7 inferior endplate to the T3 superior endplate (Fig. 7-14C).

Reconstruction

The resulting defect is measured with a caliper to determine proper cage size (Fig. 7-14D). Endplates are decorticated with the high-speed burr to gently bleeding bone. An endplate trial template is placed against the caudal-most exposed vertebral body to estimate the cage footprint and is

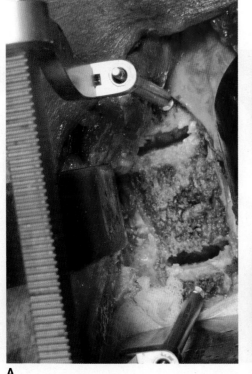

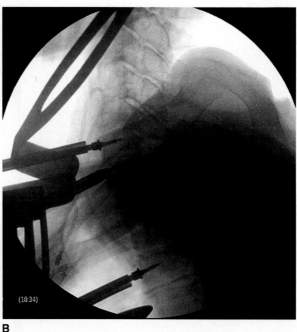

A   B

FIGURE 7-13

Discectomies are performed above and below the planned corpectomy sites. Caspar pins are placed into the vertebral bodies immediately cephalad and caudad to the level of planned corpectomy, in this case C7 and T3.

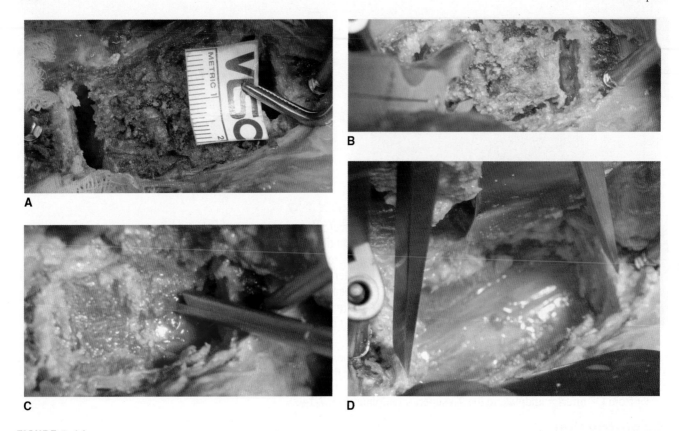

FIGURE 7-14

Corpectomy. The midline is marked and a ruler used to measure the width of the planned corpectomies **(A)**. Initial burr troughs laterally set the boundaries; then a large rongeur is used to remove the vertebral bodies down to the posterior vertebral wall **(B)**. The corpectomy is then completed with a nerve hook elevating the PLL and posterior vertebral wall carefully, while a 2-mm Kerrison punch completes the bony and PLL resection along the entire defect from C7 inferior endplate to the T3 superior endplate **(C)**. A caliper **(D)** measures the defect.

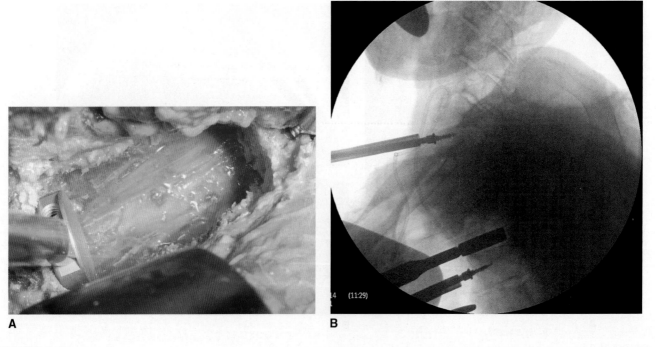

FIGURE 7-15

Template endplate size. Use of commercial endplates or a depth gauge protects against overly large or posteriorly placed implants. We often use a depth gauge as well.

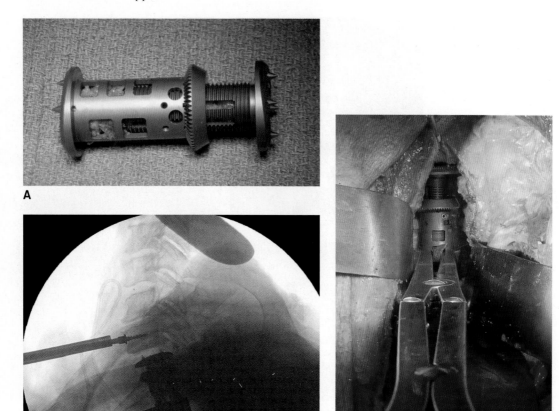

FIGURE 7-16

An expandable titanium cage (Globus Medical, King of Prussia, PA) is packed with local autologous graft **(A)**, inserted into the defect **(B)**, and using laterally fluoroscopy expanded once appropriate depth has been chosen **(C)**.

confirmed with fluoroscopy not to be in the canal (Fig. 7-15A and B). The proper-sized expandable cage is selected and packed with harvested local bone graft (Fig. 7-16A), is fastened to an inserter, and is placed into the defect (Fig. 7-16B). Prior to cage expansion, fluoroscopy confirms proper amount of depth above and below the cage (Fig. 7-16C). Once the correct depth is achieved, the cage is expanded, securing it in place. Final positioning and orientation of the cage are confirmed with fluoroscopy followed by the placement of a static titanium anterior plate with four self-drilling and self-tapping screws (Fig. 7-17A–C).

Closure

The manubrium is then wired anatomically with 16-gauge sternal wires, while we prefer suture repair of well-preserved periosteum over plate fixation of the medial clavicle (Fig. 7-18). We repair the strap muscles; typically do not repair the omohyoid; leave deep retropharyngeal space closed suction drains x2, which are stitched in place; and close in layers the platysmal, subdermal, and subcuticular layers with 2-0 Vicryl, 3-0 Vicryl, and 4-0 Monocryl. In this case, posterior supplemental fixation was added to further stabilize the construct with a hybrid pedicle screw-hook construct (Fig. 7-19A and B).

ALTERNATIVE TECHNIQUES

Low Cervical Smith-Robinson or Supraclavicular Approach Without Osteotomy

Other techniques have been utilized in the literature for accessing cervicothoracic junction pathology anteriorly. We have been able to perform corpectomy down to T2 without splitting the

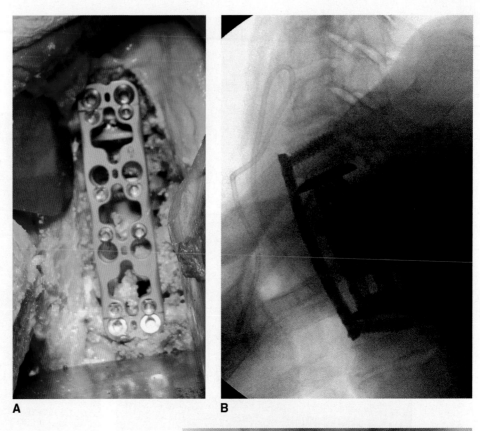

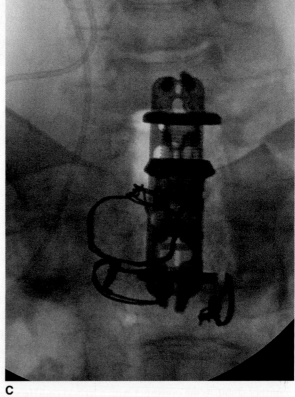

FIGURE 7-17

Cervicothoracic anterior plating. An anterior plate is anchored with variable angled screws **(A)**. The radiographs are taken in the lateral **(B)** and AP **(C)** planes. Notable is the sternal wiring reconstruction.

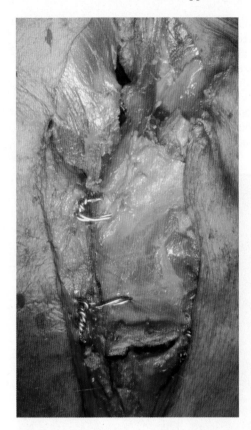

FIGURE 7-18
Sternal wiring reconstruction. Performed with sternal 16-gauge sutures.

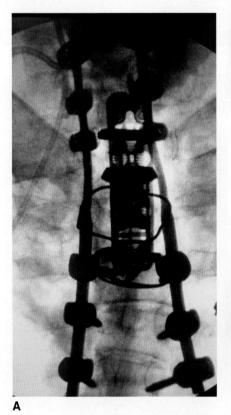

A

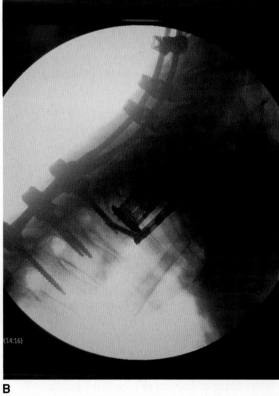

B

FIGURE 7-19
AP **(A)** and lat **(B)** fluoroscopic images demonstrate the final construct after posterior supplemental fixation from C5 to T5.

manubrium, sternum, or clavicle to decompress a postoperative anterior cervicothoracic ventral epidural hematoma after C4–C7 anterior cervical diskectomy and fusion (Fig. 7-20A–C). Alternatively, use of a supraclavicular transverse incision can allow access to T1 or T2 (Fig. 7-21). One of these techniques, the modified anterior approach, utilizes the same skin incision and initial dissection. However, the clavicle is sectioned at the medial third and disarticulated from the manubrium (in contrast to the manubrial window created in the previously discussed approach). The removal of the medial third of the clavicle allows for adequate exposure of the thoracic vertebral bodies. However, leaving the manubrium in place can create an oblique approach to the upper thoracic vertebral bodies, which may make instrumentation and screw placement difficult.

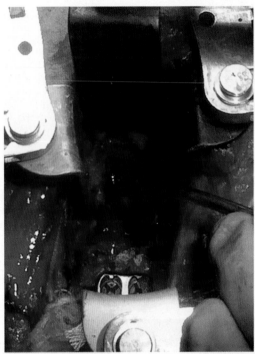

A

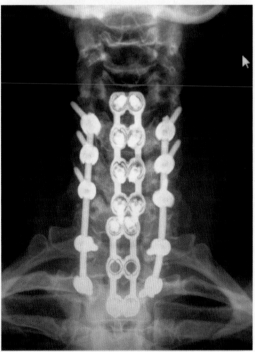

B

FIGURE 7-20

Intraoperative photo demonstrating evacuation of ventral epidural hematoma (dark compressive space-occupying lesion at tip of suction in **[A]**) via T1 and T2 corpectomy with ICBG allograft strut reconstruction **(C)** from a low anterior cervical approach without osteotomy followed by supplemental posterior fixation **(B)**. Note the caudal end of the cranial plate in C7 vertebral body. Non-FDA–approved lateral mass fixation was used in the subaxial cervical spine for fixation with T1 and T2 pedicle screw placement.

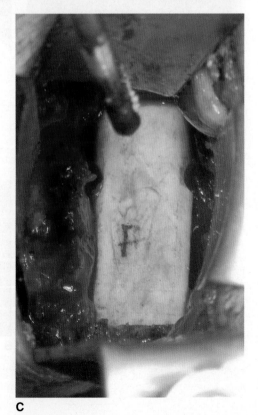

C

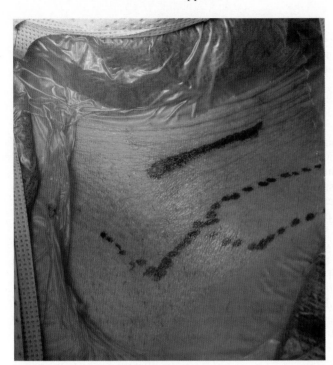

FIGURE 7-21

Left transverse supraclavicular incision for approach to ventral cervicothoracic junction.

Transthoracic (Third Rib Resection)

Another technique involves a proximal thoracotomy with removal of the third rib, typically. The patient is placed in the left lateral decubitus position and then rolled 30 degrees toward the supine position. The skin incision is made over the rib to be resected, beginning at the anterior axillary line and extending laterally and posteriorly to the lateral border of the right paraspinal muscles. The latissimus dorsi and trapezius muscles are sectioned and then retracted. Rib resection is carried out by cutting the rib as far anteriorly and posteriorly as possible. Care is taken to protect the intercostal nerve, vein, and artery. A rib cage spreader is placed, and a wet towel is used to cover the right lung before it is retracted anteriorly. We prefer to use a double-lumen endotracheal tube and let the lung down at this point. With this technique, the exposure to the first four thoracic ribs is adequate, but access to the lower cervical vertebrae is often difficult. In addition, this approach carries the added morbidity associated with chest tubes and lung manipulation. The sympathetic chain ganglion is also at risk in this exposure. Injury can lead to Horner syndrome (ipsilateral miosis, ptosis, anhidrosis).

Transsternal Approach

Another alternative is the transsternal approach. It should be noted that the sternal-splitting approach does not provide any more exposure than that obtained with the transmanubrial-transclavicular or modified anterior approach. However, it does add a substantial morbidity risk, with the potential for sternal wound infection, which could require extensive muscular flap coverage.

POSTOPERATIVE MANAGEMENT

Most patients should be immobilized routinely during the postoperative stage for a period of 6 to 12 weeks. This length of time will vary depending on the patient's physiologic status, specific pathology, and the degree of bony healing corresponding to radiography. Our practice prefers to place patient into an Aspen collar (Aspen Medical Products, Long Beach, CA) with a T extension. This is a rigid-type collar consisting of two pieces, front and back, that are attached on the sides by Velcro. It is usually worn 24 hours a day, and patients are typically more comfortable if cornstarch or a silk scarf is applied next to the skin, underneath the collar. Other alternatives to consider include the Minerva and sternal-occipital-mandibular immobilizer braces (Orthomed, Johannesburg, South Africa). A halo apparatus affords the most rigid fixation of the cervical spine available, but is used only in cases of unstable fractures or multiple-level complex cervical spine surgery. It consists of a titanium halo ring that is placed around the patient's head and is held in place by four pins in the skull. The ring is connected to four bars that attach to a vest worn by the patient anchoring the halo device and holding the neck in place.

COMPLICATIONS

The complication rate and type encountered are also similar to that of other more common superior approaches to the neck, but have the added morbidity associated with entering the lung cavity and the potential for injuring thoracic inlet vessels. The thoracic duct is in danger of being injured if the surgeon strays too far laterally from the carotid artery. Disrupting this vessel could lead to notable leakage of lymph fluid, causing a chylothorax. Staying medial to the carotid sheath will avoid this problem. The thoracic duct should be repaired primarily even though the tissues may prove to be extremely friable. Vascular injury can also occur to venous structures, including the brachiocephalic and subclavian veins, in addition to arterial structures, which consist of the carotid artery and aortic arch. Immediate attention must be given to achieving hemostasis by the primary repair of any injured vascular structures. Occasionally, pressure necrosis resulting in perforation or indirect injury to the esophagus may occur, leading to a possible life-threatening retropharyngeal abscess or mediastinitis. At the end of every procedure, it is routine practice to flood the esophagus with dilute indigo carmine (5 mL in 60-mL saline) via a retracted orogastric tube and to look for blue dye leakage to ensure no occult injury has occurred. As mentioned previously, sternal wound infections can often lead to increased morbidity requiring muscular flap reconstruction when the transsternal approach is used. Moreover, as with all neck dissections, injury to the RLN can occur and may result in hoarseness and dysphagia. More care has to be taken to keep retractors deep to the esophagus and not in the tracheoesophageal groove where the nerve can be injured by repetitive concussion with a retractor. A final note is that an extremely rare complication of shoulder girdle weakness may arise because of the resection of the SC joint. It is thought that this problem may only be substantial in younger patients who are left handed.

RESULTS

On average, neurologic results depend on preoperative status and underlying disease process. Myelopathy secondary to tumor, infection, or disc herniation can recover one to two Nurick grades. In addition, patients can expect to achieve approximately 20-degree correction of kyphosis postoperatively. Shoulder dysfunction occurs rarely, and swallowing dysfunction is usually temporary. Finally, most patients recover quite well from this procedure, with the vast majority experiencing notable pain relief and a timely return to independent ambulation.

CONCLUSION

These approaches are useful for pathologies of the difficult-to-access upper thoracic spine (T1–T4). If careful anatomic and dissection principles are achieved, then successful outcomes can be obtained and complications can be kept to a minimum.

RECOMMENDED READING

1. An HS, Vaccaro A, Cotler JM, et al.: Spinal disorders at the cervicothoracic junction. *Spine* 19: 2557–2564, 1994.
2. Birch R, Bonney G, Marshall RW: A surgical approach to the cervicothoracic spine. *J Bone Joint Surg Br* 72: 904–907, 1990.
3. Cho W, Buchowski JM, et al.: Surgical approach to the cervicothoracic junction: can a standard Smith-Robinson approach be utilized? *J Spinal Disord Tech* 25: 264–267, 2012.
4. Darling GE, McBroom R, Perrin R: Modified anterior approach to the cervicothoracic junction. *Spine* 20: 1519–1521, 1995.
5. Falavigna A: Anterior approach to the cervicothoracic junction: proposed indication for manubriotomy based on preoperative computed tomography findings. *J Neurosurg Spine* 15: 38–47, 2011.
6. Lam FC, Groff MW: An anterior approach to spinal pathology of the upper thoracic spine through a partial manubriotomy. *J Neurosurg Spine* 15(5): 467–471, 2011.
7. Garcia-Lopez A, Iborra A: Transmanubrial transclavicular approach in tumors of the brachial plexus. *Ann Plast Surg* 67(4): 387–390, 2011.
8. Jiang H, Xiao Z-M, Zhan X-L, et al.: Anterior transsternal approach for treatment of upper thoracic vertebral tuberculosis. *Orthop Surg* 2: 305–309, 2010.
9. Kumar R, et al.: Transmanubrial transclavicular approach to CTJ. *Pan Arab J Neurosurg* 15(1): 10–15, 2011.
10. Kurz LT, Pursel SE, Herkowitz HN: Modified anterior approach to the cervicothoracic junction. *Spine* 16(10 Suppl): S542–S547, 1991.
11. Luk K: Anterior approach to the cervicothoracic junction by unilateral or bilateral manubriotomy. A report of five cases. *J Bone Joint Surg Am* 84-A: 1013–1017, 2002.
12. Pointillart V, Aurouer N, et al.: Anterior approach to the cervicothoracic junction without sternotomy. *Spine* 32(25): 2875–2879, 2007.
13. Resnick D: Anterior cervicothoracic junction corpectomy and plate fixation without sternotomy. *Neurosurg Focus* 12: E7, 2002.
14. Sar C, Hamzaoglu A, Talu U, et al.: An anterior approach to the cervicothoracic junction of the spine (modified osteotomy of manubrium sterni and clavicle). *J Spinal Disord* 12: 102–106, 1999.

15. Steinmetz MP, Mekhail A, Benzel E: Management of metastatic tumors of the spine: strategies and operative indications. *Neurosurg Focus* 11(6): e2, 2001.
16. Tamura M, Saito M, Machida M, et al.: A transsternoclavicular approach for the anterior decompression and fusion of the upper thoracic spine: technical note. *J Neurosurg Spine* 2: 226–229, 2005.
17. Xiao ZM, Zhan XL, Gong de F, et al.: Surgical management for upper thoracic spine tumors by a transmanubrium approach and a new space. *Eur Spine J* 16: 439–444, 2006.

8 Posterior Cervical Microdiscectomy/ Foraminotomy

Michael P. Kelly and K. Daniel Riew

INDICATIONS

The ideal candidate for a laminoforaminotomy is one who has radicular pain without constant numbness or profound weakness. This is because, with pain, one knows immediately postoperatively if the operation was a success. With constant numbness or weakness, it can take time for the deficits to resolve, and sometimes, it never improves. During that time, one wonders if the deficits are persisting because of inadequate decompression, irreversible deficits, or insufficient time for the nerves to recover. Magnetic resonance imaging (MRI) and even computed tomography with myelography may show persistent stenosis, but there is no way to know if further anterior surgery will help or not. Therefore, while we have performed laminoforaminotomies in patients with neurologic deficits, we do so with trepidation and warn the patient in advance of the downsides to doing this procedure in such cases.

We pay particular attention to the Spurling maneuver. We have found that the ideal candidate is one in whom doing the Spurling maneuver increases the pain whereas forward flexion eliminates it. If the pain persists upon forward flexion and the patient does not have a herniated disc, a simple foraminotomy is not likely to improve the pain. This is because a laminoforaminotomy will not alter ventral root compression from an uncinate spur when the patient flexes the neck postoperatively. The exam should include provocative maneuvers for compressive neuropathies, such as cubital tunnel and carpel tunnel syndromes, and shoulder pathologies, such as rotator cuff tendinitis and impingement syndrome.

After determining the level of the pathology, we often utilize transforaminal epidural steroid injections (TESI) or selective nerve root blocks as both a diagnostic and therapeutic intervention. As the therapeutic effects are inconsistent, we remind the patient to pay close attention to the relief achieved in the first several hours, while the local anesthetics are active.

Radiculopathy due to

- Disc herniation causing foraminal stenosis
- Uncinate hypertrophy causing foraminal stenosis
- Facet joint (superior facet greater than inferior facet) causing foraminal stenosis
  - In our practice, a positive Spurling maneuver, with improvement upon flexion, predicts a successful posterior foraminotomy.

CONTRAINDICATIONS

- Central compression.
- Compressive pathology causing asymptomatic T2 signal intensity in spinal cord as seen on MRI.
- Dynamic instability at the level undergoing decompression is a relative contraindication.
- Not recommended for patients having undergone previous foraminotomy or laminectomy or those with a profound neurologic deficit.

PREOPERATIVE PREPARATION

One must understand the anatomy of the foramen, with the relations of the nerve root to the offending pathology (1,6). The lateral aspect of the spinal canal is bound dorsally by the inferior and superior lamina and the adjoining ligamentum flavum. The medial aspect of the facet joint defines the entry to the neural foramen. The superior and inferior borders of the foramen are the cranial and caudal pedicles, respectively. Ventrally, the foramen is bound by the intervertebral disc, the cranial vertebral body, and the uncovertebral joint. Dorsally, the foramen is bound by the facet joint, with 1 to 2 mm of the inferior facet of the superior vertebra and the entire superior facet of the inferior vertebra. Thus, compression can be from ventral uncovertebral hypertrophy, a soft disc, a "hard" disc-osteophyte complex, or facet joint hypertrophy.

Plain radiographs (anteroposterior [AP], lateral upright, lateral flexion/extension, obliques) (Fig. 8-1A–F) should be obtained prior to any higher-level imaging. The oblique radiographs are of particular utility when looking at the foramen, revealing both uncinate hypertrophy and facet joint osteophytes. MRI (Fig. 8-2A and B) should be used to identify areas of central and foraminal stenosis. An oblique, parasagittal view is ideal to visualize the neuroforamen (Fig. 8-2C). Often, the etiology of the stenosis can be determined as well (e.g., soft disc herniation, uncinate hypertrophy). In some cases, computed tomography scans may be used to identify disc-osteophyte complexes and ossification of the posterior longitudinal ligament. Coronal and sagittal reformats sometimes aid in surgical planning.

TECHNIQUE

We prefer to position the patient prone on an open Jackson frame (Orthopedic Systems, Inc., Union City, CA), with the neck flexed and the head held with Gardner Wells tongs in 15 pounds of axial

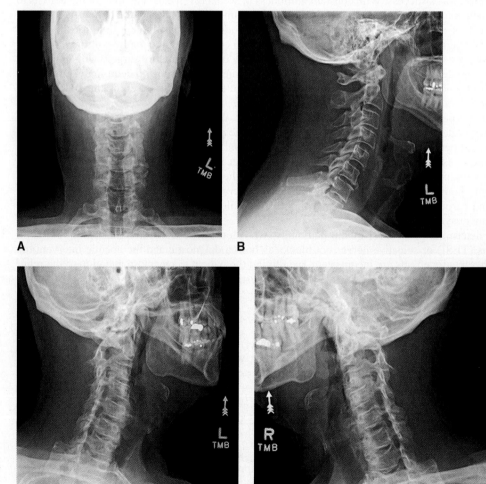

FIGURE 8-1

A: Preoperative upright, AP radiograph. The patient is a 64-year-old gentleman with a right C4 radiculopathy that failed to respond to nonoperative interventions, including TESI. **B:** Upright lateral radiograph. **C:** Right oblique radiograph. **D:** Left oblique radiograph.

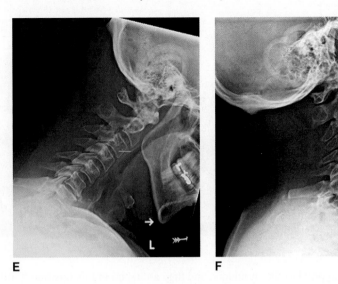

E

F

FIGURE 8-1
(*Continued*)
E: Preoperative flexion radiograph. **F:** Pre-operative extension radiograph.

traction. We will position the patient in reverse Trendelenburg, to encourage pooling of blood in the lower extremities to minimize blood loss and to bring the field into better view for the surgeon (Fig. 8-3). The support frames are placed at the top rung at the head and the bottom rung at the foot. This maximizes the reverse Trendelenburg position.

- Some have advocated positioning the patient in an upright, "beach chair"–type position, though this raises the risk of an air embolus complicating the procedure. Blood loss is less, however. The main disadvantage is that it is somewhat less comfortable for the surgeon.

The chest and pelvis are supported with bolsters, and the legs are placed in a sling. The hands, wrists, and elbows are well padded and then secured to the sides of the patient with a sheet.

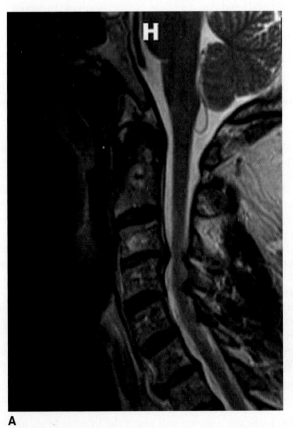

A

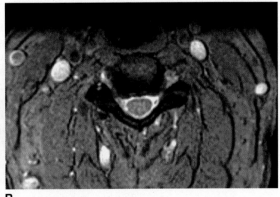

B

FIGURE 8-2

A: Midsagittal STIR MRI. **B:** Axial T2-weighted MRI at C3–C4. A right paracentral disc herniation is causing foraminal stenosis.

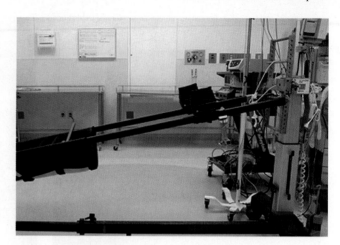

FIGURE 8-3

We position the patient on a posted, open frame table in maximum reverse Trendelenburg position.

Minimal traction is applied to the shoulders, and they are taped in this position. Pulling too hard on the shoulder will stretch the nerve and make it more difficult to mobilize the root if a discectomy is necessary.

Neurologic monitoring is accomplished with transcranial motor evoked potentials and somatosensory evoked potentials. This has alerted us to excessive traction on the brachial plexus due to positioning, so our preference is to use neuromonitoring for all cases.

Multiple techniques for visualization have been described:

1. Open
2. Open with microsurgical techniques
3. Endoscopic with tubular retractors
   - We prefer to perform the procedure in an open fashion, using the floor-mounted microscope to perform the approach and decompression. This allows excellent three-dimensional imaging and allows an assistant or trainee to see the operative field with minimal obstruction. While endoscopic techniques also work well and can decrease the incision size by about 5 mm, it requires fluoroscopic guidance, exposing the surgeon and patient to more radiation. An open technique typically requires just one localizing x-ray.

After prepping and draping in the usual fashion, we palpate the spinous processes of C2 and C7 and determine the level of our incision accordingly. Typically, a 2.5-cm incision will suffice for a single-level foraminotomy. If bilateral foraminotomies are planned, then a midline incision is made. If a unilateral decompression is needed, the incision is made 1 cm lateral to the midline. In either case, a midline dissection is carried out from the spinous process, dividing the supraspinous ligament and the interspinalis muscle in the midline. Contrary to popular belief, there is no interspinous ligament, so there should not be any attempt to preserve it. Dissecting lateral to the interspinalis muscle devascularizes it, so stay in the avascular and amuscular midline plane. Subperiosteal dissection is used to expose the lamina, but the facet capsule is preserved. The lateral aspect of the joint should be identified, but the exposure should not go past the lateral aspect of the joint, as there is a venous plexus that will bleed when disturbed (Fig. 8-4). In addition to subperiosteal dissection, muscle splitting approaches have been described, both open and using tubular retractors.

Care not to disturb the facet joint must be taken. The inferior lamina of the superior vertebra and the superior lamina of the inferior vertebra must be clearly identified. The confluence of these laminae, at the medial border of the facet joint, is termed the "interlaminar V" (Fig. 8-5A). This defines the medial border of the decompression to be performed (Fig. 8-5B). With a minimal incision (2.5 mm), one can use 2-hook retractors on a McCulloch (V. Mueller, Waukegan, IL) retractor or any of the available tubular retractors (Fig. 8-4).

Prior to starting the foraminotomy, one must ensure that the head is placed in maximal flexion. This distracts the facet joint, exposing the superior facet more clearly for resection, and allows for preservation of more of the inferior facet (Fig. 8-6).

- If one is performing a fusion in addition to the decompression, then preservation of bone stock is critical to achieve adequate screw fixation and to leave bone stock for the fusion to heal.

Using a high-speed, blunt, matchstick-shaped burr, we will resect the inferior facet, again taking care not to resect more than 50% of the joint in the mediolateral direction and preserving as much proximal bone as is possible. Resection of the inferior facet will expose the superior facet of the inferior vertebrae (Fig. 8-7). This defines the posterior border of the foramen. We prefer to resect

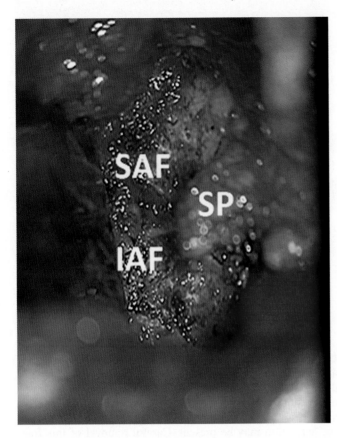

FIGURE 8-4
Subperiosteal dissection to the lateral border of the facet joint.

the superior facet with the same blunt, matchstick burr. Some advocate using a Kerrison rongeur to resect the facet and perform the decompression. We avoid this as the placement of the Kerrison tip, under the superior facet, may cause injury to an already compromised nerve root as it enters the stenotic foramen. If the majority of the decompression is complete, then a 1-mm back-angled curette or 1-mm Kerrison may be used to complete the resection of the facet. Continuous irrigation and suction will assist with visualization, removing blood and bone dust. As the foramen is bound by the pedicles cranially and caudally, the decompression must go out to the lateral border of the

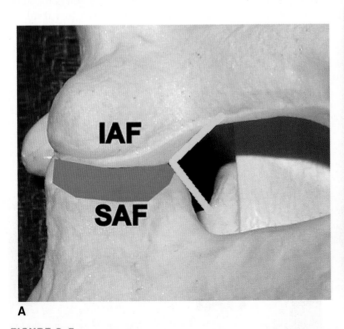

A

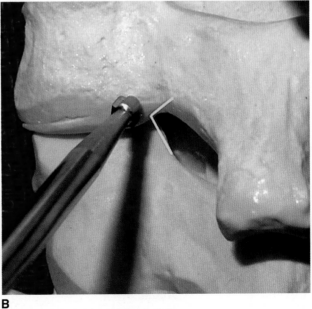

B

FIGURE 8-5
A: The "interlaminar V," which defines the medial border of the foramen to be decompressed. **B:** The decompression begins at the "interlaminar V" with a high-speed burr.

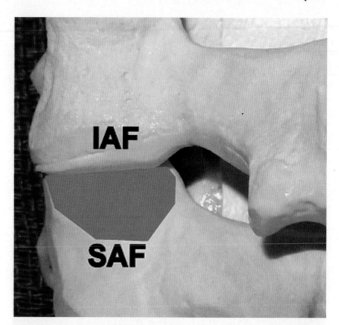

FIGURE 8-6

Flexion of the neck exposes the superior articular facet (SAF), allowing for preservation of more inferior articular facet (IAF).

pedicle. Again, one must take care not to resect more than 50% of the joint in doing so, as this may cause iatrogenic instability. We will angle the burr, to undercut the ventral aspect of the superior facet, again preserving as much dorsal bone stock as is safely possible. This will prevent leaving a sickle-shaped decompression, which may result in persistent neural compression (Fig. 8-8). At this point, the bony decompression is complete (Fig. 8-9).

In some cases, a soft, foraminal disc herniation may be present. Careful removal of this fragment through this foraminotomy is possible. To access the fragment, often one must remove the superomedial portion of the caudal pedicle. Resection of 2 mm (one burr tip head diameter) is often sufficient to provide access without weakening the pedicle. At this point, a micro ball-tipped nerve hook may be placed under the exiting nerve root to remove the fragment. Gentle manipulation is essential to avoid undue traction on the nerve root or the spinal cord medially. The hook may be used to "sweep" the fragment into the field, where it is removed with a pituitary rongeur. This same nerve root hook is used to confirm an adequate decompression. The hook should probe from the superior pedicle, laterally, and around to the inferior pedicle without difficulty.

Prior to closure, we will ensure hemostasis using bipolar electrocautery and a collagen hemostatic product. The wound is irrigated with nonpulsatile, normal saline. We then place 0.5 to 1.0 mL of

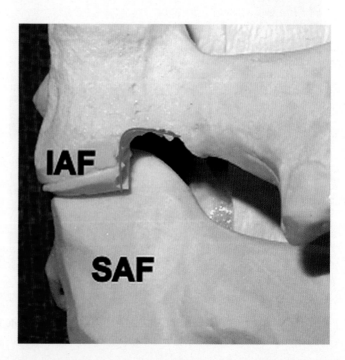

FIGURE 8-7

Medial portion of inferior articular facet (IAF) resected, exposing the superior articular facet (SAF). The entry to the foramen is exposed.

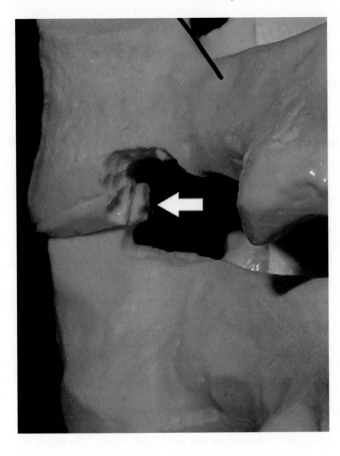

FIGURE 8-8

The SAF has been removed. Notice the sickle-shaped *(white arrow)* SAF fragment. This must be resected with a back-angled curette or Kerrison rongeur.

a particulate corticosteroid in the perineural area and 250-mg vancomycin powder in the wound prior to closure. The wound is closed in multiple layers, taking minimal "bites" of the paraspinals to approximate the muscle to the midline. In addition to improving cosmesis, reapproximating the muscular attachments restores their length-tension properties and decreases postoperative neck pain, in our experience.

PEARLS AND PITFALLS

- Not knowing the anatomy of the foramen dooms the surgery to failure.
- A positive Spurling maneuver, with improvement on forward flexion, helps define pathologies that may be successfully managed with a posterior foraminotomy.
- The ideal patient only has pain and no neurologic deficits.

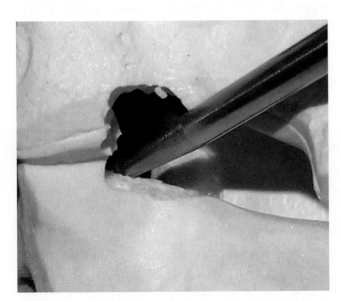

FIGURE 8-9

The "sickle" has been removed, and a nerve hook is used to palpate the lateral border of the pedicle; confirming the decompression is complete.

- Preoperative segmental kyphosis and previous posterior cervical surgery may be risk factors for a poor outcome (3).
- An intraoperative radiograph or fluoroscopic image must be obtained to minimize the risk of performing wrong-level surgery.
  - In our practice, radiographs from the office visit are hung on the wall. They are marked with the patient initials and the procedure to be performed. This is checked with the "time out" and with the intraoperative imaging.
- Flexion of the neck opens the "shingled" facet joint. This facilitates access to the foramen.
- Care must be taken not to resect greater than 50% of the facet joint, thus limiting the risk of iatrogenic instability.
- Bone wax, applied with the end of a no. 2 Penfield retractor, assists in bony hemostasis following resection of the facets.
- We prefer to resect the inferior facet with a blunt, matchstick-type high-speed burr. The footplate of a Kerrison rongeur may inadvertently injure an already irritated exiting nerve root.
- Use a nerve hook or foraminal probe to ensure the foramen has been adequately decompressed. If the probe does not pass freely, the foramen is still stenotic.
- Closure of the wound in multiple layers minimizes paraspinal atrophy, leading to better wound cosmesis.
- Foraminotomies can be performed with laminectomies and laminoplasties to decompress the central canal and foramen. If performing a laminoplasty, we will "open the door" on the side undergoing a foraminotomy.
  - Some recommend prophylactic C4–C5 laminotomies to decrease the risk of C5 palsy following laminoplasty (4).
- A soft collar is provided for comfort only. An early return to full range of motion may help minimize postoperative neck stiffness and pain.

POSTOPERATIVE MANAGEMENT

This procedure is performed both as an outpatient procedure and for 24-hour stays, depending on patient preference and pain thresholds. For admitted patients, intravenous ketorolac and acetaminophen work well to minimize postoperative pain for the first 24 hours. Opiates are given for supplemental analgesia. All patients are given a soft collar for their comfort but are encouraged to avoid its use as soon as possible. There are no range-of-motion restrictions, and patients are encouraged to resume normal activity as soon as they can tolerate.

COMPLICATIONS

- Infection
  - Irrigation with normal saline should be performed prior to closure. We routinely place 250 mg of vancomycin powder within the wound.
- Incidental dural opening
  - Treat with primary closure/patch as possible. Lumbar drains should be used for those openings for which a water tight closure is not possible. Often, 2 to 3 days of drainage, with the head of bed up, allows for the dural opening to close. Sequelae are rare.
- Nerve root or spinal cord injury
- Inadequate decompression
- Cervical kyphosis
- Instability from overresection of the facet

RESULTS

- Excellent results have been reported for relief of neck pain and arm pain associated with cervical radiculopathy (2,3,5,7).
- Though less common than after laminectomy, postforaminotomy kyphosis can develop with time. Patients with known risk factors should be followed for this complication (3).

RECOMMENDED READING

1. Barakat M, Hussein Y: Anatomical study of the cervical nerve roots for posterior foraminotomy: cadaveric study. *Eur Spine J* 21(7): 1383–1388, 2012.
2. Fessler RG, Khoo LT: Minimally invasive cervical microendoscopic foraminotomy: an initial clinical experience. *Neurosurgery* 51(5 Suppl): S37–S45, 2002.

3. Jagannathan J, Sherman JH, Szabo T, et al.: The posterior cervical foraminotomy in the treatment of cervical disc/osteophyte disease: a single-surgeon experience with a minimum of 5 years' clinical and radiographic follow-up. *J Neurosurg Spine* 10(4): 347–356, 2009.
4. Katsumi K, Yamazaki A, Watanabe K, et al.: Can prophylactic bilateral C4/C5 foraminotomy prevent postoperative C5 palsy after open-door laminoplasty?: a prospective study. *Spine* 37(9): 748–754, 2012.
5. Ruetten S, Komp M, Merk H, et al.: Full-endoscopic cervical posterior foraminotomy for the operation of lateral disc herniations using 5.9-mm endoscopes: a prospective, randomized, controlled study. *Spine* 33(9): 940–948, 2008.
6. Russell SM, Benjamin V: Posterior surgical approach to the cervical neural foramen for intervertebral disc disease. *Neurosurgery* 54(3): 662–665, 2004; discussion 665–666, 2004.
7. Woertgen C, Rothoerl RD, Henkel J, et al.: Long term outcome after cervical foraminotomy. *J Clin Neurosci* 7(4): 312–315, 2000.

9 Cervical Laminoplasty

Nikhil A. Thakur and John G. Heller

The concept of laminoplasty was introduced in 1972 by Oyama and Hattori. Their "expansive Z-laminoplasty" was developed to address the unsatisfactory outcomes of patients undergoing laminectomy for myelopathy due to multilevel cervical spondylosis. Hirabayashi then introduced the "open-door" laminoplasty technique in 1977, followed by the Kurokawa double-hinge, or "French door" technique in 1980. Subsequently described techniques for laminoplasty are modifications of these two principal concepts, with variations seen in how the laminoplasty is held open as well as the exposures used. More recently, efforts continue to refine the criteria for selecting the levels to be decompressed, appropriate sagittal configurations, and postoperative rehabilitation methods.

INDICATIONS

Laminoplasty rapidly gained popularity in Japan in the treatment of cervical myelopathy due to ossified posterior longitudinal ligament (OPLL) and multilevel cervical spondylosis. That these innovations might originate in Japan stands to reason, given the high rates of OPLL and congenital cervical stenosis in that population.

Today, indications for laminoplasty have expanded to some degree. Arguably, it remains the method of choice for treating cervical myelopathy due to OPLL and multilevel spondylosis involving three or more motion segments (Fig. 9-1). Other indications include spinal cord decompression to salvage a failed anterior cervical decompression and fusion (ACDF) procedure, recurrent myelopathy due to adjacent segment disease after ACDF, and as a primary treatment of myelopathy in hosts at increased risk for nonunions (i.e., smokers and patients with metabolic bone disease). Laminoplasty is particularly well indicated in patients with developmentally narrow spinal canals (midbody anterior posterior [AP] diameter less than 12 mm), since spinal canal expansion directly treats the underlying primary pathology. This use should be particularly appealing, as 50% of patients undergoing ACDF for cervical spondylotic myelopathy have relative (less than 13 mm) or absolute (less than 10 mm) developmental spinal canal stenosis.

CONTRAINDICATIONS

Laminoplasty is relatively contraindicated in the following situations: (a) epidural fibrosis (i.e., following infection, previous posterior spinal surgery), (b) large "hill-shaped" lesions of OPLL (8) that occupy more than 50% to 60% of the AP canal diameter, (c) axial neck pain as the patient's primary clinical complaint, and (d) fixed kyphosis greater than either 5 degrees or 13 degrees, depending on certain magnetic resonance imaging (MRI) characteristics. Additional potential reasons to select an alternative procedure include morbid obesity and diabetes mellitus, which can result in a two- to eight-fold increase in surgical site infections, particularly with a posterior cervical approach, let alone the technical challenges related to positioning these patients on the operating table and surgical exposure.

With regard to the overall alignment of the cervical spine, lordotic or straight spines have been reported to have statistically significantly higher functional recovery outcomes than kyphotic or sigmoid-shaped curves after laminoplasty (26). Suda et al. (26) recommended patients whose cervical spines range from lordotic to 13 degrees or less of kyphosis as ideal candidates for

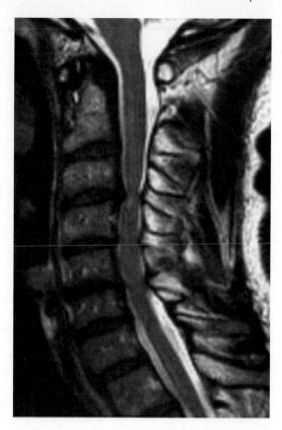

FIGURE 9-1

Sagittal T2-weighted MRI demonstrating multi-level cervical spondylosis.

laminoplasty if there is no cord signal change on the T2-weighted MRI. If there is cord signal hyperintensity on the T2-weighted MRI, then the upper limit of acceptable preoperative kyphosis is 5 degrees or less. Note that the presence of a lordotic alignment is not a prerequisite for performing a laminoplasty. This myth is born of misinterpretation of the literature, which seems to have taken on a life of its own as it is repeated in text after text without an objective review of the original studies.

TYPES OF LAMINOPLASTY

The two major schools of laminoplasty derive from the Hirabayashi "open-door" procedure and Kurokawa's "French door" laminoplasty technique. Other subsequently described techniques are variations on these themes. These techniques are illustrated in Figure 9-2. Most differ either in how the surgeon secures the laminae in their new position or in how the exposure is made (Fig. 9-2E). Initially, hinges were either tethered open with suture or wire or propped open with bone grafts or other spacers, such as ceramic or polyethylene blocks. Use of laminoplasty plates has become more frequent, particularly in the United States, and is often the mainstay at many centers. These are used either in isolation or in conjunction with bone grafts. The latter are not necessary for success since permanently maintaining the "open" position rests on healing of the hinge.

PREOPERATIVE PREPARATION

Preoperative Workup

The preoperative diagnostic imaging workup should consist of plain radiographs of the cervical spine, including AP and neutral lateral radiographs (Fig. 9-3). Flexion-extension films have been shown in some studies to be useful in determining presence of segmental instability. Sakai et al. (23) showed that presence of a retrolisthesis resulted in significantly lower Japanese Orthopaedic Association (JOA) recovery rates as compared to anterior spondylolisthesis or no spondylolisthesis (which had equivalent outcomes). Masaki et al. (16) further observed that hypermobility at the point of maximum spinal cord compression could further compromise neurologic recovery rates, which suggested that another surgical strategy might be wise, such as adding a fusion.

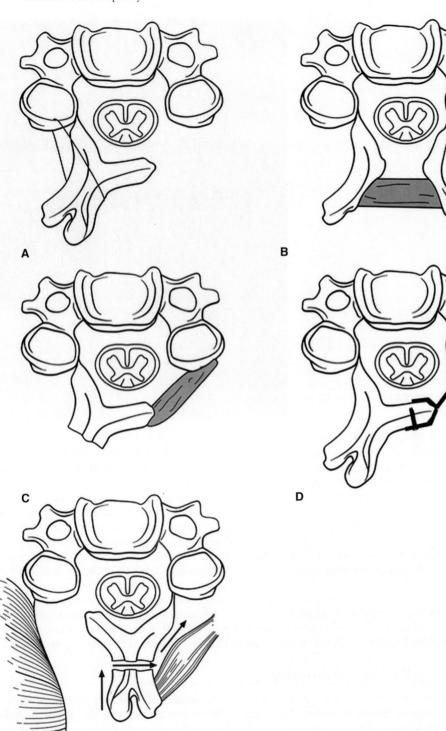

A

B

C

D

E

FIGURE 9-2

Various methods to perform a laminoplasty. (Reprinted from Rao RD, Gourab K, David KS. Operative treatment of cervical spondylotic myelopathy. *J Bone Joint Surg Am* 88(7): 1619–1640, 2006, with permission.)

The "K-line" or "kyphosis line" concept was introduced by Fujiyoshi et al. (3) as a tool to determine if laminoplasty could be used successfully in patients with OPLL. This tool can also be extended to address large ventral lesions or fixed kyphoses, which are often contraindications to laminoplasty. On a lateral cervical radiograph, the K-line was defined (3) as the line connecting the midpoints of the spinal canal at C2 and C7 (Fig. 9-4). A (+) K-line did not have an OPLL lesion crossing it, whereas a (−) K-line was present when the pathology extended dorsally beyond the line (Fig. 9-4). In K-line positive group, the average neurologic recovery rate following laminoplasty was 66% compared to 19% in the K-line negative group.

An MRI study is useful in preoperative planning to determine which levels need to be included in the laminoplasty. Moreover, an MRI allows the surgeon to determine if a C2 dome laminectomy

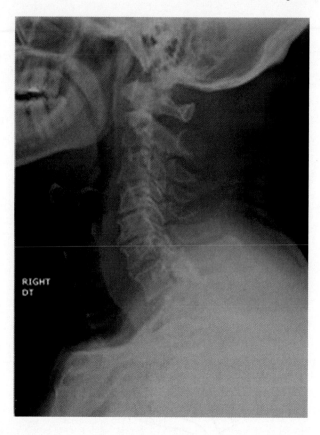

FIGURE 9-3

Neutral lateral radiograph, demonstrating multilevel spondylosis in the cervical spine.

should be included with the laminoplasty technique. Hypertrophied flavum, congenital stenosis, cervical spine lateral architecture, etc. can result in impingement of the cord at the C2 level after laminoplasty due to cord drift back and cause postoperative myelopathy.

The use of a computed tomography (CT) study or a CT/myelogram study is surgeon and patient specific. A CT scan gives the surgeon a more precise appreciation of the bone anatomy including presence of OPLL (Fig. 9-5), ossified ligamentum flavum, and foraminal stenosis due to osteophyte formation. Foraminal stenosis detected on CT and correlated with physical examination can be addressed during the surgical procedure with a foraminotomy on the affected side. The use of myelography enhances structural detail including details of patterns of compression and thickness and shape of lamina. At times, it is indicated when the patient's MRI leaves some doubt about the nature and extent of the pathology. A CT scan also helps determine the "occupation ratio" for a large ventral lesion (AP diameter of the lesion/AP diameter of the canal × 100). An occupation ratio of greater than or equal to 50% to 60% should temper any expectations about postoperative neurologic improvement. All of these additional anatomical details can be important tactical information to be used intraoperatively.

Room Setup/Patient Positioning

Laminoplasty is performed in the prone position. The authors recommend that the patient's comfortable range of motion be assessed preoperatively, so that they can be positioned in some flexion (flexed-chin-tucked position) during surgery. The advantages to this include the following:

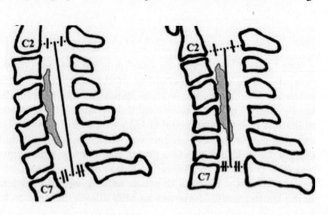

FIGURE 9-4

Depiction of the K-line concept.

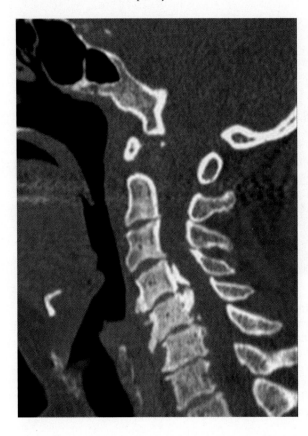

FIGURE 9-5
OPLL at the C4 and C5 vertebral bodies.

(a) cervical extension may result in worsening of canal stenosis and cord compression, and (b) the procedure is technically easier as the overlap or "shingling" of the laminae is reduced (Fig. 9-6). This also helps with excessive skin folds in some patients.

A Mayfield three-pin head holder is used to immobilize the cervical spine, as well as to protect the face and eyes. Longitudinal bolsters are placed on the lateral border of the chest to take pressure off the central chest and abdomen. Knees and ankles are flexed to reduce lower extremity neural tension. Taping of the shoulders is not necessary. Tape may be used to shift the redundant soft tissues when needed in obese patients. A reverse Trendelenburg position is used to decrease venous pressure, thereby decreasing intraoperative blood loss.

Special Instruments/Equipment/Implants

Somatosensory evoked potentials (SSEPs) are generally recommended during laminoplasty procedures for myelopathy. In the authors' opinion, the routine use of motor evoked potentials (MEPs) is open to discussion. Monitoring EMGs is an option when foraminotomies are added to the operative plan. Neuromonitoring may also serve to identify potentially significant episodes of hypotension or decreases in spinal cord perfusion. In both of these circumstances, early detection of a potential problem allows for rapid intervention and neurologic protection. More importantly, we prefer to use an arterial catheter for continuous monitoring of the mean arterial pressure, which is kept at a suitable level by whatever means necessary.

Roh et al. (22) reported the largest series of patients undergoing cervical spine procedures with SSEP monitoring. The authors found that degradation of SSEPs from baseline was seen in 17 of 809 (2.1%) patients, which prompted intervention and may well have prevented neurologic sequelae in 15 of these

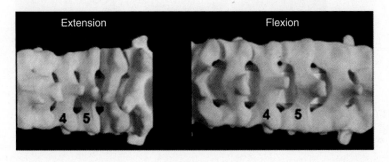

FIGURE 9-6

Depiction of shingling of laminae. (Obtained with permission from John M. Rhee, MD.)

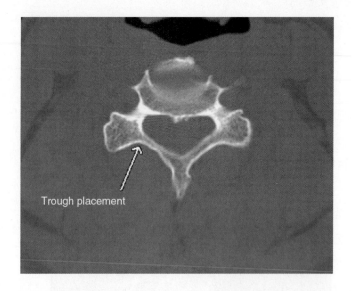

FIGURE 9-7

Placement of the trough for the open-door laminoplasty at the lamina-lateral mass junction.

17 patients (88%). The authors noted that monitoring may also help identify brachial plexopathies associated with positioning (e.g., taping down the shoulders), particularly in obese individuals (22). The use of MEPs has been shown to be beneficial in cervical spine surgery as an adjunct to SSEP. A recent article demonstrated that MEPs were more sensitive to changes associated with cervical myelopathy than SSEPs during intraoperative monitoring (4) and can be useful during laminoplasty. However, they are more susceptible to technical issues and false-positive changes. In addition, the lack of neuromuscular blockade required by MEPs and/or EMGs creates its own set of safety issues for patients due to the potential for sudden movement of the patient during critical steps of the procedure.

Technique

The authors prefer an "open-door" laminoplasty technique, as originally described by Hirabayashi. Since only two troughs are required, it is a bit more time efficient than a "French door" procedure (requiring two troughs and a midsagittal laminar splitting technique). But there may be greater degrees of frustration inherent in controlling the lateral epidural veins. In addition, it is easier to perform supplemental foraminotomies on the open side of a Hirabayashi-style operation than it is to do so with "French door" procedures.

   Intraoperatively, the hinge and open-side troughs are made at the lamina-lateral mass junction. Often, this corresponds to an inflection point where the two structures merge (Fig. 9-7). However, the landmarks may either be indistinct or obscured by facet arthrosis. Correlation with a preoperative CT scan can be quite helpful. The troughs are created using a high-speed burr with a tip of choice. The depth of the trough, which need not be any more than approximately 4 mm, should also be assessed frequently during preparation. If the surgeon is too lateral and deep, there is a potential risk of damage to the vertebral artery (Fig. 9-8). Placing the troughs too medially can result in an inadequate decompression.

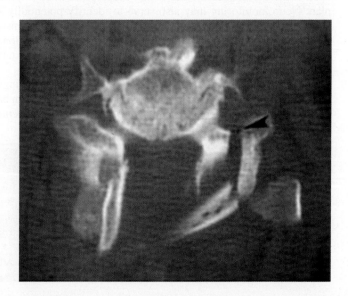

FIGURE 9-8

Far lateral placement of the trough, with violation of the vertebral foramen.

The open-side trough should be made first. It is important to exercise caution with a burr until ligamentum flavum is visualized at the inferior half of the lamina. The remaining cranial opening can be completed either with a burr or with a curette and kerosene rongeur. The authors recommend a 3-mm round diamond burr for this last step, unless one is highly experienced with more aggressive tips. Bipolar cautery should be used to coagulate and divide the plexus of veins as one opens the laminoplasty. These veins arborize dorsally from the longitudinal veins, which course over the nerve roots in the lateral spinal canal. Try to coagulate them a few millimeters dorsal to their branch point, as they are easier to control if a short stump of the vein remains on the longitudinal vein.

On the hinge side of the laminoplasty, the placement of the trough is the same. The burr should be used to remove the dorsal cortical bone and the underlying cancellous bone. The inner cortical layer is thinned until a stiff hinge is fashioned. Excessive bone removal will result in a floppy hinge, which may displace into the canal and cause either root or cord impingement.

We employ a laminoplasty plate in order to rigidly fix the laminae in their open position. It is not necessary to employ additional bone grafts with these plates. This adds technical difficulty and expense without clinical benefit. In a study looking at plate only laminoplasty in 54 patients, Rhee and Basra (20) reported a 93% hinge healing rate at 1 year, with no loss of fixation in any patient or premature closure. No revision surgery was required in any patient, and canal expansion was maintained in the unhealed group (7%, 4 patients) as well.

POSTOPERATIVE MANAGEMENT

Postoperative care consists of typical postoperative surgical wound management. The authors do not recommend any brace or collar wear. Immobilization impedes early active range of motion, which is strongly encouraged as outlined above. Evidence is accumulating to support that prolonged immobilization of any sort risks increased axial pain, loss of range of motion, and possibly kyphosis. Active neck and shoulder conditioning begin with isotonic exercises 6 weeks after surgery. In the interim, patients are encouraged to engage in daily nonimpact aerobic conditioning, such as walking or stationary cycling. The latter is more practical for those with significant preoperative gait problems.

Follow-up consists of a clinical assessment with static radiographs at 6 weeks. Isotonic exercises are initiated at that time and progressed as tolerated. Lateral flexion/extension radiographs are obtained at 3-month intervals thereafter until the patient has reached maximal neurologic improvement, which is to be expected by about 1 year after surgery. As demonstrated by Rhee (21), the hinge side of the laminoplasty procedure heals reliably by 6 months. Thereafter, provided there are no instability patterns on the dynamic radiographs, patients are free to engage in any activities without limitation, including most sports.

COST

Cost comparative effectiveness when related to surgical techniques, implant usage, and related outcomes is becoming more prevalent. Highsmith et al. (5) retrospectively compared 30 patients who underwent laminoplasty versus 26 patients who underwent laminectomy and fusion. Both groups had similar improvement postoperatively in their Nurick grades and mJOA scores, visual analog score for neck pain, and similar complication rates. However, the laminectomy and fusion group had three times the implant cost as the laminoplasty group.

COMPLICATIONS

Wound Infections

Wound infections with laminoplasty are reported to be around 3% to 4% (20), which is similar to other posterior cervical procedures. Perioperative antibiotics and good surgical technique, including watertight fascial closure, can minimize infection rates. Addition of a separate drain for a thick subcutaneous layer can also be beneficial. A postoperative cervical collar is not necessary, as early motion is encouraged, which we believe may further reduce the risk of posterior cervical wound infections.

Neck Pain

Historically, postoperative axial neck pain has been reported to occur in up to 40% of patients at 10-year follow-up (28). The sources for axial neck pain have been thought to include facet joint injury, deep extensor muscle denervation, detachment of C2 and/or C7 muscles, detachment of the nuchal ligament, and prolonged postoperative external immobilization (7).

In the past few years, there have been several studies that have looked at maintaining muscle and nuchal ligament insertions on C2 and C7. Hosono et al. (6) reported significantly improved axial pain in the postoperative period in patients who underwent a C3–C6 laminoplasty versus the traditional C3–C7 laminoplasty. The C3–C6 group reported an incidence of 5.4% axial neck pain compared to 29% of patients who were symptomatic after C3–C7 laminoplasty ($P = 0.015$). Given that both groups had equivalent neurologic improvements, the inclusion of the C7 level in a posterior laminoplasty ought to be avoided when possible. Sakaura et al. (25) also reported a 3.2% rate of axial neck pain in a 5-year prospective follow-up of patients who had a C3–C6 laminoplasty but no significant difference in neck pain when detaching the muscle insertions at C3–C6 versus maintaining these insertions.

Overall, reasonable data exist to suggest that preservation of the muscle attachments at C2 or C7 results in reduced postoperative axial neck pain. There also appears to be a correlation between neck muscle strength and axial neck pain post laminoplasty. In patients with no axial neck pain, Fujibayashi et al. (2) found neck muscle strength recovered to 120% of preoperative levels, whereas muscle strength in patients with neck pain remained at 60% and did not recover. It is difficult, however, to ascertain if muscle weakness induces neck pain or if neck pain causes limitation of motion and resultant weakness. Further prospective studies could help clarify this, which may result in increased utilization of muscle strengthening both pre- and postoperatively.

Strategies to reduce postoperative axial pain include preservation of muscle attachments to C2 and C7 when possible and muscle strengthening postoperatively. Early active range of motion after surgery may play as important a role as any other measures in reducing pain and stiffness. Kawaguchi et al. (10) emphasized early range of motion and limited brace use less than or equal to 1 m and demonstrated reduced axial neck pain in their postoperative laminoplasty patients compared to patients with prolonged brace use and restricted range of motion.

Postoperative Kyphosis and Loss of Motion

Cervical kyphosis in the postoperative period has been reported more frequently after cervical laminectomy (1,13). The incidence of kyphosis after laminoplasty is lower than reported with a laminectomy alone and is 0% to 22% based on the literature (1). The risk of kyphosis is most directly related to prolonged immobilization and extensive muscle detachment resulting in weakness and loss of motion (1). As a result, postoperative kyphosis may result in poor neurologic recovery and late neurologic deterioration (12). One possible etiology for the loss of lordosis and subsequent kyphosis is attributed to the detachment of semispinalis cervicis from its insertion at C2 (27). Sakaura et al. (24) found that by preserving C2 and C7 muscle attachments, lordosis was equally maintained in patients with or without C3–C6 muscle detachment.

Loss of motion after laminoplasty has also been reported in the early literature. Given the fact that laminoplasty is a nonfusion motion-sparing technique, loss of motion postoperatively is detrimental as a surgical outcome for the patient and can result in increased axial neck pain (28). Wada et al. (28) demonstrated 71% loss of motion in patients who underwent grafting of their hinge side and were immobilized for 2 to 3 months postoperatively. Patients with no grafting and 3 weeks of immobilization had only a 27% loss of postoperative motion.

The issues of postoperative kyphosis and loss of motion have been shown to be synergistic. Maeda et al. (15) demonstrated that postoperative kyphotic deformity occurred in stiffer spines, while lordosis was maintained in flexible cervical spines after laminoplasty. The authors concluded that maintaining range of motion postoperatively prevented stiffness and subsequent kyphotic deformity and recommended use of a soft collar only for 1 week after surgery. The authors share this observation.

Machino et al. (14) recently published a case series of 520 patients who underwent French door–style laminoplasty. They reported the following surgical techniques and postoperative modalities to preserve motion: reduced surgical soft tissue exposure, preservation of attachment of the semispinalis cervicis to the C2 spinous process, a more medial setting of the lateral gutters, immediate postoperative range of motion, and less than or equal to 2 weeks or no application of a neck collar. They reported that a mean C2–C7 alignment in the neutral position was 11.9 degrees lordotic preoperatively and increased to 13.6 degrees lordotic postoperatively. The mean total range of motion decreased from 40 to 33.5 degrees. Approximately 87.9% of patients had preservation of their range of motion. Of the patients who had a lordotic alignment preoperatively, 92.8% of them remained lordotic after surgery. Of the 63 patients who were kyphotic preoperatively, 49.2% maintained a lordotic alignment postoperatively, while 50.8% remained kyphotic.

In summary, preserving muscle attachments to the C2 and the C7 laminae plays an important role in reducing axial pain and preventing the development of postoperative kyphosis. Early range of motion and limited use of a cervical orthoses also help prevent development of postoperative kyphosis and maintenance of preoperative sagittal alignment. We do not graft the hinge side intraoperatively nor do we routinely use any cervical orthoses in the postoperative management of these patients. All of our patients are encouraged to pursue unrestricted active range of motion as soon as tolerated and also start isotonic exercises 6 weeks postoperatively.

Laminar Closure: Restenosis

Laminar closure has been reported with a wide variety of laminoplasty techniques. Matsumoto et al. (18) reported a 34% lamina reclosure rate when using early active range of motion after the traditional Hirabayashi suture method to perform the laminoplasty. However, they observed no significant changes in outcomes in short-term follow-up. In a 5-year follow-up of the same cohort (17), the authors reported that while not statistically significant, recovery rates tended to decline in the closure group as compared to the nonclosure group. They recommended considering the use of more rigid laminar fixation methods, such as plates and screws, to prevent laminar closure. Kaito et al. (9) demonstrated postoperative displacement of hydroxyapatite spacers with deformation of the enlarged spinal canal in 59% of patients after a French door laminoplasty procedure. They did not see any worsening of neurologic function in their patients. Other studies (11) have also reported reclosure after laminoplasty with traditional laminoplasty techniques, recommending use of more rigid laminar fixation techniques.

The use of laminoplasty plates (Fig. 9-9) may help to reduce the risk of laminoplasty closure. Rhee et al. (21) reported no premature closures of laminoplasty with the use of the aforementioned plate technique without hinge bone grafting in their series of 54 patients. The authors routinely use laminoplasty plates without allograft to secure the hinge side open and maintain canal expansion and do not graft the hinge side.

Hinge Fracture/Displacement

Hinge failure can result from fracture or from displacement of a floppy hinge. The ideal hinge results in a "greenstick" deformation of the bone as it is opened. If not enough bone has been removed while fashioning the "hinge," fracture can occur when attempting to "open" the laminae. If too much bone is removed from the ventral cortex of the hinge trough, it can be too floppy risking displacement. The hinge can then sag into a clinically significant displaced position. Either mode of failure could result in nerve root or spinal cord compromise.

Following removal of the dorsal cortex from the hinge side, repeated assessment of its stiffness is necessary to avoid removing too much of the ventral cortex. The use of a diamond burr may help

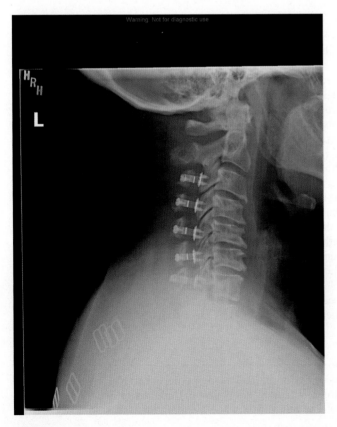

FIGURE 9-9

Use of laminoplasty plates to maintain the opening of the lamina.

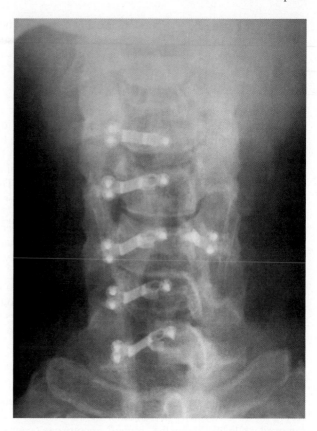

FIGURE 9-10
Use of a hinge plate to stabilize a hinge
fracture.

minimize this technical error and prevent hinge failure (20). In the event of an intraoperative hinge fracture or displacement, the use of a so-called hinge plate or a contoured mini-fragment plate can be used to stabilize the hinge fracture (Fig. 9-10). Postoperative lamina fractures from the failed hinge may require surgical decompression if any neurologic symptoms manifest.

Motor Root Palsy

The incidence of motor root palsies after laminoplasty has been reported from 5% to 12%, with the C5 nerve root being most commonly involved. While the issue of motor root palsy was initially described in detail in relation to the laminoplasty technique, such nerve root events are not unique to this operation. This complication has been reported to occur in similar frequency with other cervical myelopathy procedures, including laminectomy, laminectomy and fusion, and anterior decompression and fusion (20). This calls into question whether the issue is a by-product of the treatment or the disease itself.

There have been several theories proposed for this complication. The C5 nerve root is thought to be most susceptible as it typically exits at the apex of a lordotic curve and often has a short course that makes it vulnerable during excessive posterior cord migration. Other potential causes include spinal cord reperfusion injury, C4–C5 neuroforaminal stenosis, and C3–C4 central stenosis.

In a review of 630 patients (19) who underwent anterior- or posterior-based cervical procedures, 42 patients (6.7%) reported a postoperative C5 palsy. Of these patients, the incidence was highest for laminectomy and fusion (9.5%), followed by corpectomy with posterior fusion (8.4%), corpectomy only (5.1%), and lowest in the laminoplasty group (4.8%). These findings certainly bring into question the theory of excessive cord drift with a short course for the C5 nerve root.

Clinically, patients most often exhibit painless weakness of the deltoid and biceps muscles. A minority of patients can experience sensory dysfunction and radicular symptoms. These symptoms generally manifest 2 to 3 days after surgery but can appear at anytime from immediately after surgery up to 2 months postoperatively (19). Nassr et al. reported the time to maximum recovery ranging from 1 week to 2 years, with a mean time of 21 weeks. Residual motor deficits were lowest in the laminoplasty group (0%) and highest in the laminectomy and fusion group (27.3%).

CONCLUSION

Laminoplasty is an excellent surgical option for patients with multilevel cervical myelopathy, with or without radiculopathy. The neurologic outcomes are equivalent to anterior decompression and fusion procedures, as well as laminectomy and fusion while avoiding the issues typically seen in fusion procedures such as pseudarthroses, graft extrusion, or subsidence. Nonetheless, from patient positioning to surgical technique, the potential exists for complications. It is therefore important to be meticulous with patient selection, operative technique, and postoperative rehabilitation to ensure an optimal result.

RECOMMENDED READING

1. Cho CB, Chough CK, Oh JY, et al.: Axial neck pain after cervical laminoplasty. *J Korean Neurosurg Soc* 47(2): 107–111, 2010.
2. Fujibayashi S, Neo M, Yoshida M, et al.: Neck muscle strength before and after cervical laminoplasty: relation to axial symptoms. *J Spinal Disord Tech* 23(3): 197–202, 2010.
3. Fujiyoshi T, Yamazaki M, Kawabe J, et al.: A new concept for making decisions regarding the surgical approach for cervical ossification of the posterior longitudinal ligament: the K-line. *Spine (Phila Pa 1976)* 33(26): E990–E993, 2008.
4. Haghighi SS, Mundis G, Zhang R, et al.: Correlation between transcranial motor and somatosensory-evoked potential findings in cervical myelopathy or radiculopathy during cervical spine surgery. *Neurol Res* 33(9): 893–898, 2011.
5. Highsmith JM, Dhall SS, Haid RW Jr, et al.: Treatment of cervical stenotic myelopathy: a cost and outcome comparison of laminoplasty versus laminectomy and lateral mass fusion. *J Neurosurg Spine* 14(5): 619–625, 2011.
6. Hosono N, Sakaura H, Mukai Y, et al.: C3-6 laminoplasty takes over C3-7 laminoplasty with significantly lower incidence of axial neck pain. *Eur Spine J* 15(9): 1375–1379, 2006.
7. Hosono N, Sakaura H, Mukai Y, et al.: The source of axial pain after cervical laminoplasty-C7 is more crucial than deep extensor muscles. *Spine (Phila Pa 1976)* 32(26): 2985–2988, 2007.
8. Iwasaki M, Okuda S, Miyauchi A, et al.: Surgical strategy for cervical myelopathy due to ossification of the posterior longitudinal ligament: part 2: advantages of anterior decompression and fusion over laminoplasty. *Spine (Phila Pa 1976)* 32(6): 654–660, 2007.
9. Kaito T, Hosono N, Makino T, et al.: Postoperative displacement of hydroxyapatite spacers implanted during double-door laminoplasty. *J Neurosurg Spine* 10(6): 551–556, 2009.
10. Kawaguchi Y, Kanamori M, Ishiara H, et al.: Preventive measures for axial symptoms following cervical laminoplasty. *J Spinal Disord Tech* 16(6): 497–501, 2003.
11. Lee DH, Park SA, Kim NH, et al.: Laminar closure after classic Hirabayashi open-door laminoplasty. *Spine (Phila Pa 1976)* 36(25): E1634–E1640, 2011.
12. Liu G, Buchowski JM, Bunmaprasert T, et al.: Revision surgery following cervical laminoplasty: etiology and treatment strategies. *Spine (Phila Pa 1976)* 34(25): 2760–2768, 2009.
13. Lonstein JE. Post-laminectomy kyphosis. *Clin Orthop Relat Res* 128: 93–100, 1977.
14. Machino M, Yukawa Y, Hida T, et al.: Cervical alignment and range of motion after laminoplasty: radiographical data from more than 500 cases with cervical spondylotic myelopathy and a review of the literature. *Spine (Phila Pa 1976)* 37(20): E1243–E1250, 2012.
15. Maeda T, Arizono T, Saito T, et al.: Cervical alignment, range of motion, and instability after cervical laminoplasty. *Clin Orthop Relat Res* 401: 132–138, 2002.
16. Masaki Y, Yamazaki M, Okawa A, et al.: An analysis of factors causing poor surgical outcome in patients with cervical myelopathy due to ossification of the posterior longitudinal ligament: anterior decompression with spinal fusion versus laminoplasty. *J Spinal Disord Tech* 20(1): 7–13, 2007.
17. Matsumoto M, Watanabe K, Hosogane N, et al.: Impact of lamina closure on long-term outcomes of open-door laminoplasty in patients with cervical myelopathy-minimum 5-year follow-up study. *Spine (Phila Pa 1976)* 37(15): 1288–1291, 2012.
18. Matsumoto M, Watanabe K, Tsuji T, et al.: Risk factors for closure of lamina after open-door laminoplasty. *J Neurosurg Spine* 9(6): 530–537, 2008.
19. Nassr A, Eck JC, Ponnappan RK, et al.: The incidence of C5 palsy after multilevel cervical decompression procedures: a review of 750 consecutive cases. *Spine (Phila Pa 1976)* 37(3): 174–178, 2012.
20. Rhee JM, Basra S: Posterior surgery for cervical myelopathy: laminectomy, laminectomy with fusion, and laminoplasty. *Asian Spine J* 2(2): 114–126, 2008.
21. Rhee JM, Register B, Hamasaki T, et al.: Plate-only open door laminoplasty maintains stable spinal canal expansion with high rates of hinge union and no plate failures. *Spine (Phila Pa 1976)* 36(1): 9–14, 2011.
22. Roh MS, Wilson-Holden TJ, Padberg AM, et al.: The utility of somatosensory evoked potential monitoring during cervical spine surgery: how often does it prompt intervention and affect outcome? *Asian Spine J* 1(1): 43–47, 2007.
23. Sakai Y, Matsuyama Y, Inoue K, et al.: Postoperative instability after laminoplasty for cervical myelopathy with spondylolisthesis. *J Spinal Disord Tech* 18(1): 1–5, 2005.
24. Sakaura H, Hosono N, Mukai Y, et al.: Preservation of muscles attached to the C2 and C7 spinous processes rather than subaxial deep extensors reduces adverse effects after cervical laminoplasty. *Spine (Phila Pa 1976)* 35(16): E782–E786, 2010.
25. Sakaura H, Hosono N, Mukai Y, et al.: Medium-term outcomes of C3-6 laminoplasty for cervical myelopathy: a prospective study with a minimum 5-year follow-up. *Eur Spine J* 20(6): 928–933, 2011.
26. Suda K, Abumi K, Ito M, et al.: Local kyphosis reduces surgical outcomes of expansive open-door laminoplasty for cervical spondylotic myelopathy. *Spine (Phila Pa 1976)* 28(12): 1258–1262, 2003.
27. Takeuchi K, Yokoyama T, Aburakawa S, et al.: Anatomic study of the semispinalis cervicis for reattachment during laminoplasty. *Clin Orthop Relat Res* 436: 126–131, 2005.
28. Wada E, Suzuki S, Kanazawa A, et al.: Subtotal corpectomy versus laminoplasty for multilevel cervical spondylotic myelopathy: a long-term follow-up study over 10 years. *Spine (Phila Pa 1976)* 26(13): 1443–1447; discussion 1448, 2001.

10 Laminectomy and Posterior Fusion

Paul A. Anderson and Michael A. Finn

Posterior cervical decompression and fusion is a commonly performed surgery used to treat neurologic compression and spinal instability. Cervical laminectomy, once popular, has diminishing utilization as a stand-alone procedure secondary to its potential to lead to kyphotic deformity and recurrent symptoms (Fig. 10-1) (8,9). Early attempts at stabilization after laminectomy with wiring constructs were fraught with difficulty, required rigid postoperative orthoses, and had a poor capacity to maintain correction. Modern lateral mass and pedicle screw instrumentation has, however, enabled stable reconstruction of the unstable spine even after laminectomy. These newer stabilization techniques are simpler to implement and safer, have better clinical results, and decrease the need for postoperative orthoses when compared with prior methods of fusion.

INDICATIONS

Posterior laminectomy and fusion is indicted when posterior decompression is required for the treatment of spinal cord compression syndromes in combination with instability or kyphotic deformity. Most commonly, this is for the treatment of cervical spondylotic myelopathy associated with degenerative spondylolisthesis or kyphotic deformity. Other conditions include intradural pathology (e.g., spinal cord tumor) needing to be accessed and the potential for the creation of iatrogenic instability (22,31). In some cases of traumatic central cord syndrome requiring decompression, fusion is added if there is concomitant discoligamentous injury (Table 10-1).

There is currently no consensus on the definition of cervical instability. Although rigid radiographic criteria for cervical instability have been proposed, including more than 3.5 mm of subluxation and 11 degrees of angulation on dynamic x-rays (28), more broadly encompassing definitions are often cited. White and Panjabi defined clinical instability of the spine as the loss of the spine's ability to maintain its patterns of displacement under physiologic loads so there is no initial or additional neurologic deficit, no major deformity, and no incapacitating pain (27). Broader definitions such as this extend the indications for fusion to patients with significant axial neck pain and/or deformity who do not present with mobile listhesis.

In cases of cervical spondylotic myelopathy, it is postulated that both motion and compression are contributors to the myelopathic process (30). As such, a fusion may be more strongly considered for this indication. A recent systematic review of the literature did suggest that there is strong evidence to support the utilization of cervical laminectomy and fusion in the treatment of cervical spondylotic myelopathy (1). In cases of cervical kyphosis, fusion should be performed with a goal of reestablishing at least neutral alignment. Irreducible kyphosis may be better treated through an anterior or combined approach.

Advantages of a posterior approach over an anterior approach include surgeon familiarity, ease of exposure, shorter operative times, and reduced risk of dysphagia and recurrent laryngeal nerve palsy (14). Patients with multilevel disease are particularly well suited for posterior approaches as well as patients with ossification of the posterior longitudinal ligament (OPLL), who are at greater risk for complications, including cerebrospinal fluid (CSF) leak and neurologic injury, with an anterior approach (1). The disadvantages of the posterior laminectomy and fusion approach are

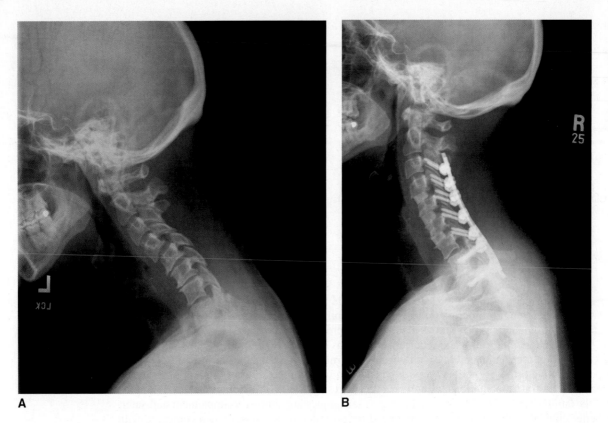

A   B

FIGURE 10-1

A: A 46-year-old female treated with C4–C7 laminectomy for congenital stenosis and myelopathy 6 years prior to presentation with increasing neck pain and myelopathy. X-ray shows postlaminectomy kyphosis. **B:** Patient underwent C3–T2 circumferential fusion with restoration of normal cervical lordosis.

the limited area for bone graft placement, need for costly instrumentation, and higher risk of infection.

CONTRAINDICATIONS

Posterior decompression and fusion is contraindicated as a stand-alone procedure in cases of significant anterior compressive pathology or in patients with irreducible kyphosis. Relative contraindications include patients at particularly high risk for infection (e.g., s/p radiation, malnutrition, prior posterior approach) who may be adequately treated through an anterior approach.

TABLE 10-1   Indications for Posterior Cervical Fusion

Instability
- >3.5-mm subluxation or >11-degree angulation
- Inability to maintain patterns of displacement under physiologic loads so there is no initial or additional neurologic deficit, no major deformity, and no incapacitating pain
- Unstable traumatic injury pattern

Cervical myelopathy with kyphosis or loss of lordosis
Cervical myelopathy with neck pain
Iatrogenic instability
- Tumor resection
- Adjacent level disease

Augment long (>3 level) anterior constructs
- Tobacco users

Pseudoarthrosis treatment

TECHNIQUE

Anesthesia

The anesthesiologist must be made aware of the nature of the patient's condition. In cases with significant canal stenosis, specific anesthetic considerations include intubation, positioning, and hemodynamic support, each of which may compromise the patient's neurologic integrity. Intubation should be performed with in-line stabilization of the neck, and we recommend consideration of awake endotracheal intubation. This has the advantage of allowing for confirmation of neurologic stability after endotracheal tube placement. Care should be taken to avoid neck hyperextension in patients with significant stenosis, as this may contribute to further canal narrowing and neurologic injury. In myelopathic and significantly stenotic patients, careful monitoring of blood pressure is essential, and intra-arterial lines for continuous blood pressure monitoring are routinely used. We maintain a mean arterial pressure of greater than 85 mm Hg to ensure cord perfusion. The use of multimodal neural monitoring is controversial and may allow for early recognition of neurologic injury (21). Similarly, the use of steroids to prevent spinal cord deterioration is controversial and unproven but is an option in patients with severe spinal stenosis or with neurologic deficits.

Positioning

Patients are typically placed in Mayfield 3-point fixation to provide stable positioning without the risk of ocular pressure. Alternatively, patients may be positioned on a padded horseshoe with Gardner-Wells tongs to provide distraction. Care must be taken to ensure that the weight of the head is not resting on the eyes when utilizing this method.

After placement of pins, the patient is rotated into the prone position onto padded gel rolls, a Wilson frame, or the Jackson table. A Jackson table is preferred for obese patients, as it allows for greater decompression of the abdominal compartment and subsequently less venous hypertension and potential for blood loss (Fig. 10-2). A vertical footboard is used to prevent downward sliding when inclining the bed, and the position of the head is fixed. The bed is placed in a reverse Trendelenburg position to aid venous drainage and reduce intraoperative bleeding. However, maintenance of mean arterial pressure after positioning is essential to prevent cord ischemia. Hyperextension is avoided in stenotic patients, as this reduces canal diameter and may predispose to injury. The head is typically positioned in a slight "military tuck" position, with the head flexed and the neck somewhat extended

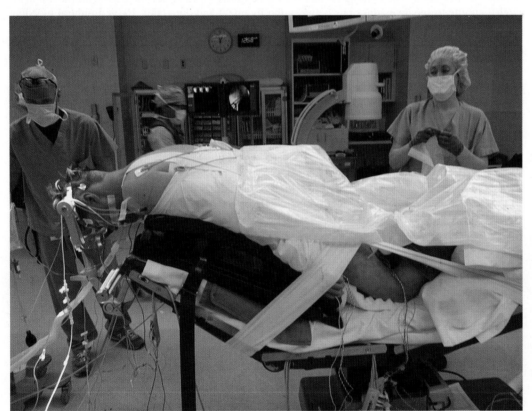

FIGURE 10-2

Patient positioned prone in 3-point Mayfield fixation on a Wilson frame. Note reverse Trendelenburg inclination of the bed, which enables the cervical spine to be positioned level to the floor and above the level of the heart, facilitating anatomic recognition and venous drainage, respectively.

to increase exposure but maintain cervical lordosis. The arms are secured by the patient's sides, and the shoulders are taped slightly inferiorly to aid in x-ray visualization of lower cervical levels.

Once secured, fluoroscopy can be used to demonstrate adequacy of positioning and maintenance of reduction if alignment is a concern. If neural monitoring is used, signals are rechecked after final positioning.

Exposure

The incision is marked utilizing landmarks, with the C2 and C7 spinous processes easily palpable in most patients. Intraoperative radiographs can aid in planning incisions for small operations.

A midline incision is created and dissected to the fascia with electrocautery. The midline avascular raphe is exploited to minimize blood loss. A self-retaining retractor is placed to maintain exposure when the spinous processes are encountered. Electrocautery is used to create a paramedian fascial incision on either side of the bifid processes. The paraspinous muscles are then elevated off the spinous process and lamina in a subperiosteal fashion, using a Cobb elevator to hold retraction and electrocautery to separate tissue adhesions and maintain hemostasis. Care is taken to avoid damaging the interspinous ligaments, particularly at the cephalad and caudal ends of the planned construct (24). Care is also taken to preserve the joint capsules of the facets at the distal ends of the planned construct. After final exposure, levels are confirmed radiographically. Unless absolutely required for adequate decompression, the nuchal ligaments attachments to C2 and C7 should be preserved or repaired to avoid the development of postoperative kyphosis.

Decompression

The laminectomy can be performed primarily with rongeurs. The cephalocaudal limits of the decompression are demarcated by using a Leksell rongeur to remove the supraspinous and interspinous ligaments. Likewise, these ligaments are removed at each level to be decompressed to facilitate processing of local autograft. Laminectomy can then be performed using a combination of Leksell and Kerrison rongeurs. In cases of severe stenosis, a "no touch technique" (no canal intrusion with instruments) should be employed. In this case, the lamina-facet junction is identified and marked with the marking pen, and a high-speed burr is used to osteotomize the lamina at the lamina-facet junction bilaterally. The trough is cut through the outer cortical and cancellous layers of bone. The final thin inner cortical bone can be removed with a 1-mm Kerrison rongeur or diamond burr under continuous irrigation. The floating lamina is then carefully elevated off the dura with the aid of an angled curette to separate adhesions between the ligament and dura (Fig. 10-3). Epidural bleeding may be brisk, especially in patients with highly stenotic canals, but this is usually easily controlled with bipolar electrocautery and topical hemostatic agents. Care should be taken to extend the laminectomy to the medial edges of the pedicle to ensure complete decompression. When possible, avoid removing the spinous processes of C2 and C7 as the nuchal ligaments attach at these sites and compromise of the integrity here may contribute to the development of a kyphotic deformity. Partial laminectomy of the cranial aspect of C7 may allow sparing of that level with adequate decompression of the C6–C7 interspace. Another alternative, which is not covered in this chapter, is to combine laminoplasty and posterior fusion (Fig. 10-4).

If foraminal stenosis is causing radiculopathy, foraminotomies may be performed. It is helpful to begin the foraminotomy with palpation of the pedicle and neural foramen with a nerve hook. This not only allows identification of the exact location of the foramen but also gives the surgeon an idea of the degree of stenosis present. A high-speed burr is then used to remove the medial half of the facet articulation overlying the foramen, leaving only a thin shell of bone dorsal to the nerve (Fig. 10-5). A small (1 or 2 mm) Kerrison is then used to access the foramen and remove the remaining bone. The nerve root is visualized, and the decompression of the foramen is confirmed with a nerve hook. Removal of more than 50% of the facet should be avoided at levels not to be fused, as this may lead to instability (31). A good rule of thumb is not to remove the facet past the lateral margin of the pedicle. The utility of a prophylactic C5 foraminotomy to reduce the risks of C5 palsy is controversial and not routinely performed by the authors (17).

Fusion

An optimal fusion environment is created by minimizing motion and preparing an optimal fusion bed. The former is supported by instrumentation, and the latter is supported by thorough decortication and facet preparation.

Modular screw and rod-based constructs offer the greatest immediate stability in the cervical spine. Lateral mass screws are most commonly used from C3 to C6 with pedicle screws being commonly implemented at C2 and C7. Although lateral mass screws can be placed at C7, long

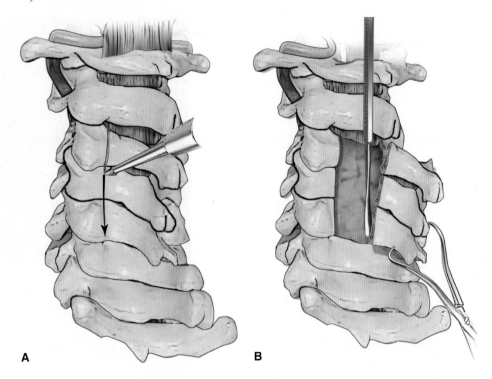

A   B

FIGURE 10-3

The laminectomy can be performed with rongeurs or in an en bloc fashion. An en bloc fashion may be safer in severely stenotic canals and is illustrated here. **A:** Trough is created at the junction of the lamina and lateral mass on either side using a high-speed burr and a "no touch" technique. Completion of the trough may be complete with a 1-mm Kerrison rongeur to minimize canal intrusion. **B:** The laminae are removed en bloc. Adhesions between the ligament and dura are anticipated and taken down with a sharp curette. Additionally, epidural bleeding can be significant but is easily controlled with topical hemostatic agents and gentle bipolar electrocautery.

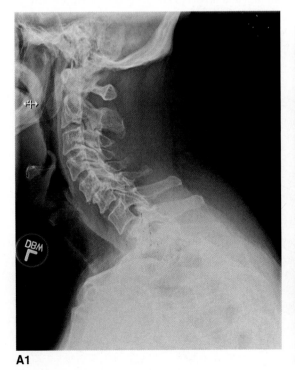

A1

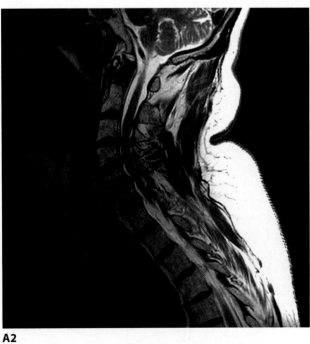

A2

FIGURE 10-4

Posterior cervical fusion can be combined with other techniques, such as laminoplasty. **A:** This patient presented with myelopathy, multilevel cervical stenosis, and spondylolisthesis.

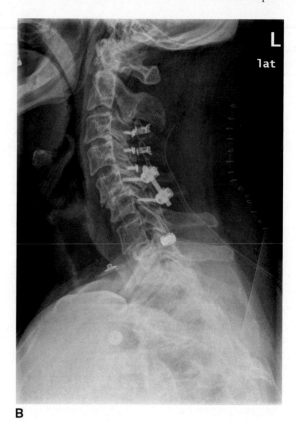

FIGURE 10-4 (*Continued*)

B: The spondylolisthetic level was treated with a fusion, while the remaining areas of stenosis were decompressed with a laminoplasty.

B

constructs ending with lateral mass screws may have a higher failure rate, and consideration should be given to pedicle screw fixation at this level. Additionally, long constructs ending at C7 are associated with a significant risk of adjacent level degeneration and may be reasonably extended across the cervicothoracic junction, typically to T1 or T2. Pedicle screws may be placed from C3 to C6, although this technique is technically demanding and involves greater risk of vertebral artery injury than lateral mass screws.

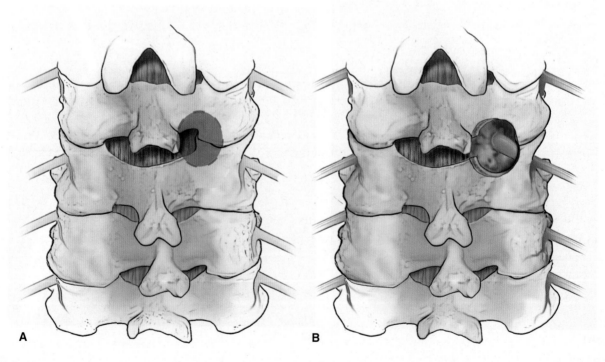

A   **B**

FIGURE 10-5

A: Schematic showing area of bone to be removed to perform a foraminotomy. Care must be taken to remove less than 50% of the facet articulation at levels not to be fused. **B:** Final foraminotomy with observation of the decompressed nerve root.

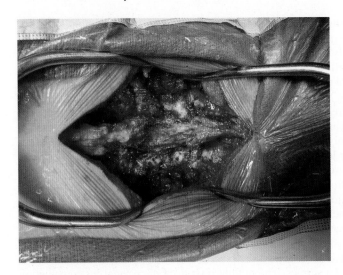

FIGURE 10-6

Intraoperative photo showing exposure and placement of screw pilot holes. Lateral mass pilot holes are created prior to decompression to protect the spinal cord and facilitate anatomic recognition of trajectory. All tracts are marked and placed in quick succession to minimize mediolateral variability and thus maximize ease of rod insertion.

We create the pilot holes for lateral mass screws before decompression as landmarks are more easily identified and the risk to inadvertent trauma to the exposed dura and spinal cord is lessened (Fig. 10-6). The decompression however is performed prior to screw insertion, decortication, and bone grafting. Where pedicle screws are placed, the pilot holes can be made after decompression, which allows for direct palpation of the pedicle to assure proper placement.

The placement of lateral mass screws requires identification of the borders of the lateral mass. The cephalad and caudal borders are defined by the articulations, the lateral is the palpable lateral edge of bone, and the medial border is defined by the transition point of the lateral mass and lamina. Usually, there is a valley or depression at this point. With the borders identified, the quadrilateral surface of the lateral mass can be divided into four equal quadrants from which to base screw trajectory. Based on technique, we identify and mark our screw entry point with a match-head burr.

Numerous lateral mass screw trajectories have been described with the Magerl, Roy-Camille, and Anderson methods being most commonly utilized. We use that described by Anderson and mark our screw entry point at the cephalocaudal midpoint approximately 1 mm medial to the center point of the lateral mass. After the starting point is created, a power drill is used to create a prospective tract approximately 30 degrees cranially and 20 degrees laterally (Fig. 10-7). These angles can be closely

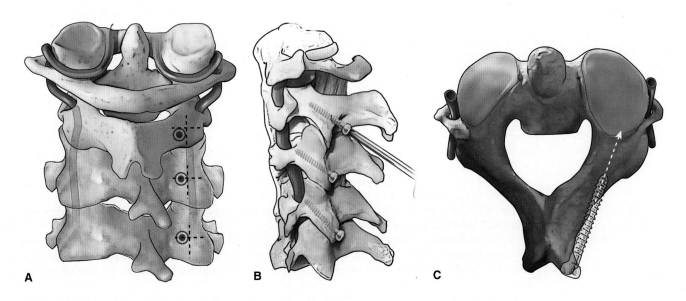

A   B   C

FIGURE 10-7

Figure showing lateral mass screw entry point and trajectory. No slightly medial of center entry point and cephalocaudal angulation in line with the facet articulation. Lateral angulation can be approximated by leaning the drill guide against the intact spinous process.

approximated by leaning the drill on the next caudal spinous process. Further clarification of the cranial angle can be obtained by removing the articular cartilage of the joint with a high-speed burr over the dorsal half of the joint and directly observing their angulation. We use a high-speed drill with a K-wire in lieu of a standard fluted drill bit as we feel that smooth edges of the K-wire may lessen the chances of neurovascular injury. We also use an adjustable drill guide set at progressively greater depths to reduce the risk of "plunging" during this portion of the procedure. A 12-mm length is initially used and increased in 2-mm increments until the ventral cortical surface is breached. Abutment of the drill against the ventral cortex can almost always be felt, but a ball-tipped probe can be used to confirm depth if there is any uncertainty. Bicortical screw purchase increases the risk of neurovascular injury and is typically reserved for long fusions and cases in which there is significant osteopenia or deformity. All screw trajectories are created in a similar fashion. It is helpful to place a ball-tip probe down the first tract created to allow that trajectory to be emulated for adjacent and contralateral screws. It is also helpful to create trajectories on a single side in fairly rapid sequence, maintaining positional alignment of the drill as each tract is created. Again, for extended fusions, marking each entry point prior to drilling ensures that each screw is uniformly placed and eases rod insertion.

If a laminectomy is to be performed, we pack the pilot holes with a hemostatic agent (Gelfoam and thrombin). Following decompression, the screws are placed, and a rod is bent to conform to the cervical alignment and secured with set screws. The pullout resistance of cervical instrumentation is relatively weak, and care must be taken when attempting to persuade the rod to the screw tulips. If deformity correction is to be attempted, thought should be given to pedicle screw placement or bicortical lateral mass screw placement. Reduction of kyphosis is obtained by changing head position into extension after decompression, lordotic rod bending, and rod compression. The latter may create foraminal stenosis, and care must be utilized.

Fusion Bed Preparation

Preparation of the fusion bed is critical for maximizing the chances of a bony fusion. A high-speed drill is used to remove the facet capsule and decorticate the proximal facet articulation at each level to be fused. The facet capsule and cartilaginous endplates are removed. The dorsal aspect of the facet is also decorticated.

Autograft obtained from the laminectomy site is the preferred grafting material, although allograft and a number of synthetic bone substitutes are available. Graft is placed within the facet joint and dorsally over the lateral mass. Iliac crest autograft may be considered in patients at a high risk of nonunion and when there is insufficient local bone. The bone graft must be stable so that it does not migrate medially toward the neural elements. Prior to closure, a lateral radiograph is obtained to assure proper alignment and placement of instrumentation.

Closure

The wound is thoroughly irrigated prior to closure. We place 1 g of vancomycin powder in the paraspinal muscles, which has been shown to significantly reduce the risk of surgical site infection after instrumented posterior fusion (23). The wound is closed in layers, with care taken to tightly reapproximate the fascia layers. It is essential to tightly repair the nuchal ligaments to the spinous processes of C2 and C7. Staples are used for the skin closure, and a sterile dressing is applied. A closed drainage system is typically used.

PEARLS AND PITFALLS

In our opinion, the major neurologic risk occurs during intubation and positioning. Collaboration with an experienced anesthesiologist is essential. Since cord compression results in ischemia, maintenance of mean arterial blood pressure of at least 85 mm Hg during the entire procedure is critical.

When an extended construct is planned, it is helpful to mark all screw entry points with a marking pen prior the creation of trajectories. This ensures that all screws will be aligned in a similar coronal plane and facilitate rod placement.

When performing decompression in highly stenotic canals, no instrument larger than a 1-mm Kerrison rongeur should be placed into the canal. The use of a "no touch" technique with a diamond burr should be considered, but constant irrigation must be employed to reduce the risk of thermal injury.

Lateral mass screws are generally safe as long as proper identification of the starting point and screw direction is considered. Marking the starting point with a burr prevents lateral migration and subsequent poor purchase. Angulation upward and outward avoids root and vertebral artery injury, respectively.

Using a K-wire instead of a traditional fluted drill bit may be used to create pilot holes and may be less prone to neurovascular injury as there are no cutting edges to grab sensitive structures.

Decorticating the facets joints prior to screw placement can aid in identifying the facet angle and facilitate placement of lateral mass screws with the correct sagittal angle.

Placement of pedicle screws is demanding. We recommend placement of a pedicle screw at C7 because of its superior biomechanical characteristics and increased safety when compared with other cervical levels. Prior to placement, the pedicle dimension is evaluated on the preoperative imaging studies, and attention is paid to the location of the vertebral artery by looking for the presence of a flow void on T2-weighted MRI sequences. In approximately 10% of cases in which the artery is present in the foramen at C7, placement of a pedicle screw may be reconsidered. Fluoroscopic visualization is often difficult here, but the trajectory can be clarified by creating a small laminotomy and palpating the pedicle with a nerve hook. The tract is then created in parallel to the C7 endplate and angulated approximately 20 degrees medially with a blunt-tipped pedicle finder. The tract is then tapped, and the screw is placed as outlined above.

Avoid removing the spinous processes and lamina of C2 and C7 to avoid postoperative kyphosis. Decompression around this lamina can usually be achieved by undercutting the lamina.

POSTOPERATIVE MANAGEMENT

The use of a rigid external orthosis is at the surgeon's discretion but is typically not employed by the authors for short (one- or two-level) constructs. Alternatively, a soft collar may be used for comfort, although use should be limited to prevent deconditioning. In longer constructs and in those with a higher risk of failure (e.g., osteopenic patients, deformity corrections, fusions extending across the cervicothoracic junction), a cervical orthosis is recommended. Patients are mobilized the day of surgery and instructed to avoid heavy lifting and pulling activities.

Pain control relies on a combination of narcotic pain medications and antispasm medications. NSAIDs are avoided for 6 due weeks to their potentially deleterious effects on bone healing (12). Likewise, smoking cessation is encouraged (5).

COMPLICATIONS

Complications related to posterior decompression and fusion may be grouped as operative or delayed.

Operative Complications

Neurologic Injury: Spinal cord deterioration is a devastating complication and occurs in 3% to 5% of patients with significant preexisting myelopathy as these patients have ischemic spinal cords at baseline. Techniques to reduce this include care in intubation, positioning, and resuscitation. Extending the stenotic spine reduces canal diameter and may predispose to injury. Neural monitoring may provide early warning of this complication although outcomes may not be influenced (21). In rare cases, the laminectomy must be performed with the patient in a flexed position prior to reestablishing cervical lordosis. Mean arterial blood pressures are maintained above 85 mm Hg to aid spinal cord perfusion.

C5 nerve root palsy occurs with a frequency of approximately 7% to 10% and has had a number of proposed etiologies and risk factors (18). Increased rates have been correlated with the use of a diamond burr, which may result in thermal injury to the nerve unless properly cooled. Decreased rates of this complication have been reported with prophylactic C5 foraminotomy (17).

Radicular injury has been reported to occur at a rate of less than 1% due to screw placement (26). Several anatomic studies have examined the safety of various techniques with differing results (15,29). Regardless of the method used, safer trajectories may lie parallel to the facet joint and with maximal lateral angulation (15).

Vascular Injury: Vertebral artery injury with lateral mass screw placement is rare (10) and may be avoided by assessing the location of the transverse foramen and vertebral artery on preoperative studies. With typical anatomy, vertebral artery injury can be avoided with proper lateral trajectory.

Spinal Fluid Leak: Dural tears may occur with greater frequency in patients who are elderly, are highly stenotic, have ossification of the ligamentum flavum, or have had prior surgeries. Primary closure of durotomies should be attempted. In rare cases, when this is not feasible, an onlay patch and a dural sealant may be utilized. In these cases, consideration should be given to lumbar drainage for 3 days postoperatively to reduce CSF leakage at the dural injury site.

Delayed Complications

Infection: Surgical site infections occur in 1.5% to 4% of all patients undergoing posterior decompression and fusion (19,25) but may be as high as 20% in high-risk individuals, such as the elderly and those being treated for trauma or malignancy (2,13,20). Risk of surgical site infections may be reduced with the administration of preoperative antibiotics, frequent intraoperative irrigation, and utilization of powdered vancomycin (3,4,23). No benefit has been shown with the utilization of more than one dose of postoperative antibiotics (7).

Pseudoarthrosis: Pseudoarthrosis rates have been reported to range from 3% to 9% (10,11). After laminectomy, the area available for bone grafting is small, and thus, careful attention must be paid to thorough decortication and autograft packing of the facet joints. Risk factors for pseudoarthrosis include smoking, age, use of allograft bone, and greater number of levels fused.

Deformity: Cervical laminectomy, particularly when performed over multiple segments or at C2 or C7, may predispose to the development of late deformity. Kaptain et al. (8) reported a 21% incidence in the development of cervical kyphosis after laminectomy for the treatment of cervical spondylotic myelopathy, with the risk being greater in those patients with reduced preoperative cervical lordosis. Kato et al. (9) reported a 47% risk of progression of kyphotic deformity in patients treated with laminectomy for OPLL. Laminoplasty or fusion may decrease the incidence of deformity (1). The addition of a fusion should mitigate this complication; however, where to end the fusion in relation to the decompression is not fully known. Our approach is to extend the fusion past the levels of decompression to avoid adjacent segment kyphosis although some surgeons will fuse and decompress at the same levels. In general, we also recommend extending the fusion across the cervicothoracic junction.

RESULTS

Neurologic improvement after laminectomy and fusion for myelopathy occurs in 70% to 95% of patients, with a recovery averaging approximately 50% of preoperative JOA deficit (1,6,16). Success of bony fusion has been sporadically reported and is incompletely documented but appears to be higher with modern screw and rod-based constructs. Likewise, prevention of long-term deformity is also incompletely described but is likely reduced with modern instrumentation.

RECOMMENDED READING

1. Anderson PA, et al.: Laminectomy and fusion for the treatment of cervical degenerative myelopathy. *J Neurosurg Spine* 11(2): 150–156, 2009.
2. Carreon LY, et al.: Perioperative complications of posterior lumbar decompression and arthrodesis in older adults. *J Bone Joint Surg Am* 85-A(11): 2089–2092, 2003.
3. Cheng MT, et al.: Efficacy of dilute betadine solution irrigation in the prevention of postoperative infection of spinal surgery. *Spine (Phila Pa 1976)* 30(15): 1689–1693, 2005.
4. Epstein NE: Preoperative, intraoperative, and postoperative measures to further reduce spinal infections. *Surg Neurol Int* 2: 17, 2011.
5. Glassman SD, et al.: The effect of cigarette smoking and smoking cessation on spinal fusion. *Spine (Phila Pa 1976)* 25(20): 2608–2615, 2000.
6. Huang RC, et al.: Treatment of multilevel cervical spondylotic myeloradiculopathy with posterior decompression and fusion with lateral mass plate fixation and local bone graft. *J Spinal Disord Tech* 16(2): 123–129, 2003.
7. Kang BU, et al.: Surgical site infection in spinal surgery: detection and management based on serial C-reactive protein measurements. *J Neurosurg Spine* 13(2): 158–164, 2010.
8. Kaptain GJ, et al.: Incidence and outcome of kyphotic deformity following laminectomy for cervical spondylotic myelopathy. *J Neurosurg* 93(2 Suppl): 199–204, 2000.
9. Kato Y, et al.: Long-term follow-up results of laminectomy for cervical myelopathy caused by ossification of the posterior longitudinal ligament. *J Neurosurg* 89(2): 217–23, 1998.
10. Katonis P, et al.: Lateral mass screw complications: analysis of 1662 screws. *J Spinal Disord Tech* 24(7): 415–420, 2011.
11. Kim SH, et al.: Early results from posterior cervical fusion with a screw-rod system. *Yonsei Med J* 48(3): 440–448, 2007.
12. Li Q, Zhang Z, Cai Z: High-dose ketorolac affects adult spinal fusion: a meta-analysis of the effect of perioperative nonsteroidal anti-inflammatory drugs on spinal fusion. *Spine (Phila Pa 1976)* 36(7): E461–E468, 2011.
13. McPhee IB, Williams RP, Swanson CE: Factors influencing wound healing after surgery for metastatic disease of the spine. *Spine (Phila Pa 1976)* 23(6): 726–732, 1998; discussion 732–733.
14. Mehdorn HM, Fritsch MJ, Stiller RU: Treatment options and results in cervical myelopathy. *Acta Neurochir Suppl* 93: 177–182, 2005.
15. Merola AA, et al.: Anatomic consideration for standard and modified techniques of cervical lateral mass screw placement. *Spine J* 2(6): 430–435, 2002.
16. Morio Y, et al.: Clinicoradiologic study of cervical laminoplasty with posterolateral fusion or bone graft. *Spine (Phila Pa 1976)* 25(2): 190–196, 2000.
17. Nakashima H, et al.: Multivariate analysis of C-5 palsy incidence after cervical posterior fusion with instrumentation. *J Neurosurg Spine* 17(2): 103–110, 2012.
18. Nassr A, et al.: The incidence of C5 palsy after multilevel cervical decompression procedures: a review of 750 consecutive cases. *Spine (Phila Pa 1976)* 37(3): 174–178, 2012.

19. Olsen MA, et al.: Risk factors for surgical site infection following orthopaedic spinal operations. *J Bone Joint Surg Am* 90(1): 62–69, 2008.

20. Rechtine GR, et al.: Postoperative wound infection after instrumentation of thoracic and lumbar fractures. *J Orthop Trauma* 15(8): 566–569, 2001.

21. Resnick DK, et al.: Electrophysiological monitoring during surgery for cervical degenerative myelopathy and radiculopathy. *J Neurosurg Spine* 11(2): 245–252, 2009.

22. Steinmetz MP, et al.: Regional instability following cervicothoracic junction surgery. *J Neurosurg Spine* 4(4): 278–284, 2006.

23. Sweet FA, Roh M, Sliva C: Intrawound application of vancomycin for prophylaxis in instrumented thoracolumbar fusions: efficacy, drug levels, and patient outcomes. *Spine (Phila Pa 1976)* 36(24): 2084–2088, 2011.

24. Takeshita K, et al: The nuchal ligament restrains cervical spine flexion. *Spine (Phila Pa 1976)* 29(18): E388–E393, 2004.

25. Weinstein MA, McCabe JP, Cammisa FP Jr: Postoperative spinal wound infection: a review of 2,391 consecutive index procedures. *J Spinal Disord* 13(5): 422–426, 2000.

26. Wellman BJ, Follett KA, Traynelis VC: Complications of posterior articular mass plate fixation of the subaxial cervical spine in 43 consecutive patients. *Spine (Phila Pa 1976)* 23(2): 193–200, 1998.

27. White A, Panjabi M: *Clinical biomechanics of the spine*. 2nd ed. Philadelphia, PA: JB Lippincott, 1990.

28. White AA III, Panjabi MM: Update on the evaluation of instability of the lower cervical spine. *Instr Course Lect* 36: 513–520, 1987.

29. Xu R, et al.: The anatomic relation of lateral mass screws to the spinal nerves. A comparison of the Magerl, Anderson, and An techniques. *Spine (Phila Pa 1976)* 24(19): 2057–2061, 1999.

30. Yuan Q, Dougherty L, Margulies SS: In vivo human cervical spinal cord deformation and displacement in flexion. *Spine (Phila Pa 1976)* 23(15): 1677–1683, 1998.

31. Zdeblick TA, et al.: Cervical stability after foraminotomy. A biomechanical in vitro analysis. *J Bone Joint Surg Am* 74(1): 22–27, 1992.

11 C1–C2 Posterior Screw-Rod Fixation

Charbel D. Moussallem, Ahmad Nassr, and Bradford L. Currier

Many traumatic, degenerative, inflammatory conditions may result in atlantoaxial instability, which, in certain circumstances, requires surgical stabilization. The C1–C2 joint is highly mobile, has a unique anatomy, and accounts for 50% of the rotation and 10% of the flexion and extension of the cervical spine (25,28), which may predispose this joint to instability. Several techniques have been described to address C1–C2 instability, including wiring techniques, transarticular screw fixation, and rod and screw fixation of C1–C2 (Box 11-1). Surgery for atlantoaxial instability can be challenging because of the unique anatomic and biomechanical considerations of this region. Methods based on C1 lateral mass screws and C2 pedicle or pars interarticularis screws, originally described by Goel and Laheri (12) and popularized by Harms and Melcher (13), have become widely used adjuncts because of their high fusion rates and construct rigidity, which eliminate the need for external halo-vest immobilization.

The modern technique, described by Harms and Melcher in 2001 (13), uses rods to connect C1 lateral mass screws and C2 screws to stabilize the atlantoaxial joint. This technique is based on the posterior C1–C2 plate and screw construct developed by Goel and Laheri (12) and described in 1994. In their original paper, Harms and Melcher (13) described 37 patients treated by this novel technique. All these patients had solid fusion without any vascular or neurologic complications and without the need for halo immobilization. In this chapter, we describe the indications, contraindications, and surgical steps involved in applying this technique.

INDICATIONS AND CONTRAINDICATIONS

The most common indication for surgery is a displaced odontoid fracture in a patient for whom direct anterior screw fixation is not feasible or is a poor choice. Other indications include less common injury patterns (e.g., displaced fractures of C1, C2, and/or ligamentous instability); inflammatory conditions with resultant instability (e.g., rheumatoid arthritis); congenital or developmental conditions (e.g., symptomatic os odontoideum, Down syndrome, fixed rotatory subluxation) (Fig. 11-1); pathologic lesions with resultant or potential instability; and iatrogenic instability (e.g,, anterior resection of the odontoid).

Surgical stabilization of the C1–C2 joint may also be considered after failure of conservative management of fractures that present with late instability, pain, or myelopathy and in patients in whom external immobilization with a halo-vest is contraindicated.

Contraindications are primarily those related to patient factors and inability to tolerate general anesthesia. In some patients, a severe deformity or erosions caused by inflammatory disorders like rheumatoid arthritis distort the anatomy. Care must be taken when anatomic landmarks for screw fixation are lost. Often, these patients can still undergo the procedure but may require intraoperative navigation to help identify safe avenues for screw passage.

Anatomic variations of the vertebral artery (VA) anatomy may make certain screws dangerous, and careful examination of preoperative images and meticulous planning can avoid a catastrophic vascular injury.

Fractures with severe comminution of the lateral masses of C1 or C2 are also contraindications to the technique.

BOX 11.1 Internal Fixation Methods of the Atlantoaxial Complex

---

Sublaminar wires, cables, interposition grafting

Interspinous wires, cables, interposition grafting

Clamps, hooks

Transarticular screws

C1 lateral mass with C2 screws (connected by a rod or plate):

Pars interarticularis

Pedicle

Translaminar

Combination of fixation methods

PREOPERATIVE PREPARATION

Imaging

Plain upright radiographs of the cervical spine, including anteroposterior, lateral, and odontoid views, can help the evaluation and surgical plan. In some patients, when instability is not already apparent, lateral flexion and extension views may be helpful to identify dynamic instability. This is not necessary and is potentially dangerous in the acute traumatic patient. A computed tomographic (CT) scan with axial, sagittal, and coronal thin-cut (1 to 2 mm) images is necessary to identify anatomic abnormalities and to help determine the optimal screw length, diameter, entry points, and trajectory. It is ideal to have the CT reconstructed in the plane of the C1 ring for accurate templating. CT angiography can be performed simultaneously to identify the proximity of the internal carotid artery (ICA) to the anterior arch of C1 and to rule out vascular anomalies of the VA (7). CT angiography can help in planning for unicortical versus bicortical C1 screw fixation. Magnetic resonance imaging (MRI) may help define ligamentous injury, the degree of cord compression and myelomalacia, and the space available for supplementary wire fixation. Careful examination of the MRI or magnetic resonance angiography (MRA) can also define the VA anatomy and dominance. Up to 20% of patients may have a VA anomaly (20), and this can be detected on a preoperative CT (or CT angiography) or MRI (or MRA). Another common anomaly is the ponticulus posticus, which can often be detected on the lateral radiograph or CT scan. It is important to recognize this anatomic variant, which is present in 15.5% of patients (32). The presence of ponticulus posticus can give a false sense that the C1 ring is large enough in the cranial-caudal direction to accept a screw placed through the posterior arch of C1 into the lateral mass, resulting in catastrophic VA injury.

Technique

Anesthesia and Monitoring   Awake fiberoptic intubation may be necessary in patients with spinal instability or when the patient does not have adequate mobility of the neck or mouth to allow standard intubation. After induction of general anesthesia, appropriate intravenous access is obtained. Often, an arterial line is placed to monitor blood pressure, which may be necessary in patients with severe myelopathy to maintain adequate cord perfusion pressure. Neuromonitoring with motor and sensory evoked potentials is often used. Prepositioning baseline tracings are obtained, and the tests are repeated after positioning and throughout the procedure. In patients with considerable instability, the head can be secured to the Jackson table with Mayfield pinions or a halo with the patient in the supine position. The patient is then sandwiched between the posterior and anterior portion of the table and then turned to the prone position through the rotating frame. Turning the patient minimizes motion through the cervical spine. Antibiotic prophylaxis should be initiated 30 minutes before incision and then readministered every 3 to 4 hours throughout the procedure.

Positioning   Under general anesthesia, the patient is positioned prone on a Jackson table (or rotated to the prone position as described above), with his or her head fixed with either Mayfield pinions or Gardner-Wells tongs and bivector traction (Figs. 11-2 and 11-3), depending on surgeon preference and the needs of the procedure (26). All bony prominences are carefully padded. The upper extremities are padded and positioned along the sides of the patient's trunk. The knees should be flexed and well padded. Fluoroscopy is used to check the reduction and alignment of the cervical

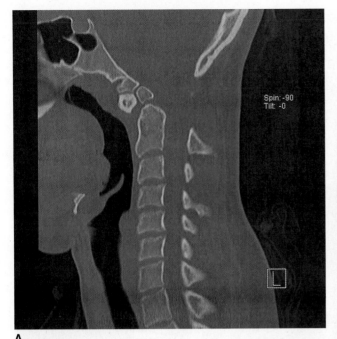

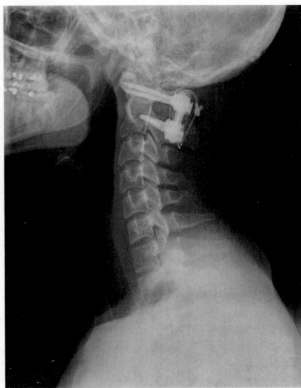

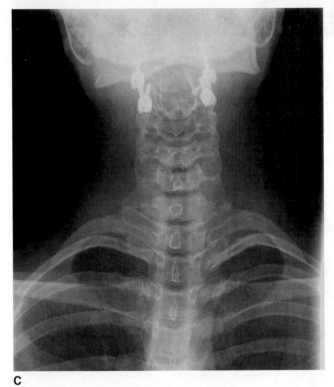

FIGURE 11-1

A: Midsagittal CT scan of the cervical spine showing an os odontoideum that was symptomatic in a young patient. **B:** Postoperative lateral radiograph showing adequate fusion with a C1–C2 screw-rod construct supplemented by wiring. **C:** Anteroposterior radiograph of the cervical spine showing the C1–C2 construct.

spine before preparing the patient. Access to the patient's head is desirable to allow for manipulation during the procedure to aid in reduction and is one advantage of the bivector traction setup as the head can be manipulated freely.

Prepping and Draping   The patient's hair is clipped to a few centimeters above the external occipital protuberance. The skin incision is planned in the midline from just distal to the external occipital protuberance to the level of the C2 spinous process. A chlorhexidine and alcohol solution is used for skin sterilization. An antimicrobial surgical adhesive is used to cover the surgical site as well as sites of possible autograft harvest. We typically include the neck as well as the patient's trunk in the surgical field to have access to the iliac crests and ribs as potential sites of autologous bone graft. This preparation can also allow for mobilization of a trapezial flap in patients who have had previous radiation or in thin patients when a muscle flap is needed to cover the instrumentation.

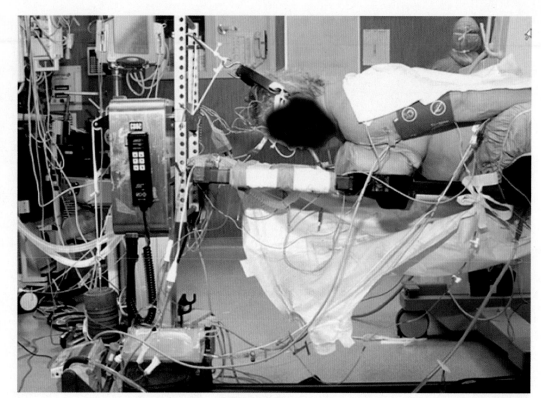

FIGURE 11-2

Positioning of a patient on the operating table in a prone position with bivector traction, with the upper extremities well padded on the sides of the trunk.

Surgical Exposure   Prior to incision, a solution of 1% lidocaine with 1:100,000 epinephrine is injected into the subcutaneous tissue to help provide hemostasis in patients with good skin vascularity and integrity. A posterior midline incision is made in customary fashion; dissection of the subcutaneous tissue is made by electrocautery to decrease bleeding. The fascia is divided in the midline. Deep dissection is carried out in the midline through the thin white median raphe of the neck to avoid excessive bleeding. Subperiosteal dissection is carried out along the posterior aspect of C1 and C2.

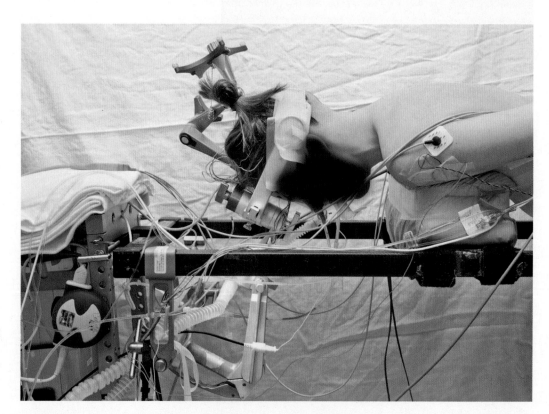

FIGURE 11-3

Positioning of a patient on the operating table with the frame for navigation attached to the Mayfield frame.

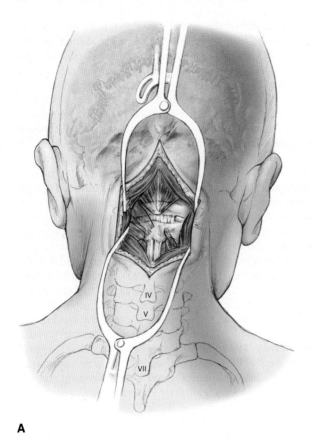

A

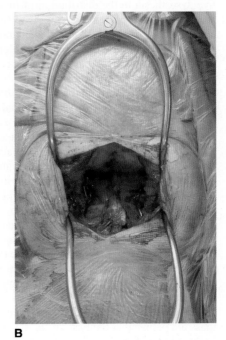

B

FIGURE 11-4

A,B: Exposure of the atlantoaxial complex after surgical preparation.

Care is taken to avoid injury to the VA along the superior surface of the C1 ring. We try to preserve the attachments of the semispinalis cervicis muscle on the caudal aspect of the C2 spinous process. If detachment is necessary, this can be accomplished by removing the muscle with a small amount of bone for later reattachment to the spinous process (Fig. 11-4). As the exposure is carried laterally, careful subperiosteal dissection should be performed to avoid inadvertent injury to the VA above the ring of C1. Generally, the dissection does not extend further than 1.5 cm laterally on either side. The exact location of the VA can be determined on preoperative MRA or CT angiography.

C1 Screw Fixation   Identification of the medial border of the pars interarticularis of C2 locates the entry point of the C1 lateral mass. The medial aspect of the lateral mass of C1 is directly cranial to this point, and this relationship helps determine where to start the dissection caudal to the C1 arch. A Penfield 4 elevator can be used to slide caudal to the arch of C1 just lateral to the location of the C2 pars interarticularis (Fig. 11-5). Hugging the bone of the pedicle analogue of C1, the instrument

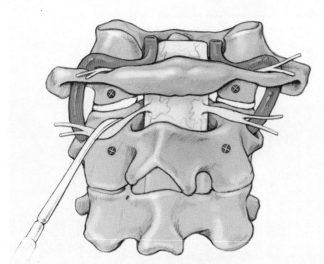

FIGURE 11-5

The entry points for the C1 and C2 screws from the posteroanterior view. A soft tissue dissector is used to gently retract and protect the C2 ganglion. Frequently, this ganglion is very large.

slides anteriorly until it docks on the posterior aspect of the lateral mass of C1. From here, the Penfield can be slid caudally on the lateral mass to the level of the C1–C2 joint. The second cervical nerve (greater occipital nerve) is retracted caudally with this maneuver. It is often possible to enter the C1–C2 joint through its capsule with the Penfield 4 and thereby maintain retraction of the C2 nerve. Some surgeons elect to sacrifice this nerve (2), but we try to preserve it to avoid postoperative dysesthesia in the distribution of this nerve (16). Surrounding the C2 nerve root and ganglion is a large venous plexus that can bleed easily and obscure the entry point of the screw. Hemostatic agents such as microfibrillar collagen and thrombin or thrombin-soaked sterile compressed sponge (Gelfoam) can be used as necessary. Gentle retraction is key for a safe insertion of the screw. A persistent first segmental artery is a vascular anomaly that is uncommon but presents frequently in patients with bony anomalies. In these patients, the VA is actually caudal to the posterior arch of C1 rather than cranial to it, and it is in the direct path of a lateral mass screw. Preoperative CT angiography or MRA can identify this anomaly and avoid injury to the artery. The venous plexus itself can bleed vigorously and give the impression that a persistent first segmental artery has been injured. Powdered hemostatic agents, a well-placed compressed rayon pad (cottonoid patties), and patience generally take care of the bleeding. In patients with a C1 pedicle analogue (portion of the bone connecting the posterior arch to the lateral mass) large enough to accommodate a screw caudal to the VA, the entry point can be on the posterior arch rather than the lateral mass (5). Care must be taken to ensure the arch is thick enough to avoid injury to the VA in the superior sulcus of C1. The anatomy can often be misleading in patients with a ponticulus posticus (32). Placement of the screw through the posterior arch of C1 can be desirable because it increases the purchase of the screw inside bone, and retracting the C2 nerve and the surrounding venous plexus can be avoided. Unfortunately, placement of this posterior arch screw can be done in only 20% to 40% of patients (5,18). Often, a small amount of the inferior arch of C1 is removed to expose the entry point and allow for an appropriate trajectory parallel to the pedicle analogue of C1. This can be performed with a Kerrison rongeur or a small bur. Care should be taken to avoid the VA, which is directly superior to this point in its sulcus. The C2 nerve is retracted caudally, and both the lateral and medial edges of the C1 lateral mass are palpated at the base of the C1 pedicle analogue. A pilot hole using a 2-mm bur is created in the middle of the lateral mass. A 2- to 2.5-mm drill is then used to create the path through the C1 lateral mass. Often, a medial trajectory of 5 to 10 degrees is made in the axial plane, slightly cephalad and aiming toward the lower half of the anterior tubercle of C1 (Figs. 11-6 and 11-7). The trajectory must avoid inadvertent penetration of the occipitocervical joint or cutout of the screw into the C1–C2 joint. These landmarks are clearly seen if image guidance is used, but when relying on lateral fluoroscopy, it is best to aim for the lower 20% to 40% of the height of the anterior tubercle (31). The path of the hole is confirmed on fluoroscopy and then tapped. A partially threaded 3.5- to 4-mm-diameter screw is then inserted, of a length long enough to allow for the polyaxial head to remain dorsal to the C1 ring. Either unicortical or bicortical purchase of the C1 screw can be performed, depending on the location of the ICA (Fig. 11-8). The ICA is in the path of the screw on at least one

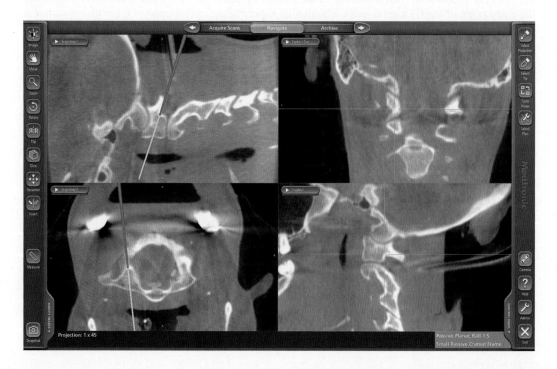

FIGURE 11-6

C1 screw trajectory as seen on the navigation screen.

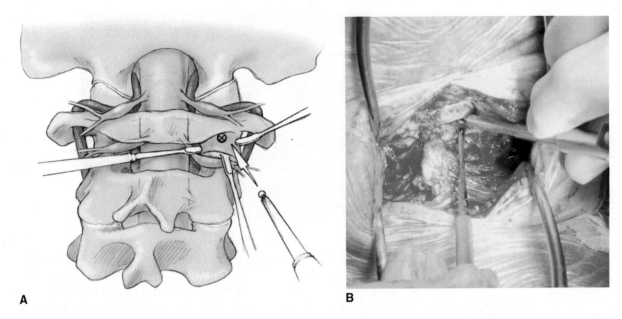

A   **B**

FIGURE 11-7

A,B: The entry point for the C1 screw has to be marked with a small-tipped high-speed bur to avoid slippage of the drill.

side and at high risk of injury in 12% of patients (7). The ICA can also be injured by a drill bit or tap that extends beyond the anterior arch of C1, and therefore, careful preoperative planning is essential (Fig. 11-9). Typically, the exit point of a bicortical lateral mass screw on the anterior arch of C1 is in the same coronal plane as the anterior aspect of the odontoid, which is clearly visible on lateral fluoroscopy. This relationship is best appreciated on an axial CT image at the level of the C1 ring (6).

C2 Pedicle Screw Fixation   First, we typically start by elevating the atlantoaxial membrane that is detached gently from the posterosuperior aspect of the neural arch of C2 to have visual control on the medial wall of the C2 pedicle. The C2 pedicle is generally defined as the portion of the C2 vertebra that is beneath the superior facet and anteromedial to the transverse foramen and connects the vertebral body to the articular process (9). The inferior articular process of C2 is then exposed. The landmark for the entry point of the C2 pedicle screw is the superior medial quadrant of the C2 isthmus (1) (Fig. 11-10). Using a bur, the entry site is marked in the upper medial quadrant of the posterior surface of the inferior articular process. A drill bit is usually used and advanced at low speed in the sagittal plane, trying to hug the medial wall of the pedicle in a slightly cephalad and medial direction. The insertion angle is 20 to 30 degrees cephalad and 20 to 30 degrees medial to the midline in the axial plane. The insertion is done under continuous palpation of the pedicle with a nerve hook. Drilling must be done in an incremental fashion toward the anterior cortex (Fig. 11-11). After drilling the path, a pedicle probe is inserted to palpate the walls of the pilot hole. Tapping is always done, even in osteoporotic bone, because it provides another opportunity to confirm that the walls of the hole have not been breached. The polyaxial screw is then inserted following the same path. Fluoroscopic guidance may be used while drilling, tapping, and inserting the pedicle screw.

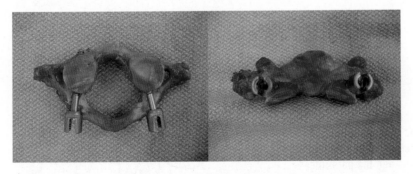

FIGURE 11-8

C1 cadaver bone showing entry points and direction of the C1 lateral mass screw. One screw is unicortical and the other is bicortical.

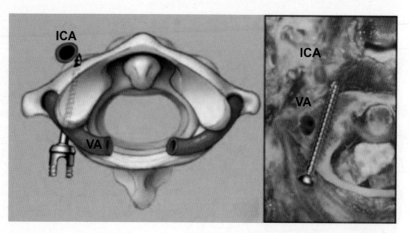

FIGURE 11-9

Axial diagram and axial section from a fresh-frozen cadaveric specimen showing the risk of C1 screw placement relative to the location of the internal carotid artery (ICA) and the vertebral artery (VA). (Adapted from Currier BL, Maus TP, Eck JC, et al.: Relationship of the internal carotid artery to the anterior aspect of the C1 vertebra: implications for C1-C2 transarticular and C1 lateral mass fixation. *Spine (Phila Pa 1976)* 33: 635–639, 2008. Used with permission of Mayo Foundation for Medical Education and Research.)

In some patients, the pedicle may be too small to safely insert a screw because of the location of the VA. In these patients, a shorter pars screw or laminar screw can be chosen.

C2 Pars Screw Fixation   Traditionally, there has been ambiguity in defining the pars interarticularis and pedicle of the C2 vertebra (4). The pars is usually defined as the narrow portion of the C2 vertebra connecting the superior and inferior articular facets (9). The entry point of the C2 pars screw is about 3 mm caudal and 3 mm lateral to the medial border of the pars interarticularis. The entry point is more cranial and medial than the starting point for a pedicle screw.

An appropriate screw entry point, trajectory, and length are determined by preoperative templating. Care must be taken to avoid injury to an atypical high-riding VA. Typically, the screws are angled 10 to 15 degrees medially and 35 degrees superiorly to avoid injury to the VA. These

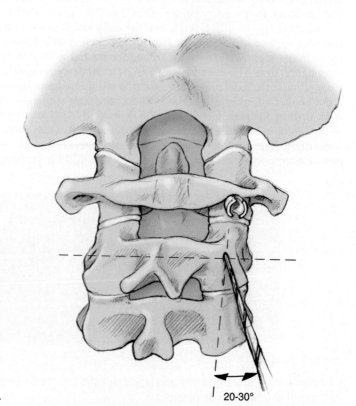

FIGURE 11-10

The correct starting point of the C2 screw is defined roughly as the intersection of the midlines of the lamina and the pars interarticularis. Some surgeons prefer to make the starting point slightly more in the upper, inner quadrant.

20-30°

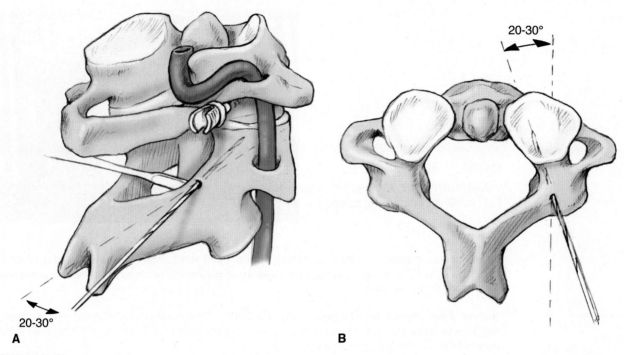

FIGURE 11-11

A,B: C2 screw trajectory is approximately 20 to 30 degrees cephalad. In the transverse direction, the orientation is also approximately 20 to 30 degrees convergent.

screws can be inserted under fluoroscopic guidance and may be used to salvage failed pedicle screws. In approximately 20% of patients, the patient's anatomy precludes insertion of a pedicle screw (2).

C2 Translaminar Screw Fixation   This technique was first described by Wright in 2004 (29). It avoids the risk of VA injury and is a good backup technique in patients with aberrant VA anatomy or after a failed pars or pedicle screw attempt. Using a high-speed bur, the entry point is marked on the junction of the posterior spinous process and lamina. The screws should be directed so the lamina can accommodate one screw on each side. A preoperative CT scan is helpful to template the screw length and width. A drill bit on a handle can be used like an awl to enter and follow the axis of the lamina. A nerve hook can be inserted on the anterior aspect of the lamina to predict the thickness of the bone and to avoid a breach in the anterior cortex of the lamina. Usually, a 20- to 30-mm screw can be placed after tapping and probing the hole. Biomechanical testing has demonstrated the superiority of lamina to pars screw fixation (8). The tip of the screw can exit from the lamina laterally to achieve bicortical purchase and also confirm that the screw has not violated the anterior aspect of the lamina (17).

Bone Grafting and Decortication   Decortication is done in areas that do not compromise screw fixation to expose bleeding bone and increase the likelihood of fusion. We normally decorticate using a cutting bur after drilling the screw paths since the screw heads can obscure a large area of the cortical bone. After insertion of the screws, we perform the arthrodesis with an autograft from the iliac crest. We prefer a structural piece of iliac crest secured to the C1 and C2 lamina using a wiring technique both to compress the graft to the lamina and to add to the biomechanical rigidity of the construct. Alternatively, an onlay technique of bone grafting without wiring can be used (Figs. 11-12 and 11-13). If the C1 ring is absent, arthrodesis can be accomplished by packing bone directly into the C1–C2 joint after removing cartilage with a curette.

Reduction and Rod Insertion   Rod contouring can be used to reduce a deformity and provide additional security to the bone graft by compressing the graft onto the lamina. Direct manipulation of the C1 and C2 segments can be achieved by manipulating the C1 ring with a Kocher clamp. Alternatively, direct manipulation of the screws can be performed to achieve reduction. Once the reduction has been achieved, the rod is secured to the screws with cap screws, and final tightening is performed. Minor compression or distraction of the screws can be performed, with care taken to prevent coronal deformity. C1–C2 deformities, including cranial settling, can be addressed by placing a graft or spacer into the C1–C2 joint (12). We have no experience with this

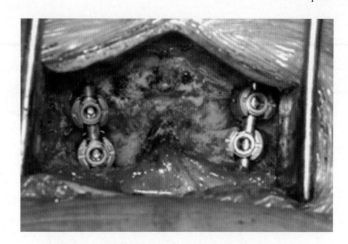

FIGURE 11-12

Intraoperative image showing the final construct with C1–C2 screw-rod fixation.

technique, but it appears to be a promising option. Goel and Laheri (12) have found it necessary to sacrifice the C2 nerve root in the vast majority of patients in order to gain enough exposure to place a spacer in the joint.

Screw Placement in Osteoporotic Patients Polymethyl methacrylate can be used to supplement screw stability when the bone quality is very poor (3,27), although we have no experience with this in the posterior cervical spine.

Closure Closure is performed in multiple layers over a deep drain. It is essential to get good fascial closure; otherwise, persistent drainage and infection are more likely. The fascia is closed with nonresorbable sutures in patients with poor wound-healing potential (those with inflammatory arthritis, postradiation, revisions, trauma, etc.). The subcutaneous tissue and skin are closed in separate layers, and sterile dressings are applied. The patient is generally placed into a rigid cervical orthosis, although some surgeons do not use postoperative immobilization.

Unicortical Versus Bicortical Screw In a study done by Eck et al. (10), a bilateral C1 lateral mass screw was inserted in 15 fresh human cadaveric C1 vertebrae to compare the pullout strength of a unicortical screw versus a bicortical screw. The mean pullout strength of a monocortical screw was 588 N (range, 212 to 1,234 N) compared with 807 N (range, 163 to 1,460 N) for a bicortical screw. This difference was statistically significant ($P = 0.008$). However, previous studies showed a mean pullout of 350 N for subaxial bicortical lateral mass screws (14), meaning that 11 of the 15 unicortical C1 screws exceeded the 350 N needed for pullout in the subaxial spine. For this reason, we recommend bicortical screws in osteoporotic patients or highly unstable conditions unless the ICA is at risk; otherwise, we typically use unicortical screws.

POSTOPERATIVE MANAGEMENT

A hard cervical collar is applied immediately after surgery and is usually kept in place for 6 weeks to 3 months, depending on the quality of fixation at the time of surgery and anticipated

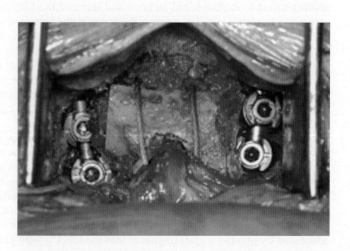

FIGURE 11-13

Intraoperative image showing the final construct with C1–C2 screw-rod fixation supplemented with a structural bone graft fixed with cables to add extra stability.

patient compliance. Drains are removed once output is less than 50 mL in an 8-hour period, typically on postoperative day 1 or 2. Postoperative antibiotic prophylaxis is given for 24 hours. The patient is encouraged to ambulate on the day after surgery, and the bladder catheter is removed as soon as the patient is walking. Typically, the patient is discharged on postoperative day 2 or 3. Upright anteroposterior and lateral radiographs are ordered before discharge. Follow-up is performed at 3 to 6 weeks postoperatively and then at 3, 6, 12, and 24 months after surgery.

COMPLICATIONS

Vertebral Artery Injury

The course of the VA through the lateral mass of the axis can be asymmetric in approximately 50% of patients, making it vulnerable to injury (20). Transarticular screws may be used to augment C1–C2 fusions in place of the Harms screw-rod technique in many patients. When there is fixed anterior subluxation of C1 relative to C2, however, transarticular screws pose an increased risk of VA injury (24). Rates of VA injury during C1 lateral mass screw placement range from 0% to 5.8% (23,30). As described previously, if a C1 posterior arch screw is intended, careful preoperative planning with a CT is required to avoid VA injury, especially when a ponticulus posticus is present (15). If the VA is injured, the bleeding may be controlled by placing the screw on that side. The screw should not be so long that it reaches the VA groove.

If a screw has not already been placed on the opposite side, it is best to avoid placing instrumentation on the contralateral side risking bilateral injury, with the possibility of stroke and death. Prompt angiographic evaluation is done postoperatively.

ICA Injury

The ICA is at risk for early or late life-threatening hemorrhage and stroke if a drill bit or bicortical screw exits the anterior aspect of the C1 lateral mass. In a radiographic study (6), 58% of patients were at moderate risk of ICA injury (due to the proximity of the artery relative to the anterior arch of C1), and 12% were at high risk, on at least one side. A greater margin of safety is provided for the ICA when the screw is angled medially relative to the axis of C1. However, some patients are at risk regardless of screw trajectory because the ICA can be tortuous and its location quite variable. Therefore, a preoperative CT scan with contrast medium is recommended before placing a screw into C1. The anterior tubercle of C1 can be used as a fluoroscopic guide during screw placement, but the surgeon must understand the anteroposterior relationship of the lateral mass of C1 relative to the tubercle. The surgeon can estimate the appropriate screw dimensions on the basis of the shape of the anterior arch of C1 in the axial plane and the location of the ICA and VA.

Other Complications

Other complications include infection, bleeding, pseudoarthrosis, paresthesia (typically in the distribution of the greater occipital nerve), adjacent level disease, pain, and medical and anesthetic complications.

RESULTS AND OUTCOME

Melcher et al. (22) conducted biomechanical testing on cadaveric cervical spine specimens and demonstrated that transarticular screws and screw-rod constructs had equivalent biomechanical properties. In addition, these constructs showed superior mechanical stability when compared with wiring. Table 11-1 outlines some of the advantages and disadvantages of each of the different C1–C2 fixation techniques.

The fusion rates of C1–C2 screw-rod constructs are usually equivalent to transarticular screw fixation and higher than wiring techniques. In their original report in 2001, Harms and Melcher (13) reported on 37 patients with a C1–C2 screw-rod construct where the fusion rate was 100% on clinical and radiologic follow-up. Only one deep wound infection was reported, and one death following pneumonia occurred. No neurovascular compromise was noted in this series. Another study done by Lee et al. (19) in 2010 compared two groups: group 1 consisting of 28 patients treated by C1–C2 transarticular fixation to group 2 consisting of 27 patients treated by C1–C2 screw-rod construct with a minimum follow-up of 2 years. At 1 year of follow-up, group 1 showed 82% fusion rates compared with 96% in group 2 ($P < 0.092$).

TABLE 11-1   Comparison of C1–C2 Instrumentation Techniques

Technique Source	Description	Advantages	Disadvantages	Risks
Gallie (11)	C1–C2 wiring	Very easy No need for special instrumentation Low cost	Cannot be done if posterior arch is deficient Low biomechanical stability	Dural tears Fracture of posterior arches
Magerl and Seeman (21)	C1–C2 transarticular fixation	Biomechanically stable	Cannot reduce C1–C2 joint Difficult technique Difficult positioning and trajectory in obese patients and patients with increased thoracic kyphosis	VA injury ICA injury Hypoglossal nerve injury
Goel and Laheri (12)	C1–C2 posterior plating	Can reduce the joint Biomechanically stable Lack of reliance on posterior arch Theoretically safer than Magerl and Seeman (21) Possibility of connection to adjacent constructs Can be used as temporary stabilization in trauma cases	Screw placement is constrained by hole spacing in the plate. More difficult to extend to additional levels with plates	VA injury ICA injury Hypoglossal nerve injury
Harms and Melcher (13)	C1–C2 screw-rod construct	Can reduce the joint Biomechanically stable Lack of reliance on posterior arch Theoretically safer than Magerl and Seeman (21) Possibility of connection to adjacent constructs Can be used as temporary stabilization in trauma cases	Difficult technique	Vertebral artery injury ICA injury Hypoglossal nerve injury

CONCLUSION

C1–C2 screw and rod fixation is a useful technique for the treatment of C1–C2 instability due to multiple pathologic conditions and has the advantage of increased stability and fusion rates compared with wiring techniques, without the need for halo-vest immobilization. It also has the advantage of being independent of patient anatomic factors that can limit the application of transarticular screw fixation. It also can be applied even with aberrant VA anatomy. Careful planning and meticulous execution of this technique often lead to excellent results, with minimal morbidity to the patient.

RECOMMENDED READING

1. Abumi K, Kaneda K, Shono Y, et al.: One-stage posterior decompression and reconstruction of the cervical spine by using pedicle screw fixation systems. *J Neurosurg* 90: 19–26, 1999.
2. Aryan HE, Newman CB, Nottmeier EW, et al.: Stabilization of the atlantoaxial complex via C-1 lateral mass and C-2 pedicle screw fixation in a multicenter clinical experience in 102 patients: modification of the Harms and Goel techniques. *J Neurosurg Spine* 8: 222–229, 2008.
3. Awasthi D, Voorhies RM: Posterior cervical fusion with methylmethacrylate, wire, and bone: technical note. *Surg Neurol* 42: 259–264, 1994.
4. Benzel EC: Anatomic consideration of C2 pedicle screw placement. *Spine (Phila Pa 1976)* 21: 2301–2302, 1996.
5. Christensen DM, Eastlack RK, Lynch JJ, et al.: C1 anatomy and dimensions relative to lateral mass screw placement. *Spine (Phila Pa 1976)* 32: 844–848, 2007.

6. Currier BL, Maus TP, Eck JC, et al.: Relationship of the internal carotid artery to the anterior aspect of the C1 vertebra: implications for C1-C2 transarticular and C1 lateral mass fixation. *Spine (Phila Pa 1976)* 33: 635–639, 2008.

7. Currier BL, Todd LT, Maus TP, et al.: Anatomic relationship of the internal carotid artery to the C1 vertebra: a case report of cervical reconstruction for chordoma and pilot study to assess the risk of screw fixation of the atlas. *Spine (Phila Pa 1976)* 28: E461–E467, 2003.

8. Dmitriev AE, Lehman RA Jr, Helgeson MD, et al.: Acute and long-term stability of atlantoaxial fixation methods: a biomechanical comparison of pars, pedicle, and intralaminar fixation in an intact and odontoid fracture model. *Spine (Phila Pa 1976)* 34: 365–370, 2009.

9. Ebraheim NA, Fow J, Xu R, et al.: The location of the pedicle and pars interarticularis in the axis. *Spine (Phila Pa 1976)* 26: E34–E37, 2001.

10. Eck JC, Walker MP, Currier BL, et al.: Biomechanical comparison of unicortical versus bicortical C1 lateral mass screw fixation. *J Spinal Disord Tech* 20: 505–508, 2007.

11. Gallie WE: Fractures and dislocations of the cervical spine. *Am J Surg* 46: 495–499, 1939.

12. Goel A, Laheri V: Plate and screw fixation for atlanto-axial subluxation. *Acta Neurochir (Wien)* 129: 47–53, 1994.

13. Harms J, Melcher RP: Posterior C1-C2 fusion with polyaxial screw and rod fixation. *Spine (Phila Pa 1976)* 26: 2467–2471, 2001.

14. Heller JG, Estes BT, Zaouali M, et al.: Biomechanical study of screws in the lateral masses: variables affecting pull-out resistance. *J Bone Joint Surg Am* 78: 1315–1321, 1996.

15. Hong JT, Lee SW, Son BC, et al.: Analysis of anatomical variations of bone and vascular structures around the posterior atlantal arch using three-dimensional computed tomography angiography. *J Neurosurg Spine* 8: 230–236, 2008.

16. Hong X, Dong Y, Yunbing C, et al.: Posterior screw placement on the lateral mass of atlas: an anatomic study. *Spine (Phila Pa 1976)* 29: 500–503, 2004.

17. Jea A, Sheth RN, Vanni S, et al.: Modification of Wright's technique for placement of bilateral crossing C2 translaminar screws: technical note. *Spine J* 8: 656–660, 2008.

18. Lee MJ, Cassinelli E, Riew KD: The feasibility of inserting atlas lateral mass screws via the posterior arch. *Spine (Phila Pa 1976)* 31: 2798–2801, 2006.

19. Lee SH, Kim ES, Sung JK, et al.: Clinical and radiological comparison of treatment of atlantoaxial instability by posterior C1-C2 transarticular screw fixation or C1 lateral mass-C2 pedicle screw fixation. *J Clin Neurosci* 17: 886–892, 2010.

20. Madawi AA, Casey AT, Solanki GA, et al.: Radiological and anatomical evaluation of the atlantoaxial transarticular screw fixation technique. *J Neurosurg* 86: 961–968, 1997.

21. Magerl F, Seeman PS: Stable posterior fusion at the atlas and axis by transarticular screw fixation. In: Kehr P, Weiner A, eds. *Cervical spine.* New York: Springer-Verlag, 1987: 327–332.

22. Melcher RP, Puttlitz CM, Kleinstueck FS, et al.: Biomechanical testing of posterior atlantoaxial fixation techniques. *Spine (Phila Pa 1976)* 27: 2435–2440, 2002.

23. Neo M, Fujibayashi S, Miyata M, et al.: Vertebral artery injury during cervical spine surgery: a survey of more than 5600 operations. *Spine (Phila Pa 1976)* 33: 779–785, 2008.

24. Paramore CG, Dickman CA, Sonntag VK: The anatomical suitability of the C1-2 complex for transarticular screw fixation. *J Neurosurg* 85: 221–224, 1996.

25. Reilly TM, Sasso RC, Hall PV: Atlantoaxial stabilization: clinical comparison of posterior cervical wiring technique with transarticular screw fixation. *J Spinal Disord Tech* 16: 248–253, 2003.

26. Rushton SA, Vaccaro AR, Levine MJ, et al.: Bivector traction for unstable cervical spine fractures: a description of its application and preliminary results. *J Spinal Disord* 10: 436–440, 1997.

27. Stambough JL, Balderston RA, Grey S: Technique for occipito-cervical fusion in osteopenic patients. *J Spinal Disord* 3: 404–407, 1990.

28. White AA III, Panjabi MM: The clinical biomechanics of the occipitoatlantoaxial complex. *Orthop Clin North Am* 9: 867–878, 1978.

29. Wright NM: Posterior C2 fixation using bilateral, crossing C2 laminar screws: case series and technical note. *J Spinal Disord Tech* 17: 158–162, 2004.

30. Yeom JS, Buchowski JM, Park KW, et al.: Undetected vertebral artery groove and foramen violations during C1 lateral mass and C2 pedicle screw placement. *Spine (Phila Pa 1976)* 33: E942–E949, 2008.

31. Yeom JS, Buchowski JM, Park KW, et al.: Lateral fluoroscopic guide to prevent occipitocervical and atlantoaxial joint violation during C1 lateral mass screw placement. *Spine J* 9: 574–579, 2009.

32. Young JP, Young PH, Ackermann MJ, et al.: The ponticulus posticus: implications for screw insertion into the first cervical lateral mass. *J Bone Joint Surg Am* 87: 2495–2498, 2005.

12 Posterior Occipitocervical Fusion

Mathias Daniels, Zachary Child, Jens R. Chapman, and Carlo Bellabarba

INDICATIONS

Occipitocervical fusion with or without neural element decompression is usually used to definitively treat craniocervical instability or deformity-related conditions. Typical indications for this procedure include patients afflicted by trauma, inflammatory disease processes, deformity, neoplasia, and more rarely infections, degenerative diseases, and congenital dysplasia (21).

Untreated instability or displacement of the craniocervical junction can result in a variety of sequelae ranging from progressive pain and neurologic dysfunction to death. Instability of the craniocervical joints in the setting of trauma is usually manifested by any translation or distraction of more than 1 mm in any plane, presence of neurologic injury, or concomitant cerebrovascular trauma (4). With respect to trauma, any injury to the atlantoaxial articulation should be evaluated for its effect on the stability of the craniocervical junction. It is important to remember that in instances of traumatic craniocervical instability, the static position of the head relative to the cervical spine is usually arbitrary and is more dependent on external forces than on any intrinsic injury characteristic. In patients with nontraumatic cranial settling or deformity, such as atlantoaxial dislocation or kyphosis, brainstem or spinal cord compression may lead to respiratory compromise, cranial nerve deficits, paresis, paralysis, and even sudden death.

GENERAL TECHNIQUE

The goal of this type of surgery is to provide permanent immobilization of the craniocervical junction and—as needed—adjacent spine segments, in a functionally useful, preferably balanced anatomic alignment. This desired result is preferably gained through a firm osseous fusion accomplished through structural bone graft in combination with morselized graft. Implants take the secondary role of securing the best possible craniocervical alignment while optimizing chances for successful osseous fusion. In this era of advanced implant fixation systems, the goal of achieving a solid fusion remains paramount to any device design, and thus, suitable attention should be placed on allowing for this important biologic healing process to take place (26). Our preferred internal fixation consists of segmental instrumentation via a rod/screw/plate construct and often involves the use of cables or wires in a supplemental fashion to secure structural bone graft that bridges the occipitocervical junction. Temporary postoperative immobilization can be supplied through a variety of modalities befitting the patient needs and range from a soft neck collar to rigid neck collars or halo-vest constructs. For very young skeletally immature patients requiring craniocervical fusion, structural bone graft alone with cables and supplemental halo-vest fixation may be sufficient.

The posterior midline approach is by far the most commonly used surgical approach to treat most craniocervical disorders. A straightforward midline exposure usually provides predictable exposure of familiar posterior anatomic landmarks and can easily be extended to an extensile approach of the lower cervical spine or the upper thoracic spine, if needed (Fig. 12-1). This

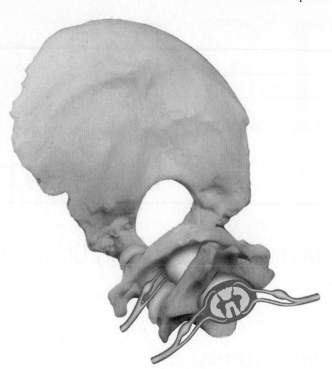

FIGURE 12-1

Posterior craniocervical exposure. For successful instrumentation of the craniocervical junction, it is critical to have a clear understanding of the complex neurovascular anatomy of this region. Anatomic norm variants and a variety of pathologic conditions can make these procedures especially challenging. Having an adequate exposure of the posterior bony structures is a first important step toward successful procedure completion.

exposure allows for posterior decompression of neural structures as well as placement of bone grafting and rigid posterior segmental fixation while it also minimizes long-term exposure-related morbidity. Indirect decompression of anterior compressive lesions caused by nonrigid upper cervical spine kyphosis can usually be gained through traction and subsequent posterior-only decompression and instrumented fusion surgery. Some anterior compressive lesions, such as retrodental pannus formation associated with atlantoaxial instability in inflammatory diseases, may also be expected to resorb with a solid posteriorly based fusion. Anterior surgery may be performed through transoral and anterolateral or direct upper neck exposures. Indications for these include fixed upper cervical deformities in need of deformity correction, neoplasia, and rarely patients with space-occupying lesions brought on by inflammatory conditions (22). Finally, so-called minimally invasive posterior stabilizing procedures relying largely on interarticular screw fixations have been described but have failed to attain greater popularity. All of these variants of craniocervical spine surgery are very limited in their indication range compared to the posterior midline approach and are highly case specific. Undoubtedly, the posterior open technique allows for superior biomechanical stabilization and controlled realignment while affording a high incidence of fusion.

PREOPERATIVE PREPARATION

As in any surgical undertaking, careful understanding of the patient anatomy and pathophysiology is an important prerequisite for a successful procedure. The craniocervical junction encompasses a confluence of multiple vital structures, which require appropriate imaging modalities for preoperative surgical planning. In addition to anteroposterior and lateral plain radiographs, it is helpful to have advanced imaging in the form of computed tomography (CT) scan and/or magnetic resonance imaging (MRI) available for comprehensive preoperative assessment as medically indicated (25). Perfusion studies, such as MR angiography (MRA) or CT angiography, may be indicated for patients with suspected vertebral artery trauma or in case of suspected vascular abnormalities (Figs. 12-2 and 12-3).

Anteroposterior and lateral radiographs are useful in assessing global sagittal and coronal alignment, as well as a number of craniocervical reference lines to measure cranial settling and instability (Harris lines, Power ratio, Wackenheim line). Ideally, a true lateral radiograph centered on the craniocervical junction is available as a valuable reference tool (20). Some understanding of preferred craniocervical alignment of the patient about to undergo permanent fusion of this articulation is helpful in order to minimize the risk of functional impairment or secondary compensatory spinal deformity. Calculation of an occipitocervical slope angle and/or occipitocervical incidence may help guide alignment determination in the future (16) (Fig. 12-4).

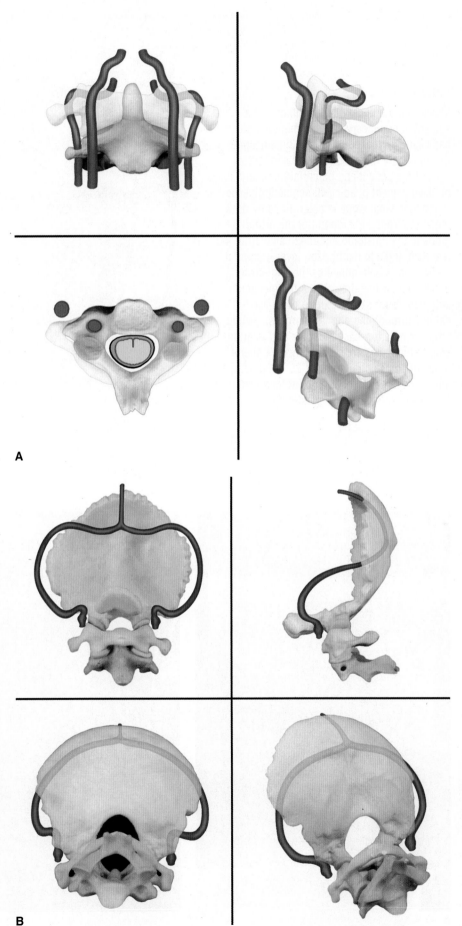

FIGURE 12-2

A,B: Hardware placement. Craniocervical instrumentation fixation has to be mindful of the vascular anatomy. The occipital and the upper cervical spine both require a specific understanding of their specific anatomy.

A: In the upper cervical spine, the arterial anatomy, especially regarding the vertebral and the internal carotid arteries, is critical. Should there be a suspicion for unusual anatomic circumstances, dedicated preoperative vascular studies may help in understanding and surgical execution.

B: For occipital part of segmental instrumentation, the location of the large venous system such as represented in the transverse venous sinus and the sagittal sinus is an important consideration. As represented in this diagram, the transverse sinus follows a lateral trajectory at the level of the inion.

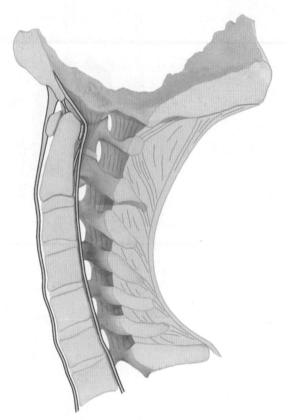

FIGURE 12-3

Measuring craniocervical alignment. The subject of craniocervical alignment angles has been overlooked for a long time despite its significant impact on overall sagittal balance of the patient and potential implications on development of adjacent segment disease. Occipitocervical slope is determined by drawing a line from the midpoint of the orbital globe to the opisthion and then calculating the resultant angle to the horizon level. Occipital inclination is determined as the angle from a perpendicular line drawn from the maximum anteroposterior skull excursion to a vertical line through the odontoid process. While larger population-based studies and relationship to outcomes are still elusive, a general range of an occipital slope of 20 to 30 degrees and an occipital inclination of 30 degrees (±5 degrees) has been suggested (19).

FIGURE 12-4

Trauma indication.
A: This is the lateral C-spine radiograph and a midline sagittal CT reformat of an 18-year-old female victim of a high-velocity car crash. She had a Glasgow Coma Score (GCS) of 13 and an ASIA motor score of 100 but complained of excruciating neck pain. The patient was placed in a halo vest for treatment of a presumed type 2 odontoid fracture. The patient continued to complain of considerable neck pain when being mobilized despite presence of the halo vest.

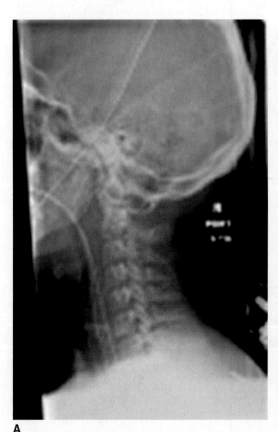

A

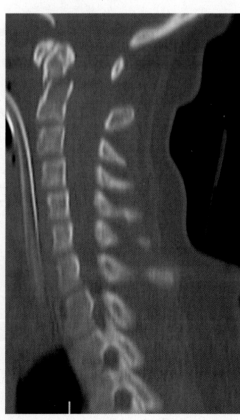

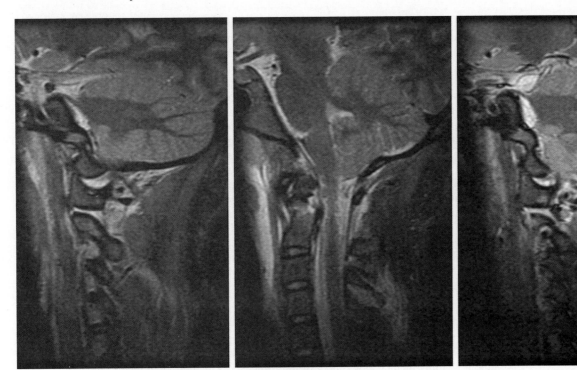

B

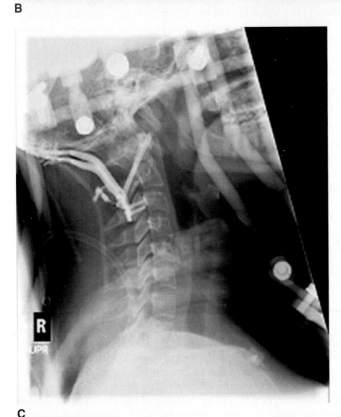

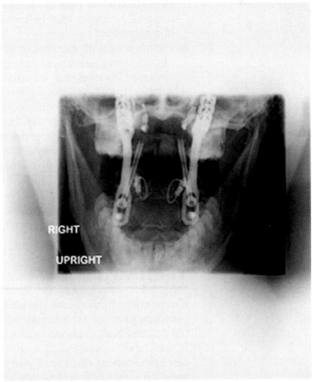

C

FIGURE 12-4 *(Continued)*

B: Due to subtle occipitocervical gapping in the parasagittal CT reformats, MRI scanning was ordered. These T2-weighted images showed clear bilateral disruption of the occipitocervical articulations. **C:** The patient experienced remarkable almost immediate pain relief following segmental instrumentation and arthrodesis as shown on the postoperative lateral and open-mouth odontoid views. The halo vest was left in place for 6 weeks after surgery as it had been put in place already. Modern segmental fixation frequently does not require more than a collar for successful fusion. The patient returned to a normal lifestyle.

CT imaging with reformatted views in sagittal and coronal planes allows for detailed assessment of bony architecture in preparation for hardware placement. This is of particular importance toward better understanding of vertebral artery anatomy, which can be quite variable. Other anatomic norm variants, such as failures of segmentation or formation in the craniocervical junction, should be assessed on CT. Finally, important insights that can be gained from preoperative CT analysis, for instance, include occipital skull thickness, the presence of associated skull and cervical segment fractures, as well as bone quality and spinal morphology in general (14).

MRI is helpful in identifying medullary signal changes in brainstem and cord, demonstrating space-occupying lesions in the neural canal and assessing for integrity of craniocervical ligaments and fluid signals in the major articulations of this critical and vulnerable transition region.

Mechanical stability of the craniocervical junction is a result of a combination of osseous, ligamentous, and muscular restraints that permit a significant degree of motion in multiple planes (7,21). For patients with questionable stability, fluoroscopically guided traction tests have been helpful adjuvants in decision making. This form of dynamic imaging has proven to be safe in our hands and can convincingly confirm either instability or ligamentous integrity (4).

For a variety of conditions, it can be very important to establish integrity of cerebral blood flow. This is probably best established with CT angiography; however, MRA can be a suitable alternative (10). In cases of flow impairment, it may be helpful to obtain cerebral Doppler monitoring to look for ongoing perfusion problems.

EXAMINATION PEARLS

- Preoperative clinical examinations of patients with suspected craniocervical abnormalities if possible preferably include assessment of long-tract signs, pathologic reflexes, and cranial nerve function 2 to 12 bilaterally in addition to the usual systematic motor, sensory, and reflex assessment. Exorbitant pain in the skull base region may indicate trauma and/or instability. Greater occipital neuralgia may be pathognomonic for chronic atlantoaxial derangement and C2 root impingement.
- Craniocervical dissociation or severe rotatory subluxation (types III or IV) should heighten the suspicion for presence of a vertebral artery injury. Fractures of the transverse foramen, especially displaced fractures, may be other tip-offs for potential vertebral artery injuries (10).
- Anterior fractures of the occipital condyles deserve scrutiny, and the potential for craniocervical dissociation should be considered (2). If in doubt, a manual fluoroscopic traction test can be performed to document stability. Presence of bilateral occipital condyle fractures invariably implies an unstable occipitocervical dissociation.
- Radiographic signs of transverse alar ligament (TAL) instability include widening of the lateral masses and bony avulsion injuries of the atlas. The TAL is considered to be the primary stabilizer of the atlantoaxial articulation.
- A preoperative/intraoperative fluoroscopic manual traction test can confirm ligamentous disruption and document cervicocranial instability.
- Preoperative CT angiography and/or MRA is recommended preoperatively for suspected vertebral artery injuries.

TECHNIQUE

Preoperative Preparation: Instability or derangement of the craniocervical junction places its neurovascular structures at risk with potential for catastrophic outcome due to a lack of substantial primary bony craniocervical stabilizers. For severe craniocervical trauma, initial stabilization is preferably accomplished with sandsacks surrounding the head with tape placed transversely across the patient's forehead. Alternatively, a primary halo-vest assembly can be considered as a temporary immobilizer. Traction is not desirable in this setting. Neither of the mentioned external immobilization options is particularly functional beyond a relatively brief temporizing period, thus placing an imperative on early definitive surgical intervention (5). For elective conditions such as craniocervical settling seen with inflammatory conditions, thought may be given to preoperative skeletal traction, usually applied through a halo ring over a course of several days, with the goal to facilitate a gradual deformity reduction over several days. Such a deformity reduction through skeletal traction is preferably accompanied by serial lateral C-spine radiographs and clinical evaluations.

Prior to actual surgery, it is important to establish a safe airway, avoiding excessive manipulation of the patient's neck prior embarking on surgery in cases of instability or major deformity. For those patients, a safe endotracheal airway can be established through awake fiberoptic or nasal intubation techniques while maintaining full spine precautions with the patient positioned prone on a radiolucent table. Baseline electrophysiologic monitoring with somatosensory evoked potentials and motor evoked potentials is completed prior to prone positioning and repeated after final positioning. Final craniocervical fine adjustment is performed under fluoroscopy shortly after turning the patient prone to assure the best possible closed reduction prior to embarking on surgery. For trauma cases, the surgeons might consider the threat of craniocervical distraction by excessive reverse Trendelenburg positioning.

Surgical Technique: The suboccipital region is prepared with an electric razor to 1 cm above the inion. Durable tape is then used to depress both shoulders to facilitate intraoperative lateral fluoroscopic visualization from the inion to the cervicothoracic junction. Depending on body habitus, tape can be helpful to retract redundant skin overlying the posterior cervical spine. Surgical exposure is gained through sharp electrocautery-aided dissection of the midline internervous plane between left and right paraspinal muscles. We make every effort to preserve the interspinous ligament anatomy emanating from the C2 spinous process to the more caudal spinous processes. Care should be taken to avoid the greater occipital nerve and terminal branches of the third occipital nerve, which are present in the fascial plane. Subperiosteal dissection is continued along the spinous processes, lamina, and facets of C1, C2, C3, as well as other lower cervical spine levels as indicated clinically. Care should be taken during dissection of the C1 arch, as the vertebral artery can be as close as 1.5 cm lateral to the midline before it penetrates the posterior atlantooccipital membrane. Dissection of the C1–C2 posterior facet is very helpful in establishing anatomic landmarks and can also help in gaining access to prepare an atlantooccipital facet arthrodesis. Dense venous plexus bleeding is to be anticipated during this portion of the dissection but can often be minimized with bipolar cauterization dissection. We prefer dissecting the C2 root bilaterally and do not routinely sacrifice this root for purposes of atlantal lateral mass hardware placement.

Decompression of neural elements is case dependent. For patients with space-occupying lesions in either the anterior or posterior extradural space, we usually have a very low threshold to perform a C1 laminectomy and a limited suboccipital decompression as well as laminotomy of the rostral edge of C2. If at all possible, we attempt to preserve a portion of the C2 lamina and its spinous process to allow for a stable caudal bony landing site for a craniocervical bone graft.

Our preferred method of cervical fixation consists of secure segmental instrumentation of the C1 lateral mass and C2 with pedicle screws, pars, or translaminar screws depending upon best available bony trajectories and bone quality. Transarticular atlantoaxial screws offer excellent bone purchase and were the previous preferred method at our institution but can be more challenging to perform and are clearly less versatile (13,27). It is encouraging to know that all these mentioned screw placement methods have shown comparable rates of biomechanical in vivo stiffness and placement accuracy in clinical series (6,17). When selecting a starting point for a C1 lateral mass screw, the surgeon should be mindful of posterior arch osseous anatomy, avoiding pitfalls such as a ponticulus posticus (posterior bone bridge over the vertebral artery) (29). If indicated, caudal extension of the construct to the subaxial C-spine and beyond is readily possible.

Prior to placement of occipital fixation, we suggest preparing for the posterior arthrodesis by selecting a suitable occipital graft landing site. It may be helpful to template a variety of occipital fixation options such as longitudinal rod plates or transverse midline crossing plates to find an optimal spatial compromise between graft and hardware in this limited space. Placement of a quality structural graft to bridge the occiput to the upper cervical spine is key to the ultimate goal of achieving a solid fusion—with the posterior arch of C2 serving as a valuable base for the structural graft (26). For this purpose, we recommend placing two small burr holes on either side of the midline about 1 cm superior to the foramen magnum. This allows for passage of a cable on either side, which can then be used to secure the occipital graft firmly against the occipital host site (26).

Fixation of the implant construct to the occiput is completed with three or four 3.5 cortical screws with bicortical purchase. Usually, midline fixation offers much better screw purchase compared to screws placed more laterally (9,12,14). Many manufacturers offer a plate construct to secure occipital screw fixation. This dictates screw fixation points to some degree but may offer biomechanical advantages if locking screws are available (9). While certainly not desirable, incidental cerebrospinal fluid leak following drilling of the occiput can be usually directly stopped by screw placement. Drilling of screw holes at or above the level of the inion is not desirable due to likely subsequent external hardware prominence and possible injury to the transverse sinus, the latter with potentially fatal consequences to the patient. A structural corticocancellous bone graft is then fashioned into a clothespin shape that can straddle the C2 spinous process and cradles the posterior occipital bulge. After decortication of the recipient bed with a high-speed burr, this clothespin-shaped structural graft is then secured to the occiput with the previously placed cables via drill holes in the graft.

Compression of the structural graft to the upper cervical spine can be accomplished with a C2 spinous process cable, sublaminar C2 cable, or cable looping the cervical component of the rod fixation. We usually will fill any gaps between posterior bony elements and the structural graft with morselized cancellous bone.

SURGICAL PEARLS

- Place the patient in not more than a slightly reversed Trendelenburg position to aid in venous outflow during surgery and minimize blood loss.
- Preoperative assessment of physiologic or otherwise desirable craniocervical angle. Transparent drapes can be used to better assess the angle clinically. Definitive normative data remain sparse, but an occipital slope of approximately 20 to 30 degrees or an occipital incidence of approximately 30 degrees (±5 degrees) has been described as normal (16). If needed, it is probably better to err toward a more downward craniocervical angle to assist the patient with an extensive occipitocervical fusion with their horizontal gaze and ground control rather than creating a hyperextended posture. Hyperextension also places the patient at a higher risk of neural element compression, while hyperflexion invites anterior subluxation of the craniocervical junction by moving the overall cranial center of gravity forward (3,19) (Fig. 12-4).
- Meticulous attention to bone grafting technique. Leave a portion of spinous process with 50% of the C2 arch intact—if possible—to allow for attachment of a structural corticocancellous bone graft and aid in fusion. Create direct compression of the structural bone graft to the occiput with transoccipital cable fixation (26).
- Consider delaying extubation after extensive upper cervical stabilization to avoid complications of airway swelling, depressed gag reflex, and airway control in the immediate postoperative period. Emergent reintubation is a possible complication of upper cervical surgery especially multilevel combined anterior and posterior approaches (3,24).
- Rigid fixation of the craniocervical junction with two separate parasagittal plates or cervical rods improves rotational stability compared to a single midline or "Y-plate" and aids in bone grafting (1,23).
- Consider placement of upper cervical spine hardware unilaterally before addressing the contralateral side as a precaution or if vertebral artery injury is suspected. Use of intraoperative Doppler ultrasound performed above the C1 arch can aid in diagnosis of an unrecognized vascular injury of the vertebral artery at C2 or below.
- Obtain a CT postoperatively if clinically indicated. This can be reassuring in identifying spatial alignment and quality of hardware placement.
- Insist on centered true lateral preoperative imaging to minimize risk of missing craniocervical derangement and to allow for referencing of intraoperative alignment changes. Reference points such as overlapping occipital condyles, C2 interarticular pedicles, and C1 lamina may help in hardware placement and determination of alignment intraoperatively.

POSTOPERATIVE MANAGEMENT

Patients undergoing craniocervical arthrodesis, as in other complex and combined upper cervical procedures, are at an increased risk for postoperative airway swelling and loss of the protective gag reflex. Premature extubation and airway obstruction from swelling can necessitate emergent reintubation with adjuvant risks. At our institution, we usually keep patients with craniocervical fusion surgery intubated until the day after surgery when the patient has been formally assessed for airway competence (24). However, airway swelling likely has peaked prior to a 72-hour postoperative time point. Keeping the patient head elevated at least 30 degrees aids in reducing soft tissue swelling of the head-neck region and will minimize the aspiration risk when there is an expected temporary diminution of the physiologic gag reflex due to retropharyngeal swelling.

Early mobilization in a cervical orthosis (Miami J, Philadelphia collar) provides adequate external support if the internal fixation is considered sufficiently strong. Infrequently, a halo can be employed for supplemental immobilization for select patients with facial fractures, multilevel cervical spine injuries, poor bone quality, or uncertain quality of the internal fixation construct (5). A cervical orthosis is usually continued for 2 to 3 months postoperatively. Flexion/extension, open-mouth odontoid, and, if necessary, traction radiographs can document stability of the upper cervical and craniocervical junction (Fig. 12-5).

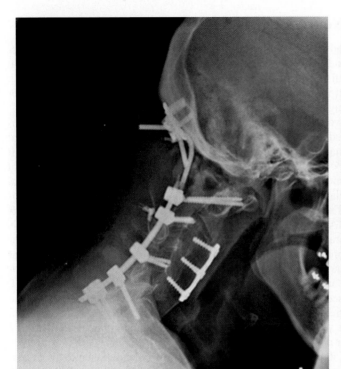
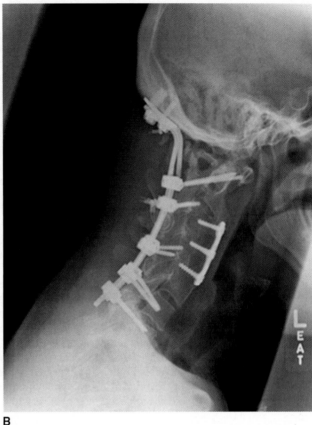

A   **B**

FIGURE 12-5

Nonunion. Advanced stable craniocervical instrumentation systems do not compensate for a stable fusion of this highly mobile transition zone. In fact, it could be argued that special attention should be paid toward achieving solid bony arthrodesis as a priority over segmental instrumentation. **A:** This lateral radiograph shows a patient who had received a craniocervical fusion for severe upper cervical cord impingement in presence of spastic cerebral palsy. This wheelchair-bound patient appeared to have a favorable symptom resolution despite an overall forward-tilted posture. **B:** Three years after his instrumentation, the patient returned with painless hardware prominence over his skull. The patient has broken his craniocervical hardware and dissolved a structural allograft due to a nonunion of the craniocervical articulations.

COMPLICATIONS

Complications from craniocervical fusion surgery can be grouped into early perioperative and late outcome-related categories. Beyond this common delineation, there are strongly divergent priorities in outcomes for trauma patients compared to patients with more elective subacute conditions, such as destructive processes involving inflammatory, neoplastic, dysplastic, infectious, or metabolic conditions.

For trauma patients, the main priority is expressed in survival and optimizing chances for recovery of neurologic injury. Injury-specific outcomes and complications of craniocervical dissociation in survivors are dependent on the type and severity of associated injuries (especially closed head injuries), neurologic injury, and the timeliness in which the diagnosis of craniocervical dissociation is made and subsequent treatment is initiated (4,30). It has been shown that early recognition and timely fixation of these injuries improve outcome by protecting against secondary neurologic deterioration. In less obvious cases of craniocervical dissociation the patients own medical comorbidities, adjuvant treatment administered and baseine functional status are felt to affect eventual outcomes. For these patients, preoperative optimization of medical comorbidities and other preparatory efforts such as traction-based realignment, embolization, and staged anterior or anterolateral surgery where indicated are aimed at minimizing perioperative complications while enhancing chances for maintenance of quality of life. However, the magnitude of initial injury and timeliness of treatment are likely the major predictors of eventual disability.

Delay in Diagnosis and Neurologic Decline

Preoperative neurologic injuries and baseline conditions play a paramount role in eventual functional outcomes. For traumatic conditions and other causes of instability, such as craniocervical insufficiency from metabolic or inflammatory etiology, delay in diagnosis may increase the risk of secondary neurologic deterioration. Recovery from manifest spinal cord injury for trauma or nontraumatic conditions has been highly inconsistent and can certainly not be counted upon.

Perhaps the most important and avoidable complication in craniocervical dissociation is the potential for neurologic decline associated with unrecognized injury and unnecessary delays in surgical stabilization. While halo/vest external immobilization is perhaps the best of the orthosis supports, it has been shown to provide overall poor stability in this highly unstable injury (5). It is therefore not recommended as stand-alone treatment (30). In the Harborview series of traumatic craniocervical dissociation, there was a clear correlation with neurologic deterioration associated with missed injuries and delays in treatment. Four of seventeen diagnosed upon evaluation with no decline in American Spinal Injury Association (ASIA) status and 5/13 patients who had a mean delay in diagnosis of 2 days suffered profound deterioration (4). Five patients in this cohort were only diagnosed after neurologic decline was noted and another five caught upon repeat ATLS screening examination at the accepting tertiary hospital. In one case of postoperative decline, a revealed malreduced occipitocervical joint, cerebellar infarction, and hydrocephalus were diagnosed. This construct was revised, the posterior fossa was decompressed, and a ventriculoperitoneal shunt placed with near-complete resolution of the patient's tetraplegia with exception of minor gait abnormalities at last follow-up. No cases of cervical pseudarthrosis were identified in our experience although one case of T1–T2 pseudarthrosis was revised at 1 year postoperative.

Based on the trauma experience, it stands to reason that every effort be undertaken to avoid secondary neurologic deterioration in patients with subacute craniocervical conditions. Recovery of myelopathy may be expected but is dependent upon factors such as age of patient, duration, as well as severity of neurologic symptoms. Overall, it appears that craniocervical reconstructive surgery seems to be affected by a very low incidence of perioperative neurologic decline.

Neurovascular Injury

Penetration of the inner cortex of the skull can lead to injury to neural or vascular structures, notably the vertebral basilar system and venous sinuses via either wires or screws. Use of the occipital "Y-plate" takes advantage of thicker midline bone and therefore longer screws but offers less rotational stability and limits application sites for structural bone graft. It is for this reason that most surgeons favor bilateral plate/rod fixation. Complications of hardware placement in the atlas and axis are described elsewhere in this textbook but include potential for screw malposition resulting in injury to the vertebral artery, spinal cord, hypoglossal nerve, and carotid artery. Placement of atlantoaxial transarticular screws has led to a reported clinical incidence of vertebral artery injury of 0% to 6%, with an associated 0.2% risk of immediate neurologic deficit and estimated 0.1% mortality. In a systematic review performed on over 2,000 patients with craniocervical fusions mainly in case reports, the authors identified a 1.4% to 4.1% incidence of vertebral artery injury mainly associated with transarticular screw fixation (18). In the event of a vertebral artery injury, local hemostasis should be achieved by placing the shorter screw on the affected side, or facilitate local hemostasis by judicious placement of local hemostatic agents and bone wax. Placement of contralateral screws should be deferred until completion of postoperative interventional angiography allows for assessment of basivertebral arterial flow and either embolization or recanalization of the affected side has been accomplished. The use of a pedicle screw at C2 if possible combined with a C1 lateral mass screw carries a lower theoretical risk of vertebral artery injury than the transarticular screw and has a more easily achievable trajectory (11,15,18). This is a viable alternative to transarticular screw fixation when there is an anomalous vertebral artery anatomy or when patient anatomy or positioning interferes with correct screw trajectory. Pars screws are frequently employed in our practice owing to their ease of placement and safety, as are translaminar screws all dependent on local anatomy (6).

Intraoperative internal carotid artery and hypoglossal nerve injury will likely not be noticed intraoperatively. Retropharyngeal soft tissue swelling on a lateral cervical radiograph can lead to the diagnosis if suspected. Angiographically aided embolization following trial occlusion with an intra-arterial balloon can be used to control local hemorrhage. The anterior cortex of the C1 lateral mass lies approximately 7 mm posterior to the anterior most portion of the C1 anterior arch and can be estimated by evaluating a preoperative lateral radiograph and CT axial images of the atlas.

Occipital numbness or dysesthesias are rare but can result from C2 nerve root injury and the posterior atlantal isthmus during posterior C1–C2 facet arthrodesis.

Nonunion/Malunion

Historically, nonunion of craniocervical fusions appeared to be quite common with rates of up to 23% having been reported with nonrigid onlay grafting and fixation using wiring-type techniques. In contrast to a large variety of nonrigid forms of craniocervical instrumentation, the current rigid segmental forms of fixation and grafting detailed in this chapter have resulted in fusion rates approaching 100%. A recent systematic review identified a nonunion rate of about 7% during atlantooccipital fusion (8).

In our trauma series of craniocervical fixation, there were no cases of cervical pseudarthrosis, although one case of T1–T2 pseudarthrosis was revised at 1 year postoperative.

Early hardware failure via screw cutout either in the atlas or of the screw shaft within the pars of the axis is uncommon but not impossible. Patient-specific anatomy such as a very shallow and arcuate isthmus can lead to limited screw purchase within the axis. Similarly, inadequate screw purchase at the anteroinferior edge of the C1 lateral mass can occur if drill trajectory is not sufficiently directed cephalad. Late hardware failure can result from a pseudarthrosis. Revision posterior atlantoaxial fusion, occipitocervical fusion, or anterior atlantoaxial arthrodesis may then be necessary.

A potential technical problem of craniocervical fusion surgery includes malreduction, which, in the Harborview series, resulted in one case of acute neurologic worsening (4). This case was emergently taken back to the operating room for craniocervical realignment, and nearly all symptoms improved. Malreduction in an excessively lordotic position can also lead to functional disability with the patient unable to reference the floor during gait. A compensatory response based on the patient's compulsion to bring their gaze to at least neutral can lead to a lower cervical compensatory kyphosis. Conversely, a kyphotic craniocervical angle can lead to subaxial hyperlordosis or induce anterior subluxation of the craniocervical junction. Craniocervical malreduction can also propagate swallowing dysfunction and can be predicted to some degree by placing a patient into a halo-vest preoperatively (3). In presence of ventral space-occupying lesions, such as a retrodental pannus formation, a flexed craniocervical position will also lead to persistent neural element impingement (Fig. 12-6).

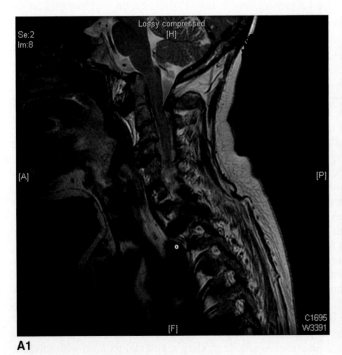

A1

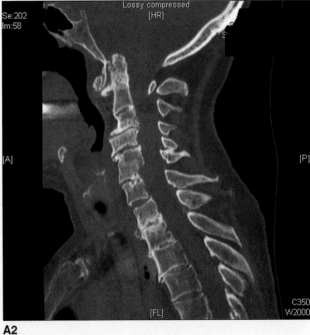

A2

FIGURE 12-6

Inflammatory indication. **A:** These are sagittal CT and T2-weighted MRI images of a 52-year-female with history of juvenile rheumatoid arthritis and substantial skeletal manifestations. Despite these, this patient leads a very active and successful personal and professional life, which was increasingly hampered by severe headaches and occipital pressure sensations with simple activities. Her physical examination showed no signs of myelopathy or focal motor deficits but was limited by joint abnormalities. These images show basivertebral invagination due to progressive destructive atlantoaxial arthropathy.

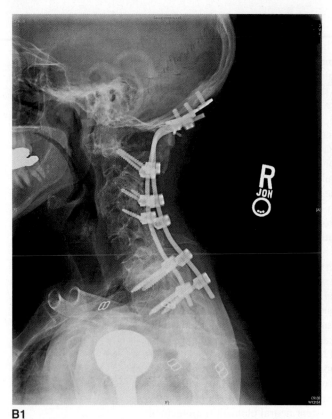

B1

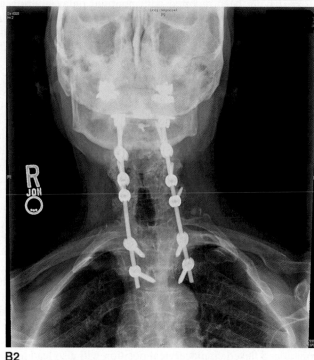

B2

FIGURE 12-6 (*Continued*)

B: Following gradually increasing skeletal traction applied over several days preoperatively, the patient returned to a symptom-free lifestyle following craniocervical instrumentation and successful fusion. Note that the caudal instrumentation was extended to the T2 segment in light of the underlying disease process of the patient.

RESULTS

Regardless of underlying conditions, most result reporting for craniocervical fusion has been limited to perioperative complications and reoperations, neurologic functional recovery, and patient survival (18). Unfortunately, there are almost no health-related quality-of-life data on affected patients living with craniocervical fusion surgery (Fig. 12-7).

For patients with preoperative neurologic compromise, some improvements may be possible following direct or indirect decompression and craniocervical stabilization surgery. In our trauma series, a mean ASIA motor score improvement of 29 points (50 to 79) was recorded, with 85% of patients improving at least one ASIA grade. Of two complete spinal cord injuries seen, one experienced substantial improvement from a high cervical to midthoracic level of function and the other maintaining a midcervical level and requiring continued ventilator dependency.

Restoration of physiologic alignment as seen on radiographs was maintained as well. The basion-dens interval (BDI) improved 6 mm (17 to 11), and the mean basion-atlantal interval decreased from 10 to 8 mm in these 17 patients. Normalization of preoperatively abnormal BDI occurred in all but two patients. One case, which presented with severe distraction that could not be completely reduced, resulted in a postoperative BDI of 18 mm.

In general, there is a much improved emphasis on timely recognition of traumatic and subacute conditions affecting the craniocervical junction. Available modern segmental fixation with modular components seems to be safe and effective. Bone healing rates require critical longer-term assessment as there may have been a lesser degree of emphasis on formal arthrodesis than in times past with less sophisticated internal fixation.

Clearly, there is a trend for increased survival in craniocervical dissociation patients. Previous reporting of these injuries documented in case reports was often notable only for their survival. Prompt diagnostic suspicion and management of these highly unstable injuries have enormous importance for patient care, and neglect can be catastrophic (11,15,28).

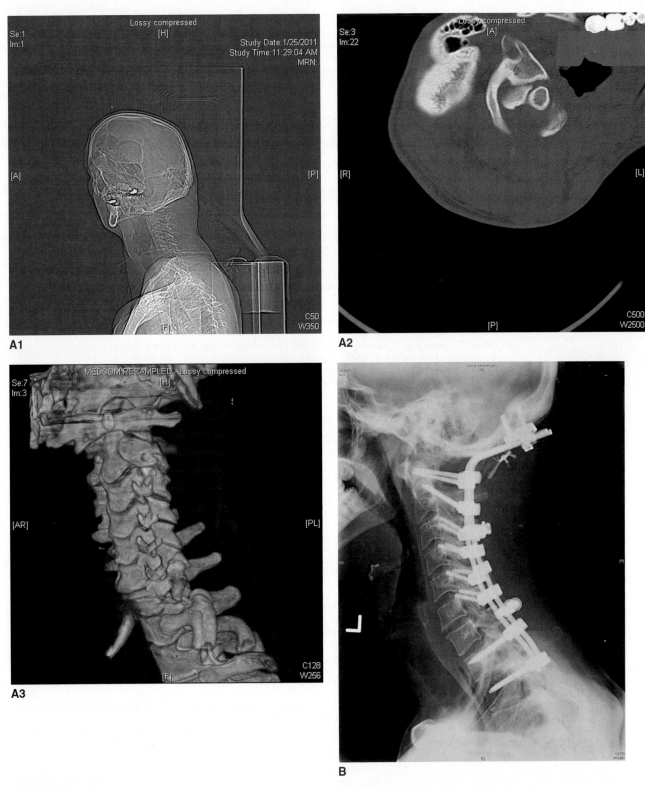

FIGURE 12-7

A: This is a CT scout, an axial CT image, and a three-dimensional CT reconstruction of a highly functional 39-year-old male with spastic torticollis secondary to cerebral palsy. He had failed extensive nonoperative care including bracing, serial Botox injections, and systemic muscle relaxant applications. His social interactions were also adversely affected by severe facial twitches, which precipitated his cervical distortions. These images demonstrate a reversible atlantoaxial rotatory dislocation and C2–C3 subluxation. **B:** After extensive counseling and following consultations with a number of nonoperative specialties, the patient elected to proceed with craniocervical fusion. In light of his neuromuscular condition, a caudal fixation to T2 was chosen. This lateral radiograph obtained at 1-year follow-up shows successful fusion in anatomically acceptable alignment. Remarkably, the severe facial contortions of the patient had also subsided to a substantial degree.

RECOMMENDED READING

1. Abumi K, Takada T, Shono Y, et al.: Posterior occipitocervical reconstruction using cervical pedicle screws and plate-rod systems. *Spine* 24(14): 1425–1434, 1999.

2. Anderson PA, Montesano PX: Morphology and treatment of occipital condyle fractures. *Spine* 13(7): 731–736, 1988.

3. Bagley CA, Witham TF, Pindrik JA, et al.: Assuring optimal physiologic craniocervical alignment and avoidance of swallowing-related complications after occipitocervical fusion by preoperative halo vest placement. *J Spinal Disord Tech* 22(3): 170–176, 2009.

4. Bellabarba C, et al.: Diagnosis and treatment of craniocervical dislocation in a series of 17 consecutive survivors during an 8-year period. *J Neurosurg Spine* 4: 429–440, 2006.

5. Bransford RJ, Stevens DW, Uyeji S, et al.: Halo vest treatment of cervical spine injuries: a success and survivorship analysis. *Spine (Phila Pa 1976)* 34(15): 1561–1566, 2009.

6. Bransford RJ, Russo AJ, Freeborn MF, et al.: Posterior C2 instrumentation: accuracy associated with four techniques. *Spine* 36(14): 936–943, 2011.

7. Crisco JJ III, Panjabi MM, Dvorak J: A model of the alar ligaments of the upper cervical spine in axial rotation. *J Biomech* 24(7): 607–614, 1991.

8. Ding X, Abumi K, Ito M, et al.: A retrospective study of congenital osseous anomalies at the craniocervical junction treated by occipitocervical plate-rod systems. *Eur Spine J* 21(8): 1580–1589, 2012.

9. Finn MA, Fassett DR, Mccall TD, et al.: The cervical end of an occipitocervical fusion: a biomechanical evaluation of 3 constructs. Laboratory investigation. *J Neurosurg Spine* 9(3): 296–300, 2008.

10. Friedman D, Flanders A, Thomas C, et al.: Vertebral artery injury after acute cervical spine trauma: rate of occurrence as detected by MR angiography and assessment of clinical consequences. *Am J Roentgenol* 164(2): 443–447, 1995.

11. Goel A, Laheri V: Plate and screw fixation for atlanto-axial subluxation. *Acta Neurochir* 129: 47–53, 1994.

12. Grob D, Crisco JJ, Panjabi MM, et al.: Biomechanical evaluation of four different posterior atlantoaxial fixation techniques. *Spine* 17(5): 480–490, 1992.

13. Grob D, Jeanneret B, Aebi M, et al.: Atlanto-axial fusion with transarticular screw fixation. *J Bone Joint Surg Br* 73(6): 972–976, 1991.

14. Haher TR, Yeung AW, Caruso SA, et al.: Occipital screw pullout strength. A biomechanical investigation of occipital morphology. *Spine* 24(1): 5–9, 1999.

15. Harms J, Melcher RP: Posterior C1-C2 fusion with polyaxial screw and rod fixation. *Spine* 26(22): 2467–2471, 2001.

16. Kim HJ, Lenke LG, Riew KD, et al.: Occipital incidence: a novel morphometric parameter for understanding occipitocervical spinal alignment. Presented at: The 40th Annual Meeting of the Cervical Spine Research Society, December 6–8, 2012; Chicago, IL. Poster no. 19.

17. Melcher RP, Puttlitz CM, Kleinstueck FS, et al.: Biomechanical testing of posterior atlantoaxial fixation techniques. *Spine* 27(22): 2435–2440, 2002.

18. Lall R, Patel NJ, Resnick DK: A review of complications associated with craniocervical fusion *surgery. Neurosurgery* 67(5): 1396–1402, 1402–1403, 2010.

19. Logroscino CA, Genitiempo M, Casula S: Relevance of the cranioaxial angle in the occipitocervical stabilization using an original construct: a retrospective study on 50 patients. *Eur Spine J* 18(Suppl 1): 7–12, 2009.

20. Noble ER, Smoker WR: The forgotten condyle: the appearance, morphology, and classification of occipital condyle fractures. *Am J Neuroradiol* 17(3): 507–513, 1996.

21. Panjabi M, Dvorak J, Duranceau J, et al.: Three-dimensional movements of the upper cervical spine. *Spine* 13(7): 726–730, 1988.

22. Reindl R, Sen M, Aebi M: Anterior instrumentation for traumatic C1-C2 instability. *Spine* 28(17): E329–E333, 2003.

23. Sasso RC, Jeanneret B, Fischer K, et al.: Occipitocervical fusion with posterior plate and screw instrumentation. A long-term follow-up study. *Spine* 19(20): 2364–2368, 1994.

24. Terao Y, et al.: Increased incidence of emergency airway management after combined anterior-posterior cervical spine surgery. *J Neurosurg Anesthesiol* 16(4): 282–286, 2004.

25. Tokuda K, Miyasaka K, Abe H, et al.: Anomalous atlantoaxial portions of vertebral and posterior inferior cerebellar arteries. *Neuroradiology* 27(5): 410–413, 1985.

26. Wertheim SB, Bohlman HH: Occipitocervical fusion. Indications, technique, and long-term results in thirteen patients. *J Bone Joint Surg Am* 69(6): 833–836, 1987.

27. Wright NM, Lauryssen C: Vertebral artery injury in C1-2 transarticular screw fixation: results of a survey of the AANS/CNS section on disorders of the spine and peripheral nerves. American Association of Neurological Surgeons/Congress of Neurological Surgeons. *J Neurosurg* 88(4): 634–640, 1998.

28. Wright NM: Posterior C2 fixation using bilateral, crossing C2 laminar screws: case series and technical note. *J Spinal Disord Tech* 17(2): 158–162, 2004.

29. Young J, Young P, Ackermann M, et al.: The ponticulus posticus: implications for screw insertion into the first cervical lateral mass. *J Bone Joint Surg Am* 87(11): 2495–2498, 2005.

30. Zavanone M, Guerra P, Rampini P, et al.: Traumatic fractures of the craniovertebral junction. Management of 23 cases. *J Neurosurg Sci* 35(1): 17–22, 1991.

PART II

THORACOLUMBAR SPINE

13 Anterior Thoracolumbar Extensile Approach

Robert A. McGuire Jr.

INDICATIONS/CONTRAINDICATIONS

The extensile approach is used to gain access to the lower thoracic spine and lumbar spine simultaneously. This approach allows spinal access for anterior soft tissue release and correction of deformities with instrumentation in the anterior position alone (5). It is also used for treatment of thoracolumbar fractures, either acute or chronic. In many patients with chronic fractures, kyphosis is often present as a result of the fracture. The extensile approach allows excellent visualization of the anterior column of the spine in a circumferential manner. This allows surgical release of the anterior soft tissue–deforming structures (such as the annulus and the anterior longitudinal ligament), vertebrectomy, and correction of the deformity. Correction of the kyphosis, reconstruction of the vertebra with placement of a graft, and anterior stabilization can be easily accomplished through this approach.

PREOPERATIVE PREPARATION

The approach can be made from either the right or the left side. The goals of the surgical procedure and the side of major pathology often dictate which side is used. If an anterior release is all that is necessary; it is most often worthwhile to work on the convex portion of the curve. It is often very difficult to work in the concave side and achieve an adequate and complete soft tissue release. For fracture decompression, reduction, and stabilization, both the right and the left sides can be used according to the surgeon's preference. Because the arterial vessels lie most often on the left side of the spine, it is often easier to approach from the left in order to mobilize the vessels and minimize risk to the inferior vena cava. It is worthwhile to determine whether there are any preexisting problems related to the pulmonary cavity, such as fibrosis from old respiratory diseases or previous abdominal procedures, that could make the approach more difficult. This extensile approach allows exposure from the distal thoracic spine all the way to the sacrum if needed.

Technique

Positioning of the patient is critical when this approach is used. Planning should be discussed with the anesthesia team because the use of a double-lumen endotracheal tube can be extremely helpful in minimizing problems with the lung. The use of the double-lumen endotracheal tube allows the lung to be deflated, which assists in visualization of the surgical field and still allows the patient to be adequately ventilated. This is most helpful for procedures at T9 and above. When the patient is positioned, great care must be undertaken to adequately pad all of the bony prominences around the knees, hips, and ankles (Fig. 13-1). An axillary roll should also be placed to minimize injury to the brachial plexus. The use of a vacuum-formed beanbag stabilizer provides individualized support and stability on the operating table and allows intraoperative radiographs to be taken (Fig. 13-2). Stability can also be augmented with the use of 3-inch-wide tape secured to the operating table on one side, brought over the shoulder and hip, and then secured to the opposite side of the table. It is preferable to flex the hip in order to relax the psoas muscle. A Foley catheter and a nasogastric tube are inserted to decompress the bladder and minimize the risk of intra-abdominal gas formation from the anesthetic. If the iliac crest is to be used for bone harvesting, draping of the surgical site should be performed in such a manner as to allow exposure of the crest. Once the patient is securely stabilized on the table, the surgical site is draped and the skin sterilely prepped.

Surgical Procedure

The incision can be made through the 9th, 10th, or 11th rib, depending on the length of exposure needed in the thoracic region. Once the determination of the rib level is made, the proposed skin incision is drawn over this rib, beginning posteriorly and extending anteriorly and distally to the level of the pubic symphysis if necessary. It can be made in a curvilinear manner, which would allow full exposure of the distal thoracic and lumbar spine as needed (Fig. 13-3). The skin incision is then made sharply through the skin and subcutaneous tissues.

The latissimus dorsi muscle is split, as is the posterior serratus if necessary, which exposes the rib (Fig. 13-4). The rib can also be used as bone graft. The rib periosteum is split, and the rib is then removed in a subperiosteal manner. It is important to make the incision of the periosteum in the cephalad half of the rib to prevent injury to the neurovascular bundle, which lies in the rib groove caudally.

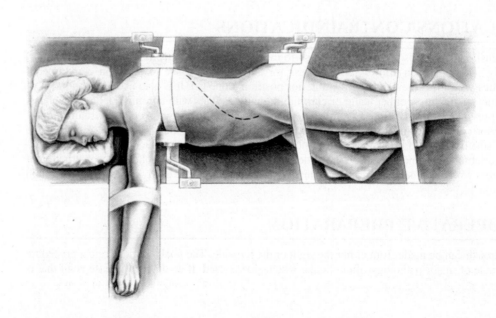

FIGURE 13-1

Positioning the patient in the appropriate manner allows good visualization of the surgical site and allows all bony pressure areas to be adequately protected.

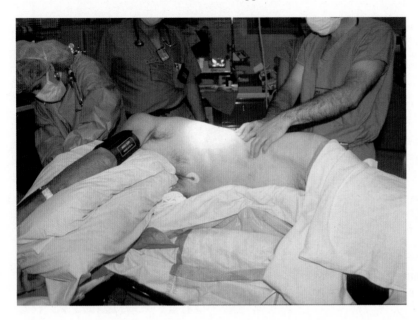

FIGURE 13-2

The use of a beanbag stabilizer provides support of the patient and allows intraoperative radiographs to be taken for verification of the operative level and to assess adequacy of reduction or decompression.

Dissection is carried as far posteriorly as needed, usually to the posterior angle, and the rib is then transected (Fig. 13-5). The pleural cavity is then opened through the periosteal rib bed. The retroperitoneal space is then entered bluntly through the cartilaginous portion of the 10th or 11th rib.

The peritoneum is identified and swept off the deep abdominal muscles in the direction from anterior lateral to posterior medial with a gauze sponge either on the surgeon's fingertip or on a sponge stick. Once the peritoneum has been reflected off the abdominal musculature, the internal oblique and transversus abdominis muscles are then incised as needed for the exposure.

Once the incision for the entire length necessary for the procedure has been made, the peritoneum is bluntly swept off the psoas muscle and from the undersurface of the diaphragm, which exposes the retroperitoneal space. Once this has been accomplished, the diaphragm is incised circumferentially, leaving approximately 1 cm of muscle cuff laterally (Fig. 13-6).

The diaphragm is innervated centrally in a radial manner; therefore, the cuff, even though it is denervated, provides an attachment for a diaphragmatic repair; the majority of the diaphragm remains functional after surgery (6). It is extremely helpful at this point to tag the ends of the

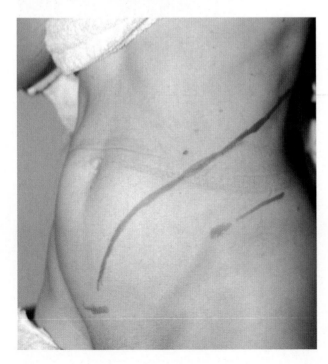

FIGURE 13-3

The skin incision is made in a way to expose as much of the spine as needed. The curvilinear exposure allows visualization of the distal thoracic spine to the lumbosacral junction if necessary.

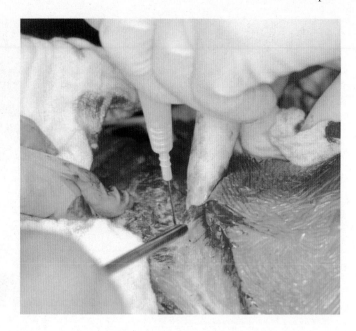

FIGURE 13-4

The latissimus dorsi muscle and external oblique muscle are split, exposing the rib.

anterior musculature as well as the diaphragm with a suture so this can be repaired in an anatomic position after the procedure. Because the diaphragm is swept anteriorly, a portion of the crus of the diaphragm may need to be reflected to gain better exposure of the spine.

Once the spine is visualized, the segmental vessels are then identified (Fig. 13-7). These can be found in the concave portion of the vertebral body; the disc spaces are the convex portion of the vertebral column when palpated. If an anterior release is all that must be performed, the vessels can sometimes be left in position and do not necessarily have to be ligated.

If corpectomy or instrumented correction is needed, then the vessels are ligated as necessary. It is important to ligate the vessels approximately 1 cm from the intervertebral foramen to allow collateral vessels to supply the spinal cord. If exposure to the sacrum is desired, vessels of the lumbar venous network often need to be ligated and sectioned. This allows mobilization of the vessels anteriorly to expose the lumbosacral junction. It may be necessary to skeletonize the iliac artery

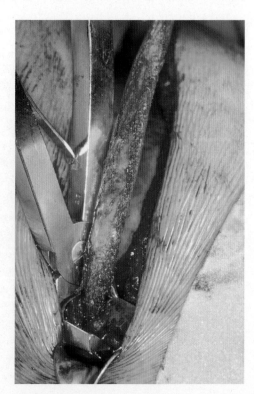

FIGURE 13-5

The rib is transected posteriorly, and the cartilage is split anteriorly to allow entrance into the retroperitoneal space.

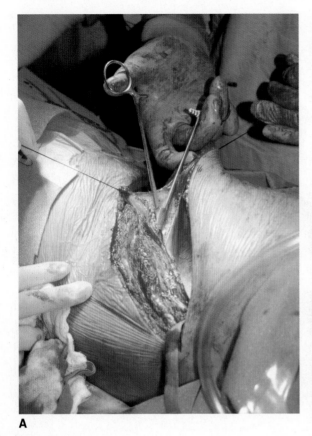 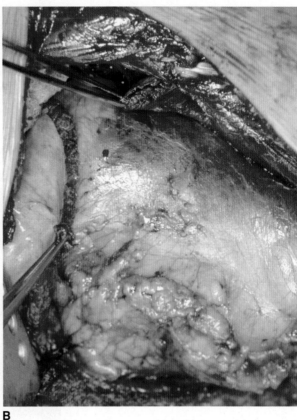

A   B

FIGURE 13-6

A: The retroperitoneal space is entered through the interval of the transected cartilaginous portion of the rib bed, the diaphragm, and the anterior abdominal musculature intersection, as shown by the scissor placement. It is important to close this interval tightly at the termination of the procedure, to minimize the risk of a hernia. **B:** The diaphragm is incised in such a manner as to leave a lateral cuff of tissue to repair after completion of the spinal portion of the case.

and vein and work between the bifurcations in order to visualize the L5–S1 segment in certain situations. The psoas muscle is mobilized in a subperiosteal manner, with great care taken not to work through the fibers of the muscle, because potential injury to the lumbar roots can occur. Retraction can also be accomplished by the use of a Kirschner wire driven into the posterior aspect of the distal vertebral body. Malleable retractors protecting the anterior vessels are then placed to allow adequate visualization while the surgeon works at either the disc space or corpectomy level of the procedure.

Once the procedure is complete, the retractors are removed; the wound is then thoroughly irrigated with warm saline. The appropriate-size chest tube is then selected and placed. The diaphragm is then repaired with large, nonabsorbable sutures. The rib bed is then closed with Prolene sutures, and the lung is reinflated. At this point, a malleable retractor can be placed intra-abdominally to protect the viscus while the muscular layers are repaired. Leaving one end of the retractor out of the skin while closing minimizes the risk of leaving this tool in the abdomen. The muscle layers are then closed individually while the peritoneum is protected. It is extremely important during closure to make sure the apex of the distal aspect of the incision, as well as the junction of the diaphragm and the abdominal musculature, are adequately addressed to minimize the risk of a hernia. The skin is then closed by the use of sutures or staples, and a sterile dressing is applied.

Extreme Lateral Approach

The extreme lateral approach to the thoracic and lumbar spine also can be used to gain access to the thoracolumbar and lumbar spine using less soft tissue dissection (1,3,4). This technique can provide visualization of the spine through a smaller skin incision but still provide access to multiple levels allowing anterior release for sagittal alignment correction, corpectomy and vertebral body reconstruction, and multilevel discectomy and interbody fusion (Fig. 13-8A–D). Great care should

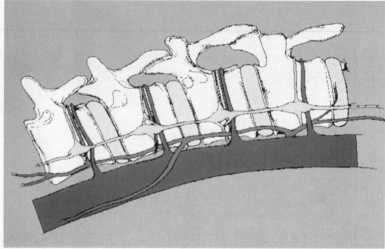

A

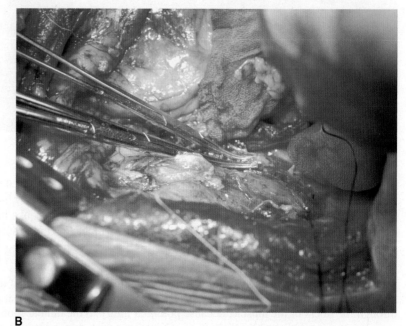

FIGURE 13-7

A: The segmental vessels are identified in the concave portion of the vertebral body. There is a paired artery and vein at each level. **B:** The disc can be identified as the convex portion of the spinal segment.

B

be utilized in the lower lumbar region to protect the lumbar roots and vascular structures. With the patient in the lateral position, I have found that by flexing the upper hip, the psoas can be relaxed making it possible to dissect the anterior border of the psoas muscle and retracting it posteriorly, which still allows access to the disc spaces but offers better protection for the lumbar roots.

This approach allows relatively easy access to the lower thoracic, the thoracolumbar junction, and the lumbar spine. The L5–S1 junction is extremely difficult to reach via this approach due to the position of the neurovascular structures that overlie this area and the iliac crest blocking direct lateral access to this segment due to the deep set position in the pelvis.

COMPLICATIONS

Closure of the wound should be done in layers to minimize the risk of hernias. Great care should be used in handling the soft tissues in the thoracic cavity to minimize the risk of injury to the lymphatic vessels, which could lead to chylothorax (2).

Complications can occur with this approach. The right-sided approach can potentially lead to damage to the liver from overaggressive retraction. The left-sided approach can lead to damage to the spleen. In men, there is the possibility of retrograde ejaculation; therefore, this should be discussed with all male patients before surgical intervention. The possibility of injury to the femoral nerve can be minimized by slightly flexing the hips.

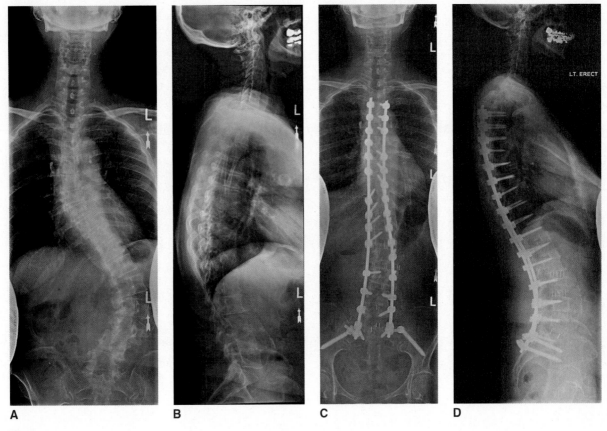

A   B   C   D

FIGURE 13-8

A,B: AP and lateral radiographs of this 55-year-old female who presents with severe scoliosis and back pain that have not been responsive to conservative management. **C,D:** Postoperative AP and lateral radiographs revealing good correction of both the sagittal and coronal alignment of the spine using the extreme lateral approach to allow access to multiple segments with the placement of interbody cages anteriorly and then stabilization posteriorly.

Potential injury to the genitofemoral nerve can also be minimized by attention to detail during dissection over the psoas musculature. If this nerve is injured, painful neuromas can develop. Attention to dissection in the region of the psoas muscle can minimize the risk of injury to the sympathetic chain. Injury to this structure often leads to sensations of differences in temperature of the lower extremities. If this potential problem is discussed with the patient before the procedure, their concerns can often be alleviated.

When the vessels are manipulated, it is important to minimize repetitive trauma to the venous structures because this can potentially lead to deep vein thrombosis and pulmonary embolus. The use of sequential compression stockings both intraoperatively and postoperatively can minimize the risk of deep vein thrombosis. It is important to visualize the ureter during the exposure, in order to minimize the risk of injury to this structure during surgery. It is critical that this structure be identified in individuals who have repeat surgery in the retroperitoneal space, to prevent injury. In this group of patients with previous retroperitoneal surgical exposures, it is worthwhile to have a urologist insert a stent into the ureter to make it more visible in the scar.

RECOMMENDED READING

1. Dakwar E, Ahmadian A, Uribe JS: The Anatomical relationship of the diaphragm to the thoracolumbar junction during the minimally invasive lateral approach. *J Neurosurg Spine* 16: 359–364, 2012.
2. Eisenstein S, O'Brien JP: Chylothorax: a complication of Dwyer's anterior instrumentation. *Br J Surg* 74: 339–341, 1977.
3. Karikari IO, et al.: Extreme lateral interbody fusion approach for isolated thoracic and thoracolumbar spine diseases: initial clinical experience and early outcomes. *J Spinal Disord Tech* 24: 368–375, 2011.
4. Patel NP, et al.: The mini-open anterolateral approach for degenerative thoracolumbar disease. *Clin Neurol Neurosurg* 112: 853–857, 2010.
5. Riseborough EJ: The anterior approach to the spine for correction of the axial skeleton clinical. *Clin Orthop Relat Res* 93: 207–214, 1973.
6. Scott R: Innervation of the diaphragm and its practical aspects in surgery. *Thorax* 20: 357, 1965.

14 Endoscopic and Anterior Approaches for Spinal Deformity Surgery in the Adolescent and Young Adult

Mark B. Dekutoski, Mark Pichlemann, and Jeremy L. Fogelson

INDICATIONS

Contemporary open thoracolumbar approaches for anterior scoliosis correction and fusion have been modeled after the early technique popularized by John Hall from Boston Children's Hospital in the late 1980s. The typical curve patterns for which this technique is most appropriate are thoracolumbar curves, which we now classify as Lenke V or VI curves. Patient selection and informed patient choice in choosing anterior versus posterior approaches need to be thoughtfully and thoroughly reviewed with the family. The patient depicted in Figure set 14-1 has a Lenke Vb thoracolumbar curve as depicted in Figure 14-1A and B radiographically and clinically in Figure 14-1C and D. Confirming that the patient's proximal and distal curves are nonstructural is critical for restoration of the trunk shift demonstrated in Figure 14-1C. Her significant rib hump demonstrated in Figure 14-1E also responds favorably to the derotation effected by 270-degree annulotomy and discectomy and deliberate orthogonal placement of the screws relative to the native rotational axis of the vertebrae. Figure 14-1F and G demonstrate the contralateral locking nut that enhances proximal screw fixation. This concept and implant design was popularized by Dr. Izzy Liebermann while at the Cleveland Clinic in the late 1990s to address the troublesome rate of proximal screw pullout, loss of correction, and potential nonunion noted with the widespread adoption. Figure 14-1G demonstrates osseous union and the patient's 1-year sagittal profile. Figure 14-1H and I demonstrate the 1-year clinical correction of coronal balance, level shoulders, waist symmetry, and reduction of rib hump on posteroanterior (PA) and forward bend photos. For this patient, a T9 to L2 anterior approach was utilized, whereas with a typical posterior approach, an additional distal segment may have been necessary.

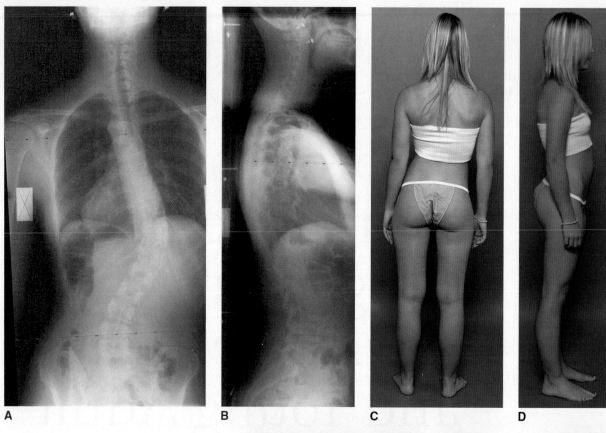

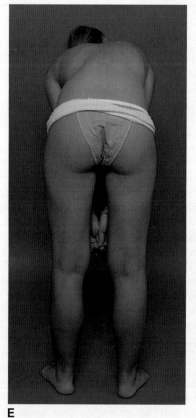

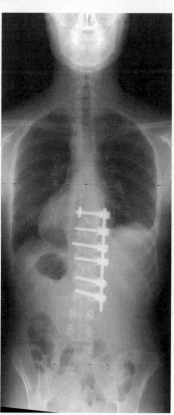

FIGURE 14-1

A: Standing PA radiograph of a postmenar-chal 14 + 6-year-old female demonstrates a right Lenke VB curve measuring 46 degree from T9 to L2. **B:** Standing lateral radiograph of patient with the Lenke VB curve with moderate pelvic incidence and sagittal balance. **C:** Standing clinical PA demonstrates trunk shift to the right and waist asymmetry. **D:** Standing clinical lateral demonstrates that sagittal balance is intact. **E:** Standing PA with forward bend demonstrates the thoracolumbar rib hump. **F:** One-year postoperative (PO) standing PA radiograph demonstrates waist symmetry, shoulder balance, and neutral coronal balance.

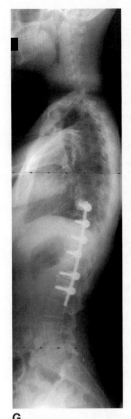

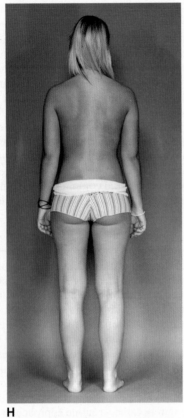

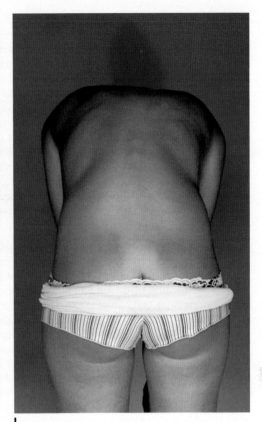

G

H

I

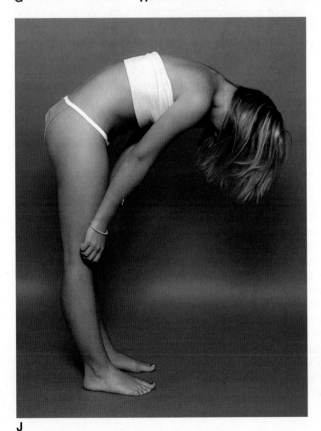

J

FIGURE 14-1 *(Continued)*
G: One-year PO standing PA radiograph
demonstrates neutral sagittal alignment.
H: One-year standing clinical PA
demonstrates waist symmetry and
coronal balance. **I:** One-year standing
PA forward bend demonstrates reduction
of rib and chest wall deformity.
J: One-year PO forward bend side view.

CONTRAINDICATIONS

Delivery of the appropriate surgical intervention with expected outcome and limited complications requires surgeon training and experience coupled with development of clinical and hospital-based teams. Surgical intervention for spinal deformity surgery is one of the most demanding technical and resource-driven procedures in tertiary medical centers. While outstanding results are published from mature centers, these results and outcomes are not generalizable to all orthopedic surgeons or neurosurgeons in spine practice. Specific patient selection, indications, informed patient consent, and technical execution of the breadth of deformity procedures require specialized training. Individual patient counseling needs to be based upon the experience and outcomes of the surgical team.

Use of endoscopic techniques in North America for anterior scoliosis is challenged by the limited number of surgeons and centers that have developed this expertise and the resource consumption associated with the increased surgical times and potential complications. That said, outstanding clinical outcomes have been published by several mature scoliosis centers for endoscopic anterior fusion.

PREOPERATIVE PREPARATION

Patient education and informed patient choice require careful discussion of the known outcomes, and breadth of treatment choices is an obligation of the surgeon team. Discussion of the specific limitations and outcome expectations for the breadth of procedures and evolution of techniques and outcomes should be presented to the patient by the patient care team.

Through the 1980s and 1990s, correction of scoliotic and kyphotic deformity evolved from in situ fusion to use of distraction and nonsegmental fixation. Anterior fusion and early anterior fixation were commonly used in deformity centers to enhance fusion rates, treat pseudoarthrosis, and limit potential for occurrence of crankshaft phenomenon. North American deformity practices represented by the founders of the Scoliosis Research Society and their fellows became adept at open techniques for thoracic and lumbar fusion (3). The commonplace thoracolumbar "sharkbite" with reflection and reconstruction of the diaphragm became a routine approach to adult and neuromuscular deformity. When compared to the high rates of pseudoarthrosis in that era, the morbidity of the anterior approach was quite favorable in the balance of risks and benefits.

In the late 1990s and early 2000s, several international and North American centers became interested in the immediate and long-term pulmonary effects of scoliotic deformity (1,2,4,13). Long-term follow-up of treated and untreated deformities confirmed the deleterious effects to pulmonary function (PFT) due to chest wall stiffening. The least impairment of PFTs was noted with brace treatment, but much more substantial impairment was effected with posterior correction and fusion. The worst pulmonary outcomes were noted with deformities treated utilizing a thoracotomy. Ongoing work by the Washington University Department of Orthopedic group in St. Louis has added granularity to these observations and noted the progressive improvement during the first 2 PO years with measurable differences at the final follow-up. The challenge to PFT-based studies is that while PFT changes were demonstrated, clinically, relevant improvements to activities of daily living or aerobic activities were not demonstrated between the various groups (7).

With advances in surgical and endoscopic techniques, many surgeons transitioned their practices to incorporate endoscopic release, discectomy, fusion, and instrumentation in an effort to generate less postthoracotomy symptoms. These techniques were advanced by Picchetti, Sucato, Newton, and others through the 1990s and early 2000s (8,9,10,12). Challenges due to high technical demand, learning curve, higher nonunion rates, and ultimately increased surgical time and expense were noted. Enthusiasm and market share for these advanced techniques have waned. However, more recent data on PFT from patients undergoing thoracoscopic scoliosis surgery have demonstrated less PFT decline than those undergoing open thoracotomy at 2 years post-op (5).

Further reducing the indication for anterior release and fusion is the strong documentation that pedicle screw fixation will overcome the crankshaft phenomena in Risser zero or one patient seen with hook or Luque constructs in these growing spines (11). As additional evidence, multicenter series and quality data have been forwarded from leading international and North American spine deformity centers and confirmed that the prevalence of anterior approaches performed has diminished significantly in the last decade (6).

TECHNIQUE

Application of anterior scoliosis techniques requires specific individualized patient assessment and curve characterization. The patient depicted in Figure 14-2 has a more typical Lenke Vb curve pattern for which the decisions for classification include focused assessment of the flexibility of the thoracic curve. Careful preoperative planning is required in order to balance the structural curve reduction with the residual curves proximally and distally. In addition, attention to obliquity of the lumbosacral (LS) takeoff and leg-length inequality is critical to obtaining a clinically acceptable outcome. Figure 14-2A and B and the thoracic side-bending film in Figure 14-2C demonstrate the Lenke VIb curve pattern. In the preoperative discussion of treatment options, one needs to include the risk of proximal curve progression. Additionally, it is important to discuss the issues of distal-level

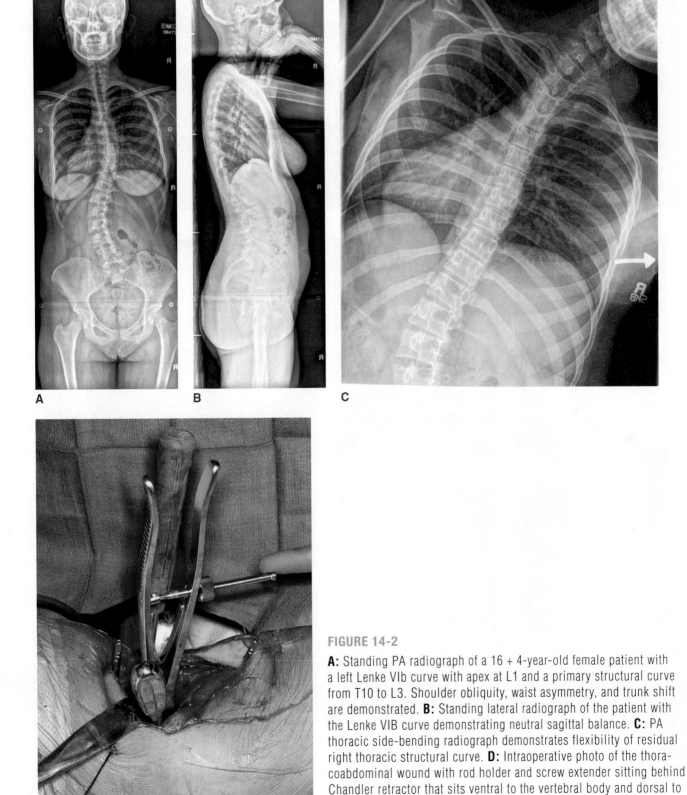

FIGURE 14-2

A: Standing PA radiograph of a 16 + 4-year-old female patient with a left Lenke VIb curve with apex at L1 and a primary structural curve from T10 to L3. Shoulder obliquity, waist asymmetry, and trunk shift are demonstrated. **B:** Standing lateral radiograph of the patient with the Lenke VIB curve demonstrating neutral sagittal balance. **C:** PA thoracic side-bending radiograph demonstrates flexibility of residual right thoracic structural curve. **D:** Intraoperative photo of the thoracoabdominal wound with rod holder and screw extender sitting behind Chandler retractor that sits ventral to the vertebral body and dorsal to the aorta.

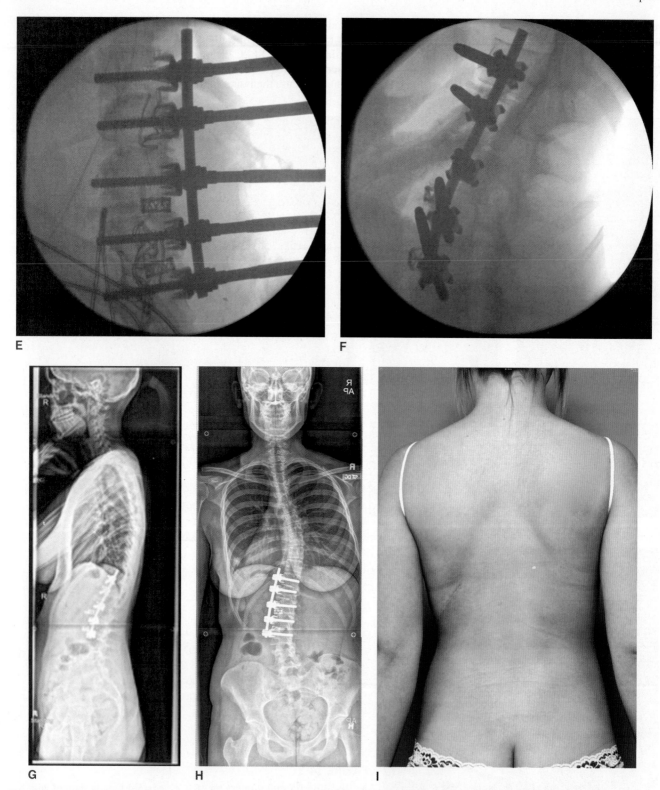

FIGURE 14-2 *(Continued)*

E: Intraoperative PA radiograph of the T11 to L3 screws, staples, and single rod in reduced position is demonstrated. Small cages are placed eccentrically within the L1 and L2 disc space to maintain lordosis. **F:** Intraoperative oblique radiograph demonstrates screw trajectory on the coronal plane with rod in position. Note screw extenders project from screws ventrally. **G:** Lateral standing radiograph at 2 months PO demonstrates maintenance of lordosis and sagittal balance.
H: Standing PA radiograph at 2 months demonstrates balanced LS and thoracic curves with improved coronal balance and residual shoulder obliquity. **I:** Demonstrates 1-year clinical follow-up with restoration of coronal balance and waist symmetry with residual left shoulder depression.

selection on flexibility and function, balanced with the potential for reoperation secondary to coronal imbalance if the residual curves "add on." Figure 14-2D depicts the single incision technique wherein the muscle-sparing window between the latissimus and trapezius is developed.

The spine is accessed proximal to the diaphragm via an intercostal window and the retroperitoneum via the typical window off the distal tip of the 12th rib. The proximal discs are excised. Implants are placed above the diaphragm, and the dorsal crus is elevated along the 11th, 12th, and 1st lumbar bodies for access and rod passage from the chest into the retroperitoneum. Figure 14-2E and F depict the implant placement neutral to the vertebral segments so as to allow for derotation with the fixed angle screws. Lumbar lordosis for the L2–L3 and L1–L2 segments is maintained with small cages in order to balance the patient's native pelvic incidence. These anterior cages have also been placed so as to avoid overcorrection of the curve. Intraoperative radiographs are limited by the lateral patient position but are used to monitor the intended curve correction. Overcorrection of the thoracolumbar curve leaving the residual stiff thoracic curve can result in shoulder obliquity. This is demonstrated in Figure 14-2G and H wherein at the 2-month PO period the patient had shoulder obliquity. A temporary thoracolumbosacral orthosis (TLSO) has been used in some cases with resultant improvement in balance. For this patient, the family deferred a TLSO, and at 1 year, the patient had excellent overall balance with slight left shoulder depression as demonstrated in Figure 14-2I.

Variations of thoracolumbar curves can also be addressed in select Lenke VIa and VIb curves. Figure 14-3 depicts a young lady with a Lenke VIb curve for whom lower instrumented vertebra – level selection is a critical issue, given the distal extent of her curve and apparent obliquity of the LS curve. Her standing radiographs, clinical photos, and bending films are depicted in Figure 14-3A–F. For this patient, posterior instrumentation from T4 to L4 or L5 was suggested. In this situation, incomplete reduction of the curves and balancing reduction of the primary thoracolumbar curve to the residual stiffness of the proximal and distal curves can be accomplished with a selective anterior release, fusion, and instrumentation. The hybrid solution of anterior release and interbody fusion as seen in Figure 14-3G–I was mated to a posterior percutaneous reduction and instrumentation

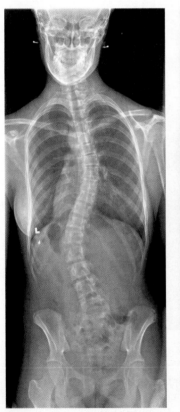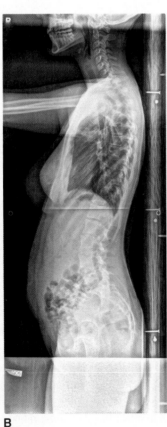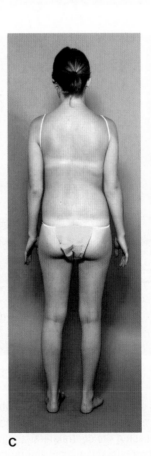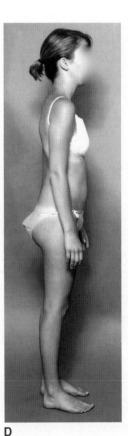

A   B   C   D

FIGURE 14-3

A: PA standing radiograph of a postmenarchal 14 + 2-year-old female with significant trunk asymmetry, coronal imbalance, and a Lenke VIB curve from T11 to L2. **B:** Standing lateral radiograph demonstrates sagittal balance. **C:** Standing clinical PA demonstrates coronal imbalance waist asymmetry and shoulder obliquity. **D:** Standing clinical lateral demonstrates sagittal balance.

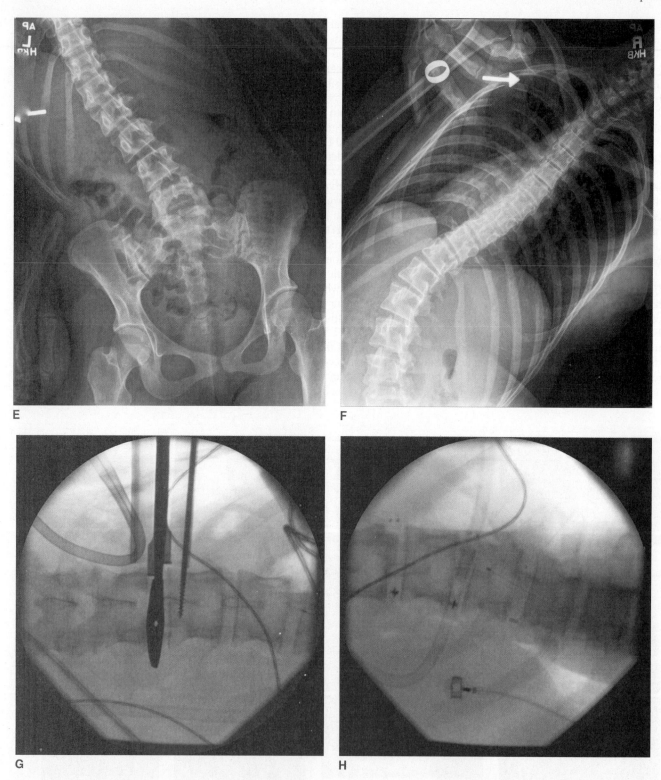

FIGURE 14-3 *(Continued)*

E: PA side-bending radiograph demonstrates LS curve flexibility. **F:** PA thoracic right side-bending radiograph demonstrates the residual structural thoracic curve with rotation. **G:** Intraoperative PA fluoroscopy view of a lateral access discectomy demonstrates the instrument crossing the contralateral annulus to affect the segmental release. **H:** Intraoperative PA fluoroscopy view of undersized implants placed within the released and debrided disc spaces.

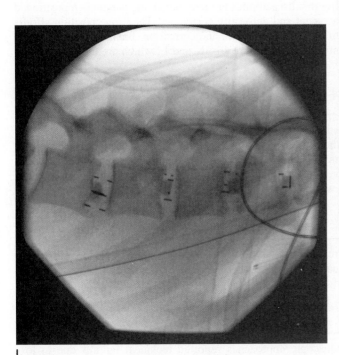

I

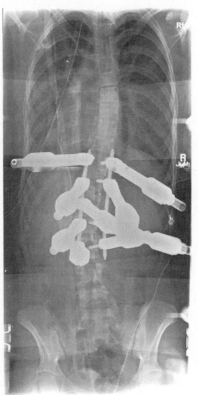

J

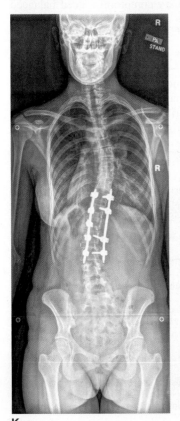

K

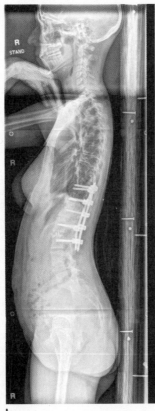

L

FIGURE 14-3 *(Continued)*
I: Intraoperative lateral fluoroscopy view of the undersized interbody spacers placed ventrally in the lower lumbar spine so as to effect maintenance of lordosis and more neutrally in the lower thoracic spine. **J:** Intraoperative prone radiograph with implants rods and reducers in place demonstrating residual coronal imbalance. **K:** Six-month PO standing radiograph demonstrates balanced curves and restoration of coronal balance with some residual left shoulder depression. **L:** Six-month PO standing radiograph demonstrates sagittal balance and avoidance of excessive kyphosis.

demonstrated in Figure 14-3J. A key technical point that achieves increased reduction is completion of the lateral interbody discectomies and annulotomy in a more thorough fashion than when one is only attempting fusion without correction. Undersizing the interbody spacers is important to allow for easier derotation. Furthermore, after the discectomies are completed, the patient is repositioned prone for the percutaneous screw placement and deformity correction. The prone position affords an optimal environment for 36-inch films to assess balance and correction. Balancing of the curves and reduced levels of fusion are demonstrated in Figure 14-3K and L, which are the 6-month PO standing radiographs.

PEARLS AND PITFALLS

Advances in technology with open pedicle screw constructs as well as minimal access and percutaneous approaches have scaled back the usefulness of open and thoracoscopic anterior approaches. Further challenge with delivery of anterior deformity technique is the unique technical and experience demands of an uncommon procedure. With ongoing development of less invasive approaches, it is clear that use of anterior surgery will continue to decline.

POSTOPERATIVE MANAGEMENT

Anterior deformity procedures require attention to chest tube management and postoperative pain management specific to chest wall pain. Use of intercostal nerve blocks and non-steroidal anti-inflammatory drugs (NSAIDs) has afforded significant gains in patient comfort and mobilization.

COMPLICATIONS

Early data on anterior open and endoscopic approaches reported technical failures due to loss of fixation and nonunion. These issues and potential late pulmonary compromise need balanced presentation to the patient and family.

RESULTS

Clinical outcomes from mature deformity centers approach the union rate of posterior approaches and result in fewer levels fused and avoid the paraspinal muscle denervation and atrophy associated with posterior thoracolumbar fusion. The degree and durability of rib hump reduction with anterior approaches exceeds that obtained and maintained by posterior approaches.

RECOMMENDED READING

1. Faro FD, Marks MC, Newton PO, et al.: Perioperative changes in pulmonary function after anterior scoliosis instrumentation: thoracoscopic versus open approaches. *Spine* 30: 1058–1063, 2005.
2. Graham E, Lenke L, Lowe T, et al.: Prospective pulmonary function evaluation following open thoracotomy for anterior spinal fusion in adolescent idiopathic scoliosis. *Spine* 25: 2319–2325, 2000.
3. Harms J, Jeszenszky D, Beele B: Ventral correction of thoracic scoliosis. In: Bridwell K, DeWald R, eds. *The textbook of spinal surgery*, 2nd ed. Philadelphia, PA: Lippincott-Raven, 1997.
4. Kim YJ, Lenke LG, Bridwell KH, et al.: Pulmonary function in adolescent idiopathic scoliosis relative to the surgical procedure. *J Bone Joint Surg Am* 87: 1534–1541, 2005.
5. Kishan S, Bastrom T, Betz RR, et al.: Thoracoscopic scoliosis surgery affects pulmonary function less than thoracotomy at 2 years postsurgery. *Spine* 32(4): 453–458, 2007.
6. Lenke LG, Betz RR, Haher TR, et al.: Multisurgeon assessment of surgical decision-making in adolescent idiopathic scoliosis: curve classification, operative approach, and fusion levels. *Spine* 26: 2347–2353, 2001.
7. Lenke LG, Bridwell KH, Blanke K, et al.: Analysis of pulmonary function and chest cage dimension changes after thoracoplasty in idiopathic scoliosis. *Spine* 20: 1343–1350, 1995.
8. Newton PO, Parent S, Marks M, et al.: Prospective evaluation of 50 consecutive scoliosis patients surgically treated with thoracoscopic anterior instrumentation. *Spine* 30(Suppl): 100–109, 2005.
9. Newton PO, Wenger DR, Mubarak SJ, et al.: Anterior release and fusion in pediatric spinal deformity: a comparison of early outcome and cost of thoracoscopic and open thoracotomy approaches. *Spine* 22: 1398–1406, 1997.
10. Picetti G, Pang D, Beuff H: Thoracoscopic techniques for the treatment of scoliosis: early results in procedure development. *Neurosurgery* 51: 978–984, 2002.
11. Sarlak, AJ Atmaca H, Buluç L, et al.: Juvenile idiopathic scoliosis treated with posterior arthrodesis and segmental pedicle screw instrumentation before the age of 9 years: a 5-year follow-up. *Scoliosis* 4: 1, 2009. doi: 10.186/1748-7161-4-1.
12. Sucato DJ: Thoracoscopic anterior instrumentation and fusion for idiopathic scoliosis. *J Am Acad Orthop Surg* 11: 221–227, 2003.
13. Vedantam R, Lenke LG, Bridwell KH, et al.: A prospective evaluation of pulmonary function in patients with adolescent idiopathic scoliosis relative to the surgical approach used for spinal arthrodesis. *Spine* 25: 82–90, 2000.

15 Hemivertebrae Excision

Serena S. Hu and David S. Bradford

INDICATIONS/CONTRAINDICATIONS

Congenital scoliosis can be categorized into deformities that are (a) secondary to failure of formation, (b) secondary to failure of segmentation, and (c) mixed lesions (13). Hemivertebrae are examples of failure of formation, whereas congenital bars and blocked vertebrae are examples of failure of segmentation. A unilateral unsegmented bar, especially one associated with a contralateral hemivertebra, has the worst prognosis for progression. Isolated hemivertebrae are less predictable in their growth potential, and consequently, the magnitude of the deformity that may result from continued spinal growth is uncertain. Hemivertebrae in the cervicothoracic and lumbosacral junctions are more likely to result in more noticeable deformity because of the inability of the spine above or below to compensate adequately (8). Surgery is indicated in children presenting with a significant deformity greater than 40 degrees with coronal imbalance secondary to a hemivertebra, in patients with a deformity that has shown progression on sequential radiographs, and in patients presenting with a lumbosacral hemivertebra associated with pelvic obliquity or lumbar scoliosis or both. There are several surgical options: (a) posterior spinal fusion, (b) combined anterior and posterior fusion, (c) hemiepiphysiodesis, and (d) hemivertebra excision.

Posterior spinal fusion has been reported as a gold standard in managing spinal deformity. It is a relatively straightforward procedure with minimal risks. However, in young patients with a hemivertebra, an isolated posterior fusion carries a high probability of worsening deformity because anterior vertebral growth may lead to bending and rotation of the fusion mass. A combined anterior and posterior fusion improves the fusion rate, may permit some correction if instrumentation is used and/ or a postoperative cast is added, and decreases the likelihood of bending and rotation of the fusion mass with further growth. Hemiepiphysiodesis is a useful procedure if performed in a young patient, preferably younger than 6 years, with mild-to-moderate curvatures (less than 30 to 40 degrees). However, even when convex fusion includes the involved segments of the curvature and not just the apical segments, correction of the deformity with growth is unpredictable. The early improvement may deteriorate with the adolescent growth spurt.

Excision of the hemivertebra can achieve a more reliable and greater degree of correction, as well as improvement in coronal balance. The optimal age range for hemivertebra excision is 3 to 10 years, after the growth potential of the hemivertebra has been demonstrated and before compensatory curves become structural. In older patients, a resection is still feasible even after the compensatory curves become less flexible, but the corrective surgery may require including these compensatory deformities in a more extensive fusion with instrumentation.

Hemivertebra excision is most optimally carried out at the thoracolumbar, lumbar, and lumbosacral area. Patients with hemivertebrae associated with minor curvatures (20 to 30 degrees) above the lumbosacral joint, without documentation of progression, should not be considered candidates for this procedure. Hemivertebra excision in the cervical spine poses a greater degree of difficulty and complexity and should only be performed by experienced spine surgeons. In the thoracic spine, rib resection is required and has higher risks to the spinal cord.

PREOPERATIVE PREPARATION

A routine history and physical examination should be obtained, as would normally be done for any patient with spinal deformity. A careful examination of the spine for evidence of a hairy patch, skin discoloration, or a sacral dimple or sinus is important. Evidence of pelvic obliquity, leg-length inequality, trunk decompensation, or neurologic dysfunction should be noted. Routine standing anteroposterior (AP) and lateral radiographs of the spine from occiput to sacrum are necessary on all patients. At the lumbosacral junction, Ferguson views (an AP view of the L5–S1 interspace, performed by tilting the beam of the x-ray machine about 30 degrees cephalad) are often needed to better visualize the bony anatomy. Bending films are important to determine flexibility of the compensatory curvatures proximally and distally. Widening of the interpedicular distance is suggestive of intrinsic spinal cord abnormalities such as diastematomyelia. Routine myelography or computed tomography (CT) scanning is not carried out; however, CT scanning with coronal reconstructions may be useful for better defining the bony abnormalities. However, magnetic resonance imaging (MRI) evaluation of the cervical, thoracic, and lumbar spine should be done in patients who have abnormal neurologic findings, in patients being prepared for operative intervention, and in patients with demonstrated widening of the interpedicular distance on routine radiographs. The MRI is important in order to rule out intracanal abnormalities such as a tethered cord, syringomyelia, diastematomyelia, or diplomyelia, or Arnold-Chiari malformation, any of which may be present in 10% to 50% of patients with congenital scoliosis (3). It is also useful in the MRI study to obtain a coronal view in the region of interest to delineate exactly where the segmentation has occurred and whether a bar exists on the contralateral side. Finally, as with other patients who have a congenital spine deformity, genitourinary abnormalities are not uncommon. Patients should be evaluated with ultrasonography or intravenous pyelography to rule out pathology. Cardiac abnormalities, although less common, may be associated as well, and any patient with a heart murmur should have an echocardiogram and/or a cardiology consultation.

TECHNIQUE

Hemivertebra resection can be performed via a posterior-only approach or a combined anterior and posterior approach. The posterior approach is increasingly commonly performed and is described below. The more traditional combined approach is recommended for the younger child with open growth plates, vertebra too small for posterior instrumentation, or a more tenuous spinal cord that may not tolerate even the gentle retraction that can occur with a posterior-only approach. We find that complete removal of the anterior cartilaginous growth plates is best performed by the combined anterior and posterior approach as described (2).

For combined anterior and posterior resection of the hemivertebra, the patient should be positioned first for the anterior resection. The patient is brought to the operating room and prepped in a routine manner. After the induction of anesthesia, a Foley catheter is inserted, and the patient is placed in the lateral decubitus position with the convex side up. A roll may be placed under the patient at the level of the deformity to facilitate the approach (Fig. 15-1). The table is flexed to open up the level and facilitate exposure. For lumbosacral excision, the patient should be prepped and draped down to the pubis.

It is advisable to prep and drape from the anterior midline to the posterior midline. A standard retroperitoneal thoracoabdominal or thoracic approach is used, depending on the level of the hemivertebra. Lumbosacral lesions may be approached through a retroperitoneal incision (Fig. 15-2), whereas hemivertebra lying at the thoracolumbar junction down to L2–L3 should be approached

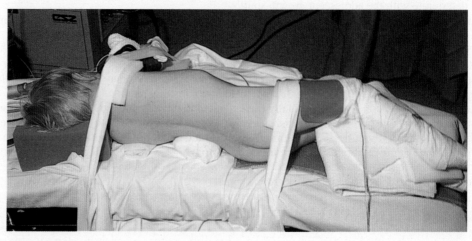

FIGURE 15-1

A patient positioned in the lateral decubitus position with a roll under his waist at the level of his lumbosacral hemivertebra.

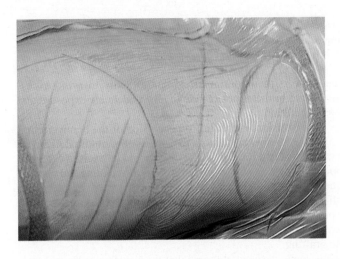

through a thoracoabdominal approach, with removal of the 10th or 11th rib. In the thoracic spine, the rib removed is the one lying one or two levels above the hemivertebra to be excised.

After rib removal, it may be possible to stay extrapleural with the approach by carefully and bluntly dissecting off the pleura from the chest wall and vertebral bodies. A pediatric-sized chest retractor is used to retract the chest or abdominal wall. Once the vertebral bodies are identified (Fig. 15-3), the

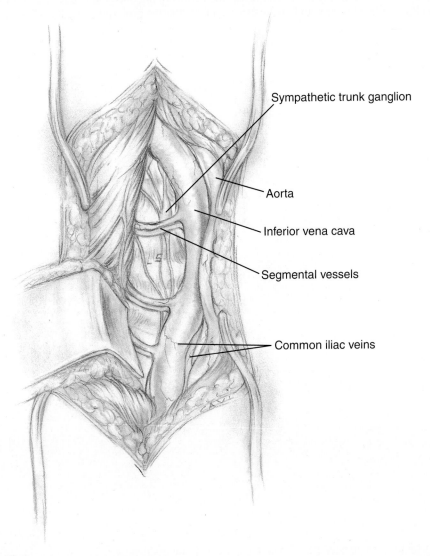

Sympathetic trunk ganglion

Aorta

Inferior vena cava

Segmental vessels

Common iliac veins

FIGURE 15-3

The segmental vessels before ligation. The inferior vena cava and the common iliac veins are seen, and the intervertebral discs and vertebral bodies are palpable.

pleura is incised, and the segmental vessels above and below the level of the excision are carefully identified and then clipped with vascular clips or tied and divided. It is useful at this stage to take a radiograph with metal markers in both the proximal and distal disc spaces to better delineate the level and margins of the hemivertebra (Fig. 15-4).

The dissection of the pleura off the spine is then continued extraperiosteally to avoid excessive bleeding. Dissection must proceed around to the opposite side to allow adequate exposure and prevent damage to the arterial or venous circulation.

Excision of the hemivertebra begins with excision of the disc on each side of the hemivertebral body. The disc is first incised (Fig. 15-5) with a scalpel along with the anterior longitudinal ligament and then removed with a combination of curettes and rongeurs. The disc should be excised carefully across the vertebral interspace to the opposite concave side, with removal of the annulus and nucleus back to the posterior longitudinal ligament, along with the cartilaginous growth plates. It is desirable to leave a small portion of the annular fibers on the concave side to act as a tether, preventing translation during the second-stage posterior procedure. After the disc has been totally removed back to the posterior longitudinal ligament, the vertebral body is excised with rongeurs and curettes (Fig. 15-6). This bone is saved for later use in bone grafting.

If the surgeon is operating in the thoracic spine, the head of the rib that is articulating with the hemivertebra and interspace is removed to facilitate exposure as well as eventual closure of the space once the vertebra has been excised. It must be stressed that the disc should be removed all the way back to the posterior longitudinal ligament. The outer disc fibers are quite fibrotic and cartilaginous, particularly posterolaterally, and during the process of deformity correction, they may retropulse into the spinal canal if the cartilaginous rim is not completely removed. It is also desirable to smooth down or shave the endplates of the vertebrae above and below the hemivertebra once the hemivertebra is excised, in order to allow better closure with bone-to-bone contact after the posterior procedure (Fig. 15-7).

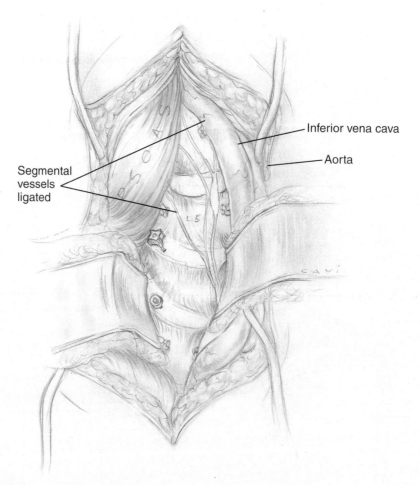

FIGURE 15-4

After segmental vessels have been ligated and divided, the great vessels are swept to the contralateral side of the disc space and vertebral body. Metallic markers are placed in the superior and inferior disc spaces for radiographic confirmation of the level.

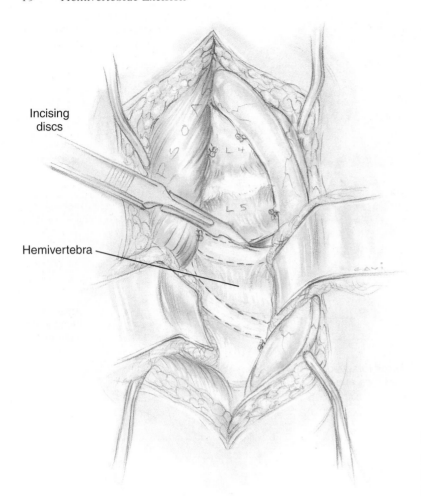

Incising
discs

Hemivertebra

FIGURE 15-5
A sharp scalpel blade
is used to incise the
superior most disc.

If excessive bleeding is encountered from epidural veins, hemostasis is achieved with Gelfoam (Pharmacia & Upjohn) soaked in thrombin solution. Topical collagen (Oxycel; Becton, Dickinson and Company, Franklin Lakes, NJ) is also helpful. It is very important to remove all the cartilage from the vertebral body above as well as below to ensure arthrodesis. Partial removal of the pedicle is performed with a high-speed bur; the more that can be removed safely during the anterior procedure, the easier the completion of the resection will be for the posterior resection (Fig. 15-8).

Gelfoam is placed loosely over the posterior longitudinal ligament, and then the space between the two vertebral bodies created by the excision may be filled partially with very finely cutup pieces of the excised vertebral body. The space obviously must not be packed too tightly with bone because it may jeopardize correction, but bone may be placed in the space loosely to facilitate arthrodesis (Fig. 15-9).

If the deformity is substantial, and if it is unlikely that anatomic correction will be achieved from the excision alone, it is desirable to perform a hemiepiphysiodesis at the segments above and below the site of hemivertebral excision. In this case, the convex half of the disc of the motion segment above is excised with a scalpel and rongeurs back to the bony endplate from the anterior ligament back to the posterior ligament, and the space is packed loosely with residual bone from the hemivertebra that was removed. By performing an epiphysiodesis in this manner above and below the site of vertebral excision, with eventual arthrodesis, a tethering effect is created, allowing improvement of the deformity with continued growth.

If in the thoracic spine, the pleura overlying the vertebral bodies is then closed with a running 2-0 absorbable suture, and the chest tube is placed in position through a stab incision and put to underwater seal suction. The chest is closed in a routine manner. If only a retroperitoneal approach has been used, no drain is necessary. The skin is closed cosmetically with a subcuticular 3-0 stitch.

The patient is then positioned for the posterior approach. This may be facilitated by transferring the patient to an additional operating table on which a four-poster frame has already been applied. If the patient is small, however, it is very easy to turn the patient in the prone position and slide a four-poster frame or rolls under the patient (Fig. 15-10). It is important to adequately pad the chest and the iliac crest bilaterally and allow ample space for the abdomen to hang free, to prevent increased venous pressure. We prefer to perform both stages of the surgery under one anesthetic. We have seen no complications from this protocol, and in fact, the morbidity is decreased with hospitalization

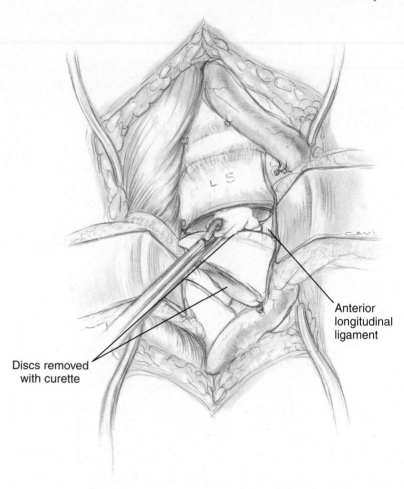

FIGURE 15-6

Curettes and rongeurs are used to remove the superior most disc. Note visualization of the inferior disc space as it intersects with the superior disc.

Discs removed with curette

Anterior longitudinal ligament

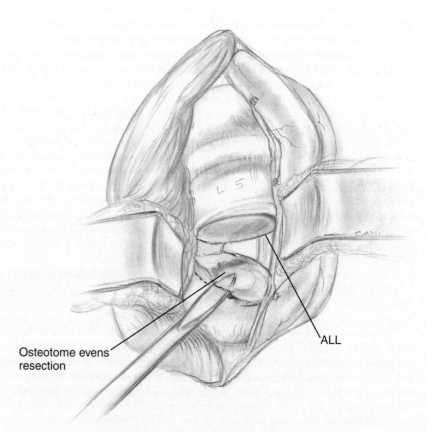

FIGURE 15-7

Because the hemi-vertebra is partially incarcerated, a curved osteotome is used to even the resection so as to leave a triangular defect that can be smoothly closed down.

Osteotome evens resection

ALL

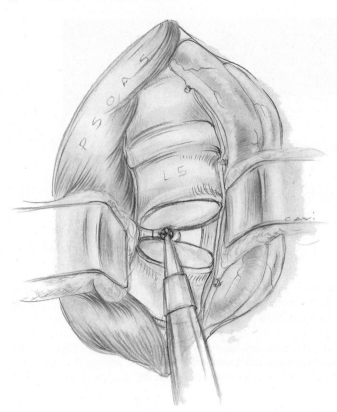

FIGURE 15-8

The resected area has been smoothed out to form an isosceles triangle. After adequate resection of the contralateral annulus has been performed, partial removal of the pedicle is performed with the high-speed bur.

time shortened and the overall cost is substantially less. The instrument trays are kept sterile during the repositioning process, and the patient is reprepped and draped in a routine manner. A routine midline exposure overlying the hemivertebra is then carried out, and after subperiosteal exposure, a radiograph is taken to determine the proper level.

Once the level has been adequately identified and complete exposure posteriorly obtained, the hemivertebra (laminae) is excised with a variety of rongeurs and curettes. Removal of the posterior arch is greatly enhanced by removing most of the pedicle during the anterior procedure. If during the anterior procedure the pedicle has not been drilled down flush to the nerve root, the removal is a bit more difficult from the posterior approach. Once the laminae, facets, and transverse process have

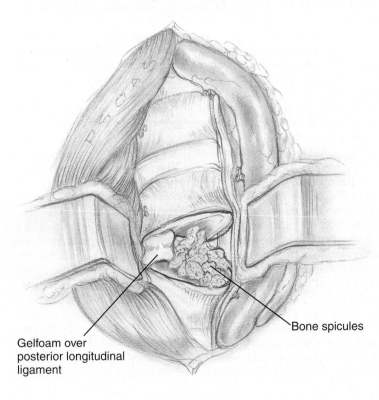

Bone spicules

Gelfoam over posterior longitudinal ligament

FIGURE 15-9

The area of the resection is loosely filled with fragments of resected bone.

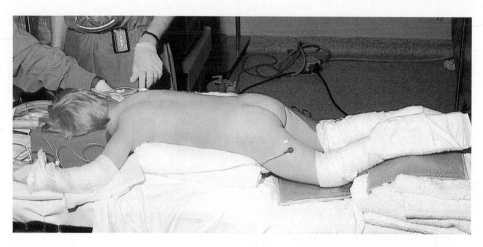

FIGURE 15-10

The patient is prone on a roll with the abdomen free.

been completely removed, the laminae above and below are decorticated carefully with a high-speed burr, and local bone graft is laid over the posterior elements one level above and one level below the excised laminae. If a hemiepiphysiodesis has been performed anteriorly, more than one additional level above and below the excised segment, then the posterior fusion should be added to the convex side over these additional segments. If a thoracotomy has been performed, sufficient bone usually exists for the fusion from the rib. If the procedure has been performed in the retroperitoneum only, as in the case of a lumbar hemivertebra, it may be necessary to expose the iliac crest and to obtain iliac crest bone or to use allograft bone.

If the patient has sufficient bone stock, it may be possible to use a short compression rod on the convex side to correct the deformity and provide adequate fixation. A compression implant on the convex side prevents the slight tendency toward kyphosis that often occurs with hemivertebra excision. In these cases, we have found that the pediatric lumbar hooks or the smallest 4.75-mm pedicle screws with the pediatric rod are adequate for compressing the two vertebrae together. The procedure may be performed with motor evoked potentials or somatosensory evoked potentials per the surgeon's preference. A wake-up test can be performed if desired or if neurophysiologic monitoring is not reliable.

If the patient's bone stock is not adequate to secure an implant, the wound is closed, and after a dressing is applied, the patient is placed on a pediatric spica frame. Anesthesia is maintained, and a plaster body spica cast that includes both legs from the ankles to the upper chest is applied. The cast is placed with the patient bent toward the convexity to maximize correction. Slight overcorrection is desired. A radiograph is taken with the patient under anesthesia to ensure closure of the wedge and adequate correction of coronal deformity. It is very important during the application of the plaster to be certain that the patient's spine does not drift into kyphosis; this is a normal tendency after hemivertebra excision. This can be avoided by maintaining posterior pressure over the apex of the deformity while the plaster is drying. A wake-up test is again performed, and/or monitoring continued, and prior to extubation radiographs obtained.

If correction is not thought to be sufficient, the cast can be wedged, and additional correction can be obtained. It is very important to pad the cast adequately, particularly over the iliac crest and the area of the deformity, to prevent skin ulceration from excessive pressure.

Posterior-based resections are increasingly performed and may be utilized if the surgeon has experience with this approach and the neurologic risk is acceptable. The patient is positioned prone on a four-poster frame or, for smaller patients, on chest rolls as described above. The exposure and radiographic confirmation is similarly performed. The intended instrumentation above and below the resection should be inserted prior to commencing the resection. This may be supra- and sublaminar hooks placed in a compression construct, but if the size of the anatomy permits, pedicle screws above and below are preferred. A laminectomy of the hemivertebra is performed, along with removal of the posterior elements including facet joints and transverse process. If in the thoracic spine, the rib heads must be removed. The anterior resection is performed from the posterior approach, working through the unilateral pedicle and around laterally as one would for a vertebral column resection. The discs above and below the hemivertebra are incised and removed, with curettes and pituitary rongeurs, as part of the resection. The hemivertebra should be decancellated completely, using a high-speed burr as well as curettes. Then, the endplates above and below are removed and the lateral vertebral body walls resected, usually with a small rongeur. The posterior wall of the vertebral body should be preserved until the final portion of the resection. A temporary rod should be placed before removal of the posterior wall, or the spine will collapse before the surgeon has completed the resection and be unstable, with potential translation of the spinal segments and neurologic injury. As with a combined anteroposterior approach, the endplates above and below should be evened out so they can collapse into bone on bone contact. When the resection is near complete and the posterior vertebral body wall is thin enough, a reverse curette can be used against it to implode this downward into the resected area. The thecal sac can be gently retracted to check the adequacy of resection and the posterior body wall palpated, to identify areas where it has not collapsed. Small fragments of the resected vertebra can be placed in the defect for fusion. Once the surgeon is satisfied with the resection, the temporary rod can be removed, or alternatively, one end of the construct can be released and compression applied to it to correct the angular deformity that had been caused by the hemivertebra. Radiographs should be obtained in AP and lateral views to assess the correction of the focal deformity, of the compensatory curves, of the sagittal alignment, and of the overall truncal balance. The instrumentation and therefore the correction can be adjusted if needed, usually requiring more compression on the side from which the hemivertebra has been resected.

The fusion levels are decorticated with a high-speed burr and/or gouge and resected bone placed over the fusion bed. Wound is closed routinely. Most children undergoing hemivertebra resection have smaller bones, and so supplemental external fixation using a brace or cast may be desirable for up to 6 months, depending upon the age and size of the patient.

Hemivertebra resection has reliably greater correction than fusion alone or hemiepiphysiodesis (15), although with a resultant higher complication rate (6). Not surprisingly, this study also found that more experienced centers performing hemivertebra resections have lower complication rates than those that perform fewer of these procedures. Posteriorly-based hemivertebra resections can have similar outcomes (10,11,12,16). It has been reported that posterior-only hemivertebra resections have lower blood loss, complication rates, and hospital stays than combined surgery (9). However, the significantly longer follow-up period for the combined surgery patients suggests that the surgeons were more experienced during the period of posterior-only surgery and does not account for differences in anesthetic and perioperative management during the time frames compared.

PEARLS AND PITFALLS

1. Overcorrection is preferred to undercorrection. Surgeons tend to judge the amount of correction achieved overly optimistically. However, if the hemivertebra resection is done at an older age where there is not full flexibility of the compensatory curves, undercorrection should be performed to maintain coronal balance.
2. It is not unusual for patients with lumbosacral hemivertebra to have some pelvic asymmetry as well. This asymmetry should be taken into account when planning the amount of correction needed. However, the correction should be planned so that the spine is perpendicular to the floor when corrected, not perpendicular to the pelvis if the pelvis is not horizontal to the floor. Asymmetric growth of an already asymmetric pelvis or lower extremities may affect the coronal balance over time; however, this is less likely to be significant if the spine is coronally balanced after fusion.
3. Beware the development of kyphosis in the uninstrumented case. Casting should be performed in uninstrumented cases with the spine held in lordosis for the lumbar and lumbosacral hemivertebra. When these patients are converted to a brace, maximum lordosis should be applied as well.
4. Although resection of an isolated hemivertebra is more likely to be definitive spinal surgery than fusion for congenital bars or other more complex congenital scoliosis conditions, the patients should still be followed through skeletal maturity to assess for other abnormal or asymmetric growth in the spine.

POSTOPERATIVE MANAGEMENT

The patient is maintained in a double spica cast with the abdomen and chest, as well as perineal area, cut out to allow for proper nutrition and hygiene. The chest tube for thoracic cases can generally be removed in 48 hours and the patient discharged in approximately 5 to 7 days. If internal fixation has not been used, the patient is kept at bed rest for 3 to 4 months, being allowed only to semirecline in a wheelchair or chaise lounge during this period. A local patient is seen in 6 to 8 weeks for repeat radiographs and inspection of the cast for any pressure sores. If a return visit at this time is not possible, radiographs are sent to the surgeon from the patient's hospital for evaluation to ensure there has been maintenance of correction. At the 4-month visit, the patient's cast is removed, radiographs are obtained to ascertain the status of the fusion, and a brace is fabricated, as a body jacket without leg extension, to be worn for an additional 2 to 4 months. If the fusion appears solid at that time, progressive activities can be undertaken. The patient should avoid competitive sports for at least 8 months after surgery.

If internal fixation has been used, then the patient is fitted for a brace shortly after operation. The postoperative activity level permitted should be directly related to the security of fixation. As a general rule, even with internal fixation, we prefer to keep the patient sedentary for 2 to 4 months after surgery in order to ensure solid fusion.

The magnitude of correction is directly related to the level of the deformity and the age of the patient. In general, deformity secondary to a lumbar hemivertebra can be corrected up to 70% to 80%. Certainly 100% is possible. In the thoracic spine, however, we have not found the correction to be as good, although substantial improvement is nonetheless possible. The advantages of the procedure include the fact that correction is obtained over a short segment. Hence, a greater degree of spine flexibility is maintained after this procedure than is possible with standard spinal fusions over multiple segments. It is important to stress to the patient's family, however, that although correction is substantial, it is nonetheless essential to continue monitoring the patient through skeletal maturity, because progression above or below the area of hemivertebra excision is still possible during the stage of active growth. Additional surgery may therefore be necessary in select patients who demonstrate the progression of compensatory curves after hemivertebra excision.

COMPLICATIONS

Complications inherent in hemivertebra excision are similar to those expected with any spinal procedure. Theoretically, there may be a greater risk of neurologic injury as a result of excision. That has not been our experience, however. In fact, transient root injuries have occurred only rarely (7,14), whereas several other series have reported no neurologic deficits (1,4,5,8).

Incomplete correction secondary to inadequate excision or loss of correction may occur and hence is more likely to lead to progressive deformity with growth. Compulsory follow-up with repeat radiographs is therefore essential in order to identify this condition. Should it occur, additional surgery with extension of the fusion and instrumentation may be the treatment of choice.

Pseudoarthrosis may occur after this procedure and is more likely to occur in patients who do not undergo instrumentation. However, adequate cast correction, restricted activities, and continued immobilization until the fusion is solid should prevent this complication.

Junctional kyphosis at the site of hemivertebra excision may occur as the spine drifts into slight sagittal deformity. This may be prevented by internal fixation or postoperative casting in an extension mode to counteract the kyphotic tendency. It is also less likely to occur when the fusion extends posteriorly on the convex side two segments above and two segments below the hemivertebra excision. Finally, it is important to remember that these patients often have multiple congenital anomalies, particularly intrinsic spinal cord pathology. Adequate evaluation with MRI studies of the spine confirms or rules out intrinsic cord pathology, which if present should be addressed and treated before hemivertebra excision.

RECOMMENDED READING

1. Bergoin M, Bollini G, Taibi L, et al.: Excision of hemivertebrae in children with congenital scoliosis. *Ital J Orthop Traumatol* 12: 179–184, 1986.
2. Bradford DS, Boachie-Adjei O: One-stage anterior and posterior hemivertebral resection and arthrodesis for congenital scoliosis. *J Bone Joint Surg Am* 72: 536–540, 1990.
3. Bradford DS, Heithoff KB, Cohen M: Intraspinal abnormalities and congenital spine deformities: a radiographic and MRI study. *J Pediatr Orthop* 11: 36–41, 1991.
4. Carcassonne M, Gregoire A, Hornung H: L'ablation de l'hémi-vertèbre (libre): traitement préventif de la scoliose congénitale. *Chirurgie* 103: 110–115, 1977.
5. Deviren V, Berven S, Smith JA, et al.: Excision of hemivertebra in the management of congenital scoliosis involving the thoracic and thoracolumbar spine. *J Bone Joint Surg Br* 83: 469–500, 2001.
6. Jalanko T, Rintala R, Puisto V, et al.: Hemivertebra resection for congenital scoliosis in young children: comparison of clinical, radiographic, and health-related quality of life outcomes between the anteroposterior and posterolateral approaches. *Spine (Phila PA 1976)* 36(1): 41–49, 2010.
7. Lazar RD, Hall JE: Simultaneous anterior and posterior hemivertebra excision. *Clin Orthop Relat Res* 364: 76–84, 1999.
8. Leatherman KD, Dickson RA: Two-stage corrective surgery for congenital deformities of the spine. *J Bone Joint Surg Br* 61: 324–328, 1979.
9. Mladenov K, Kunkel P, Stuecker R: Hemivertebra resection in children, results after single posterior approach and after combined anterior and posterior approach: a comparative study. *Eur Spine J* 21: 506–513, 2012.
10. Ruf M, Harms J: Hemivertebra resection by a posterior approach innovative operative technique and first results. *Spine (Phila PA 1976)* 27(10): 1116–1123, 2002.
11. Ruf M, Jensen R, Letko L, et al.: Hemivertebra resection and osteotomies in congenital spine deformity. *Spine (Phila PA 1976)* 34(17): 1791–1799, 2009.
12. Shono Y, Abumi K, et al.: One-stage posterior hemivertebra resection and correction using segmental posterior instrumentation. *Spine (Phila PA 1976)* 26(7): 752–757, 2001.

13. Winter RB, Moe JH, Eilers VE: Congenital scoliosis: a study of 234 patients treated and untreated. *J Bone Joint Surg Am* 50: 1–15, 1968.
14. Shono Y, Abumi K, Kaneda K, et al.: Lumbosacral hemivertebrae: a review of twenty-four patients, with excision in eight. *Spine (Phila PA 1976)* 5(3): 234–244, 1980.
15. Yaszay B, O'Brien M, Shufflebarger HL, et al.: Efficacy of hemivertebra resection for congenital scoliosis: a multicenter retrospective comparison of three surgical techniques. *Spine (Phila PA 1976)* 36(24): 2052–2060, 2011.
16. Zhang J, Shengru W, Qiu G, et al.: The efficacy and complications of posterior hemivertebra resection. *Eur Spine J* 20: 1692–1702, 2011.

16 Anterior Thoracolumbar Corpectomy and Stabilization

Thomas A. Zdeblick

INDICATIONS/CONTRAINDICATIONS

Anterior thoracolumbar corpectomy and stabilization is most often indicated for the treatment of trauma or spinal tumors (1–4,6,11). Less frequently, it may be indicated for pseudoarthrosis, chronic instability, disc herniation, or disc degeneration. In rare instances, corpectomy may also be used for the treatment of severe scoliotic spinal deformity; however, this is addressed in a separate chapter.

With trauma, the most common indication is burst fracture with neurologic deficit. Thoracolumbar burst fractures with marked comminution or fractures of both endplates may also be suitable for anterior stabilization (4). Patients with burst fracture malunions and a kyphotic angle exceeding 25 degrees, those with persistent pain, and those with neurologic worsening are also suitable for this procedure. Contraindications in trauma include fracture dislocations or multilevel involvement.

Both metastatic and primary spinal tumors may be treated anteriorly. For metastatic disease, the indication for anterior treatment is one- or two-level vertebral body involvement with pathologic fracture and bone and/or tumor retropulsion that causes canal compromise. Typically, these cases involve neurologic deficit. Obviously, factors such as patient age, concomitant disease, bone quality, and tumor type affect a surgeon's decision to perform corpectomy. Primary tumors are amenable to en bloc excision if they are contained within the vertebral body. En bloc corpectomy is outlined at the conclusion of this chapter.

PREOPERATIVE PREPARATION

Preoperative review of the computed tomography (CT) scan or magnetic resonance imaging (MRI) scan or both is helpful (Figs. 16-1 to 16-4). Unless the pathology is unilateral, I prefer the approach from the left side. This obviates the need to retract the liver. However, the position of the aorta should be visualized on the CT and/or MRI scan. On occasion, the aorta is in a far left-sided position. In these cases, a right-sided approach is preferable. In addition, should anterior stabilization be contemplated, preoperative measurements of the screw or bolt lengths can be obtained from the CT scan. By measuring the width of the vertebral bodies above and below the fractured vertebra on the CT scan template, the surgeon can accurately choose screw length in order to obtain bicortical purchase.

The patient is positioned in the lateral decubitus position (Fig. 16-5). The hips and knees are flexed on the ipsilateral side to relax the psoas muscle. The surgeon should ensure that a true lateral position is obtained. Multiple pillows between the patient's arms or a suspended arm holder for the ipsilateral arm helps maintain the lateral position. I typically utilize gel padding and a beanbag with suction

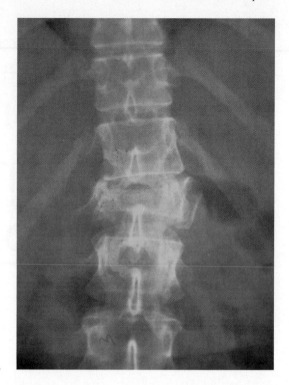

FIGURE 16-1

AP radiograph of an L1 burst fracture.
The widening of the pedicles in the lateral
deformity is visible in this asymmetric fracture.

and wide adhesive tape to maintain position. An axillary roll should be placed just superior to the beanbag. The operative incision can then be marked carefully before the patient is draped. The gibbus deformity and the ribs should be palpated to plan the incision. I generally plan to use the rib two levels above the involved vertebra. However, an anteroposterior (AP) radiograph or fluoroscopy can be used to confirm this. Typically, for an L1 burst fracture, the bed of the eleventh rib is used for access.

TECHNIQUE

An oblique skin incision 4 to 6 inches long is made along the 11th rib (if there is an L1 fracture). This usually extends proximally to the proximal angle of the rib and distally to the tip of the rib. Dissection with cautery is carried out to isolate the eleventh rib. Care should be taken on the inferior

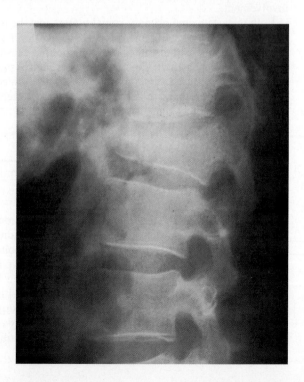

FIGURE 16-2

Lateral radiograph of an L1 burst fracture.
Marked kyphosis, loss of height, and
posterior retropulsion of bone are present.

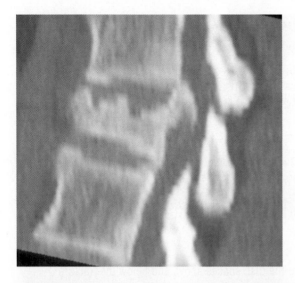

FIGURE 16-3

Sagittal CT scan reconstruction of an L1 burst fracture. The marked comminution of the superior endplate and the severe retropulsion of the "culprit" fragment into the spinal canal are apparent.

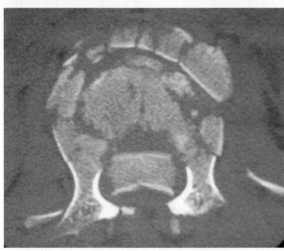

FIGURE 16-4

Axial CT scan of a severe L1 burst fracture; again, the marked comminution of the endplate and the severe retropulsion of the fragment are apparent. The patient had presented with nearly complete motor paralysis below the L1 level.

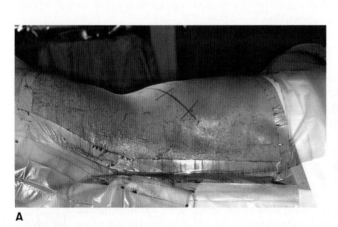

A   B

FIGURE 16-5

A: Intraoperative photograph showing the positioning in the operating room. The patient is in the lateral decubitus position, and in this photograph, the head is to the right and the feet are to the left. An axillary roll has been placed, and the arms are well padded in front of the patient. An oblique incision is marked out along the bed of the eleventh rib. **B:** Photograph showing intraoperative exposure of the lateral aspects of T12, L1, and L2. The diaphragm has been divided near its periphery, and the psoas muscle has been retracted in an anterior-to-posterior direction. The vertebral bodies are exposed anteriorly to the midline and posteriorly back to the lateral aspect of the pedicle. In this photograph, the patient's head is to the right, and the feet are to the left. The stay sutures within the divided diaphragm can be seen at the upper right. The anterior aspect of the vertebral body is at the bottom of the photograph.

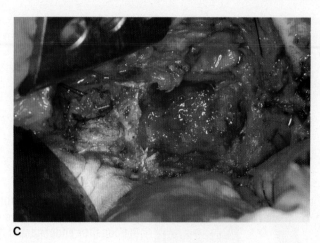

C

FIGURE 16-5 (*Continued*)

C: The corpectomy is performed by first incising the disc spaces above and below the fracture vertebrae. These discs are then removed by using a combination of elevators, curettes, and rongeurs. The corpectomy is performed first with rongeurs and then with a high-speed bur. The final posterior fragments are then removed with a curette. The dura is then seen bulging into the decompression trough. The surgeon needs to ensure that the decompression has been completed across the width of the spinal canal. The dura is visible within the corpectomy defect at the superior aspect of the photograph.

border of the rib to avoid the underlying neurovascular bundle. It is then subperiosteally exposed and divided at its proximal angle. Distally, it is divided near its cartilaginous juncture. The surgeon then enters the pleural cavity by sharply dividing the pleura along the bed of the rib. The superior surface of the diaphragm is easily visualized. Blunt dissection can be carried out near the cartilaginous distal tip of the 11th rib. With blunt dissection, the retroperitoneal space is entered just beneath the diaphragm. This plane can then be developed bluntly with sponge sticks. Once both superior and inferior surfaces of the diaphragm are well visualized, the diaphragm should be marked with cautery at points approximately 2 cm from its periphery, along the chest wall. I then divide the diaphragm with cautery along this line and between multiple stay sutures. As the division proceeds medially, the crus of the diaphragm is encountered and is divided from its spinal origin using cautery. The surgeon should then be able to place self-retaining rib retractors, and visualization of the lateral aspects of the T12, L1, and L2 vertebral bodies is possible.

Alternatively, only the posterior 4 to 6 cm of the diaphragm can be divided and the remaining diaphragm retracted. Care needs to be taken to place a suture at the apex of the diaphragmatic division to prevent propagation.

At this point, a radiograph is obtained with spinal needles placed in the disc space above and below the suspected pathology. Often, this pathology is obvious secondary to hematoma or deformity. After radiographic confirmation, the pleura overlying the vertebral bodies of T11 to L1 is divided vertically, and the segmental vessels overlying T11, T12, and L1 are isolated. I prefer to isolate these vessels by using cautery to incise in a parallel manner above and below the segmental vessels down to bone. A fine right-angled clamp is then passed beneath each segmental vessel, and each vessel is ligated. Typically, ligation is performed with silk ties, metallic clips, or both. Each of the segmentals overlying each of the three vertebral bodies is then divided. It is important to ligate these vessels in the midportion of the vertebral bodies. This allows the intersegmental anastomoses, which are present posteriorly and provide blood flow to the spinal cord, to remain intact.

Once the segmental vessels are divided, subperiosteal dissection is carried out along the lateral aspects of the vertebral body above and below the pathology. It is important to make sure that the vertebral body is exposed to the anterior midline. The anterior longitudinal ligament can be lifted off the vertebral body using a sharp elevator and cautery. Bleeding points from the vertebral body itself can be controlled with bone wax. Posteriorly, the lateral aspect of the vertebral body needs to be exposed to the lateral aspect of the pedicle. At this point, the foramen should be palpable with a Penfield elevator. Proximal to T11, this exposure may require resection of the rib head overlying the disc space. At L1 and below, it requires retraction of the psoas muscle in an anterior-to-posterior direction. With L1 fractures, this is not usually difficult. However, with fractures in the midlumbar spine, retraction of the psoas muscle can become quite difficult. It is important to begin at the anterior margin of the psoas muscle and work along the vertebral body, retracting this muscle posteriorly.

This method protects the nerve roots, which run within the psoas muscle. In rare cases, a portion of the anterior psoas muscle may be divided using cautery if visualization is inadequate. However, this must be done carefully to protect the nerve roots within.

Exposure of the involved vertebra is performed after exposure of the vertebral bodies above and below is complete. Once again, the midline should be exposed anteriorly, and exposure should continue posteriorly to the vertebral foramen. In cases of tumor involvement, this may be difficult because of the weakening of the surrounding bone. However, orientation to the foramen helps the surgeon locate the spinal canal. In difficult cases, it may be advantageous to find the lateral aspect of the pedicle of the involved vertebra and remove this with a Kerrison punch. This allows the surgeon to visualize the exiting nerve root and more easily locate the dural sac.

Once exposure is complete, the discs are removed above and below the pathology. This is done by incising the lateral annulus with a no. 10 blade all the way to the anterior midline. A fine sharp Cobb elevator can then be passed between the endplate and the disc to separate disc from the intact endplate. This maneuver is more difficult along the fractured endplate. The disc can then be removed by using a combination of curettes and pituitary rongeurs. Typically, the contralateral disc annulus is left intact. In cases of chronic kyphotic deformity, the entire anterior and contralateral annulus, as well as the anterior longitudinal ligament, needs to be incised with a no. 10 blade to release the deformity.

Once the discectomies are complete, the corpectomy is begun. I typically use a large rongeur to begin removing the vertebral body that is fractured. This is done in a piecemeal manner, and the fracture fragments are saved for later use as bone graft. A trough in the central and anterior portion of the vertebral body is created by removing these bone fragments. This trough is deepened down to the contralateral cortex of the vertebral body. The depth of this trough across the vertebral body can be estimated from the preoperative CT scan. The trough is complete when only a thin shell of bone anteriorly and on the contralateral side is remaining. At this point, only the posterior retropulsed fracture fragments and the attached disc annulus remain. As the posterior cortex is approached, bleeding from the basivertebral sinus is often seen.

The decompression of the spinal canal is performed by removing the retropulsed fracture fragments. This can be done by first thinning these fragments with a high-speed burr; I prefer a 5-mm ball-tipped burr. Then, a fine, sharp, long curette is used to peel the fragment away from the dura and into the created trough. This gives the surgeon a landing area in which to peel the retropulsed fragment. Care must be taken to protect the aorta at this step. The fragments are sequentially removed from the spinal canal using a combination of curettes and pituitary rongeurs (Fig. 16-6). There typically is a great deal of epidural bleeding at this step, and the surgeon must work rapidly and control bleeding by using thrombin-soaked sponges. Typically, the posterior longitudinal ligament is torn, and the decompression continues to the dura. The most difficult portion is where the retropulsed fragment remains attached to the posterior annulus of the superior disc. These attachments are tenacious, and sharp dissection is necessary to divide the annular attachments. It is advisable to remove the posterior cortical fragments from the contralateral (deep) side of the spinal canal first. This way, as the dura bulges into the decompression trough, it will not obscure the remainder of the retropulsed fragments.

The decompression is adequate when the dura can be seen bulging into the corpectomy trough across the entire width of the spinal canal. The surgeon can check this by palpating the pedicle on the opposite side from within the spinal canal. This is done with a fine no. 4 Penfield elevator. Finally, the intact endplates are prepared. This is performed first with a curette, all endplate cartilage being removed from the inferior endplate of T12 and the superior endplate of L2. A burr is then used to lightly decorticate these endplates but not to remove them or puncture them. Ideally, the endplates should be prepared so that they are flat. The surgeon is then ready to perform the reduction and stabilization maneuvers. Alternatively, with some fixation systems, fixation bolts may be applied first, before reduction.

Kyphosis is reduced manually. The prime reduction maneuver is to manually push on the apex of the kyphosis overlying the spinous processes. The surgeon's assistant can use a fist for this maneuver. Concomitantly, a vertebral body distracter can be placed between the vertebral endplates of T12 and L2. This should be done anteriorly near the midline. This combination of maneuvers should reduce the kyphosis until the endplates of T12 and L2 are parallel (Fig. 16-7). A distractor placed against the bolt heads, if present, can be used to hold the reduction. Alternatively, an expandable cage may be utilized to assist in reduction. At that point, a caliper is used to measure the distance between the endplates. A bone strut or cage can now be prepared to the exact length. Typically, the bone strut is filled with cancellous bone, which has been harvested from the broken vertebra and the rib. My preference is to use allograft humerus or femur, although titanium mesh, carbon fiber, or PEEK cages have also been used successfully. The strut is impacted with a bone tamp. Care should be taken to control tilting during insertion and to place the strut as far as possible across the vertebral column. Once the cage or strut is fit in place, the distracter can be removed, and the reduction is then held in place by the strut (Fig. 16-8).

The stabilization of the vertebral body above and below depends on the exact instrumentation system used. Most stabilization systems involve either a bolt-and-plate combination or bolt-and-dual-rod

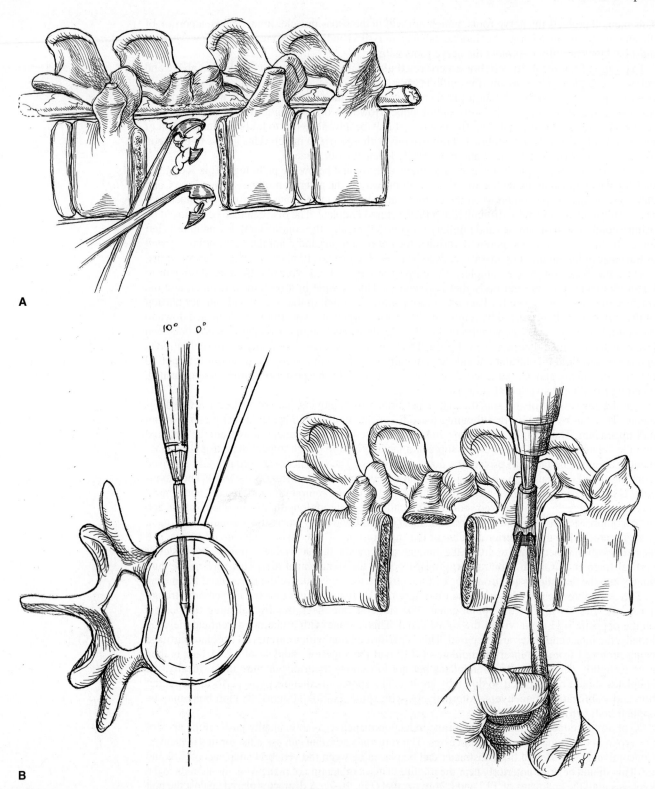

FIGURE 16-6

A: Drawing showing the corpectomy. A curette is used to remove the final culprit fragment from within the spinal canal. The vertebral endplates are then lightly prepared with a high-speed bur into flat parallel surfaces. **B:** Once the corpectomy is complete, fixation can be initiated. I prefer to use a plate-and-bolt system (Z-plate). However, other anterolateral fixation systems are available. A surgeon should consult specific technique manuals for specific instrumentation systems. Bolt placement is performed first. I prefer a starting point for the bolts that is posterior and near the endplate furthest from the corpectomy site. This bolt is angled from 0 to 10 degrees away from the spinal canal. The bolt should engage both cortices. Bolt lengths can be obtained preoperatively from the computed tomography scan.

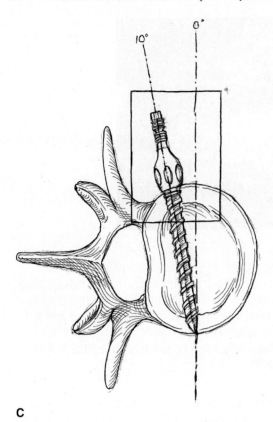

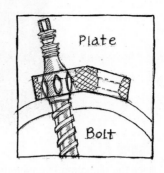

C

FIGURE 16-6
(*Continued*)

C: Drawing demonstrating the appropriate position of the posterior bolt.

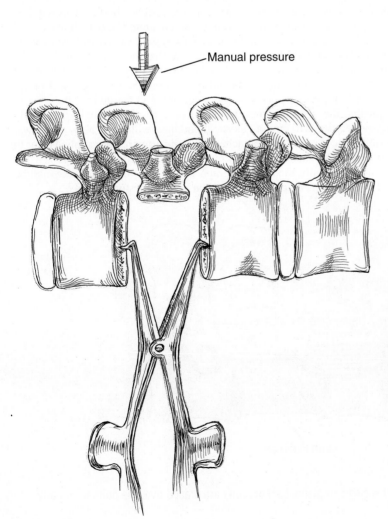

Manual pressure

FIGURE 16-7

Once the bolts are in place, reduction of the fracture can be performed. This is done predominately by the surgeon's assistant, who places manual pressure over the apex of the kyphosis posteriorly. In addition, a vertebral body distractor can be placed along the endplates anteriorly near the midline. This combination of maneuvers can reduce the fracture in terms of both height and kyphosis.

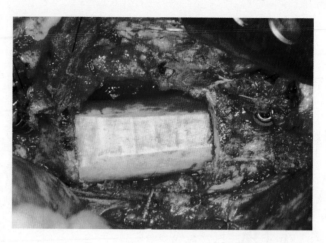

FIGURE 16-8

Once the reduction is complete, it is maintained by placement of bone graft. I prefer humerus or femur allograft. This is cut to length, and the edges are smoothed with a bur. The site may be filled with bone that has been removed from the corpectomy site or from the rib. While the reduction is maintained, this graft is impacted into place. Maintenance of reduction can be performed with a distraction device placed along the bolts. This photograph shows the spine reduced and with an allograft strut in place. Care should be taken so that the dura can be visualized to ensure that no dural compression has been caused by the bone graft.

combination. Single-rod systems have not been stable enough to use with thoracolumbar fractures. Before bolt placement, the lateral aspects of the vertebral body of T12 and L2 should be smoothed ("gardened") so that the plate fits snugly along the lateral aspect of the vertebral bodies. This requires removal of the lateral endplates near the strut graft, as well as the creation of a trough above and below the bolts, near the intact disc annulus above and below. This is to create room for the plate. The bolts are then placed across the vertebral body. It is imperative that the patient remain in the lateral position so that the surgeon is oriented with regard to the vertebral body. The posterior bolt should be placed directly perpendicular to the floor to avoid penetrating the spinal canal. I prefer a screw pattern with the superior bolt placed superiorly and anteriorly and the inferior bolt placed inferior and posteriorly. Typically, the anterior screw is placed at a 15-degree angle posteriorly toward the posterior bolt. My preference is to obtain bicortical purchase with these bolts or screws.

The plate or dual-rod fixation devices can now be attached and mild compression applied prior to final tightening (Figs. 16-9 to 16-14). AP and lateral radiographs are taken intraoperatively to ensure graft placement and plate placement. Ideally, the AP radiograph should show the graft in the midline or even near the contralateral pedicle. This helps prevent angular settling postoperatively.

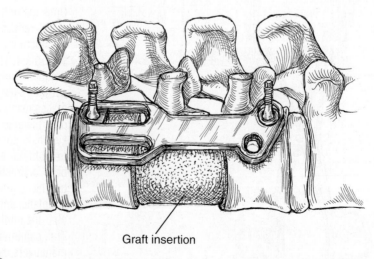

Graft insertion

FIGURE 16-9

The plate may be placed and secured in place. Locking nuts are placed over the bolts to initially lock the plate in place.

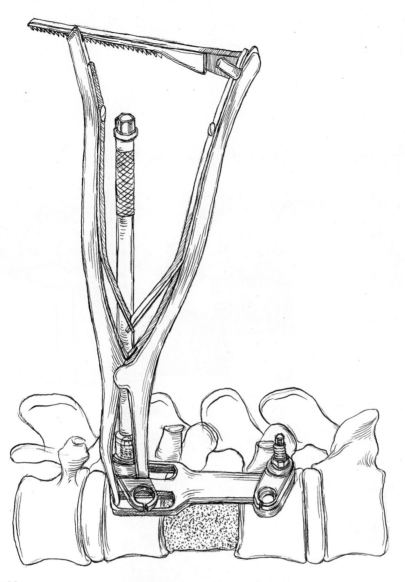

FIGURE 16-10

The graft may be compressed by use of the single-handed compression device. Once the graft is compressed, final tightening of the locking nuts is performed.

Once films are complete, the surgeon should ensure that there are no prominent areas that might affect local vascular structures. The wound is then closed over a chest tube placed in the chest cavity. The diaphragm is repaired first, usually with a running suture as well as the interrupted stay sutures. I use a resorbable no. 1 suture. Rib-to-rib approximation is then carried out with a large nonresorbable suture, followed by a separate layered closure of the intercostal, serratus, and latissimus muscle layers and the skin. Postoperatively, an orthotic brace is fit after chest tube removal. Ambulation is progressively increased, and the brace is worn for 6 to 8 weeks (Figure 16-15A–C).

RESULTS

Many authors have shown that the results of primary anterior decompression and stabilization offer benefits in terms of neurologic recovery (1,2,5,7,8,10). Kaneda et al. reported a 95% rate of neurologic improvement of at least one Frankel grade (7,8). Zdeblick et al. showed that in patients with an incomplete neurologic deficit, 100% had at least one grade of neurologic improvement (5). In this series, the rate of complication was low; only 3% of patients required additional posterior instrumentation, and final radiologic results showed an improvement of mean kyphotic angle from 18 to 6 degrees. Thus, there do appear to be certain real advantages in the use of the anterior approach for the treatment of thoracolumbar burst fractures, particularly in patients with preoperative neurologic deficit.

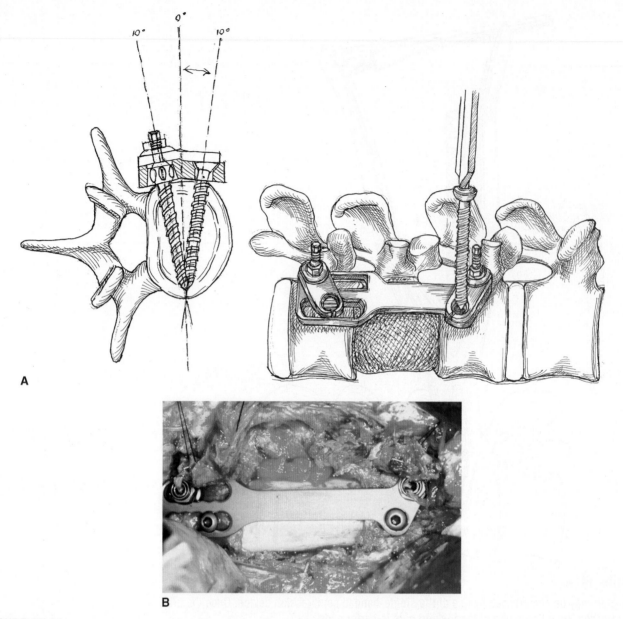

FIGURE 16-11

A: The anterior screws are placed. These are at a 10-degree angle toward the spinal canal, thus forming a triangulation pattern between the bolt and the screw. The screw should also engage the opposite cortex. Typically, the screw is 5 mm longer than the bolt. **B:** Final position of the plate and graft in an intraoperative photograph. Gelfoam (Pharmacia & Upjohn) has been placed overlying the dura. Additional graft may be placed anterior to the strut graft if space is available.

COMPLICATIONS

Inadequate exposure is a common complication. The surgeon must choose the appropriate rib level to work through so that he or she works directly on the involved vertebral body. If the spine surgeon is not performing the actual approach, he or she should be present during the approach to ensure adequate visualization. Inadequate exposure might also lead to placement of the fixation devices too anteriorly on the vertebral bodies. This could lead to impingement of vascular structures. The surgeon must ensure that the complete lateral aspect of the vertebral body is exposed posteriorly to the neural foramen, allowing lateral placement of fixation hardware.

Inadequate decompression occurs when retropulsed fragments are left within the spinal canal. The surgeon can ensure adequate decompression by palpating across the spinal canal to feel the medial edge of the contralateral pedicle. The decompression should also extend superiorly to the edge of the superior intact endplate and inferiorly to the edge of the inferior intact endplate.

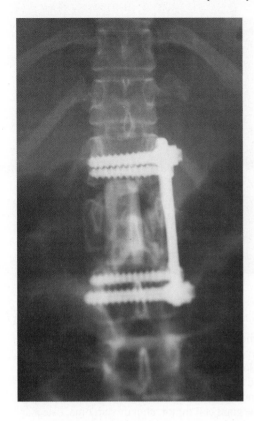

FIGURE 16-12

Postoperative anteroposterior radiograph with plate, screws, bolts, and graft. Note the reduction of the angular deformity. Note also the bicortical purchase of screws and bolts. If possible, the strut graft should be placed centrally or to the side opposite the plate.

Intraoperative imaging, including axial tomography, may be helpful in determining adequacy of decompression.

Postoperative instability occurs with inadequate strut grafting or poor fixation (10). Strut grafts must be substantial in size and have adequate weight-bearing surfaces both superiorly and inferiorly. Thin grafts, such as fibula or rib grafts, are inappropriate for use in thoracolumbar corpectomies. With osteoporotic bone, intraoperative vertebroplasty should be performed before screw or bolt placement. This greatly enhances the vertebral body fixation and helps prevent postoperative hardware failure.

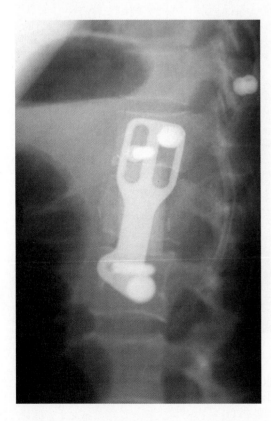

FIGURE 16-13

Postoperative lateral radiograph with plate and graft in place. Note the reduction of the kyphotic deformity and return of the spine to a neutral position.

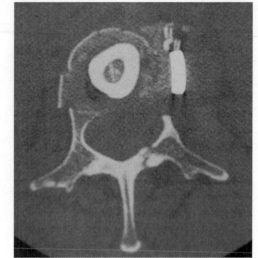

FIGURE 16-14

Postoperative computed tomography scan showing the decompression of the spinal canal, the central placement of the strut graft, and the lateral placement of the plate. In order to avoid any potential for vascular complications, the plate, bolts, and screws must be placed on the lateral, not the anterior, aspect of the spinal column.

En Bloc Corpectomy

For cases of primary vertebral body tumor, the best chance at a curative resection is to perform an en bloc vertebral body resection. This implies that the entire vertebral body is removed as a single structure, without violating its periphery. In order to do this, careful preoperative staging and planning must be performed. CT scanning and MRI are advisable to ensure that the tumor is contained within the vertebral body margins. Usually, the diagnosis will have been made by needle biopsy. Tumors most amenable to this type of resection include giant cell tumor, chondrosarcoma, osteosarcoma, and chordoma.

A posterior spinal approach is performed first. Under fluoroscopic guidance, pedicle screws are placed in the pedicles two levels above and below the involved vertebra. A wide laminectomy of

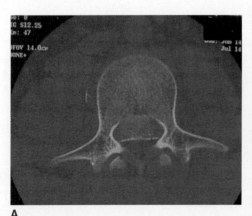

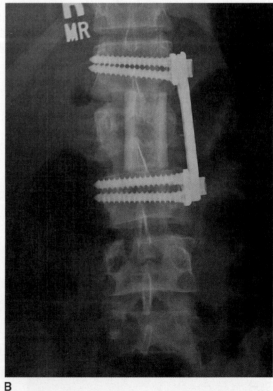

A   B

FIGURE 16-15

A: Axial CT image showing burst fracture with significant canal compromise from retropulsed bone.
B: AP image postoperatively showing fixation with lateral plate/staple/screw construct.

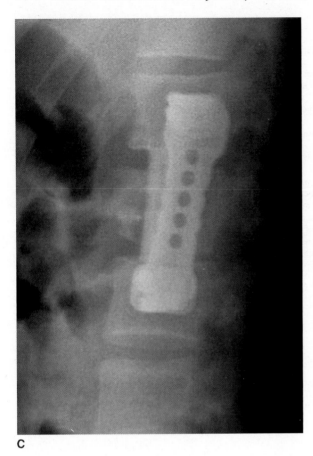

FIGURE 16-15 (*Continued*)

C: Lateral image postoperatively showing fixation with lateral plate/staple/screw construct postoperatively showing fixation with lateral plate/staple/screw construct.

C

the involved vertebra is then performed in a standard manner. Wide exposure is required so that the pedicles at the involved level can be adequately visualized. By gently retracting the dura side to side, all epidural vessels anterior to the dura are coagulated using bipolar cautery. A no. 15 blade is then used to incise the posterior longitudinal ligament and the posterior disc annulus at the levels above and below the involved vertebral body. This incision must extend to the midline on either side so that a continuous posterior incision of the disc is performed. On the right side, this disc annulus incision should extend as far laterally as possible. Facetectomy is usually necessary to expose this lateral annulus. Discectomy can then be performed through this lateral transforaminal exposure to remove as much of the posterior and right-sided lateral disc material as possible. Care should be taken not to violate the involved vertebral endplates.

The pedicles of the involved vertebral body then need to be resected at their base. This can be done either with a fine Gigli saw or in a piecemeal manner using rongeurs and a high-speed bur. Care should be taken to protect the nerve root during pedicle resection. The transverse process on the right side can also be resected at this time. A fair amount of bleeding occurs during pedicle and transverse process resection and is controlled with bipolar cautery and thrombin-soaked sponges.

Posterior spinal fixation is then completed by placing longitudinal rods between the pedicle screws above and below the resection site. A single crosslink is usually placed centrally to insure torsional stability. The fixation is tightened, and the posterior wound is then closed in layers.

The patient is turned to the lateral position, and an extensile left-sided lateral exposure of the spine is performed. This exposure proceeds much as has been outlined previously in this chapter. Once the segmental vessels have been ligated at the involved level, as well as above and below, dissection proceeds anteriorly around the vertebral bodies. Using a combination of Cobb elevators and sponge dissectors, the surgeon elevates the segmental vessels off the contralateral aspect of the vertebral body. If possible, this vessel should be ligated far on its contralateral side. The disc spaces above and below the involved vertebra are then incised with a no. 10 blade laterally and anteriorly. The anterior longitudinal ligament is divided, and the contralateral lateral annulus is divided from within the disc space. Finally, dissection of the contralateral psoas muscle off the vertebral body is performed with sharp elevators. The entire vertebral body can then be rolled away from the spinal canal. Epidural adhesions are transected bluntly, and attachments along the epidural posterior longitudinal ligament are dissected sharply. In this manner, the vertebral body can be rolled away from the spinal canal and removed in its entirety. Strut grafting and plate placement then proceed as previously outlined.

RECOMMENDED READING

1. Bradford DS, McBride GG: Surgical management of thoracolumbar spine fractures with incomplete neurologic deficits. *Clin Orthop* 218: 201–216, 1987.
2. Dunn HK: Anterior stabilization of thoracolumbar injuries. *Clin Orthop* 189: 116–124, 1984.
3. Esses SI, Botsford DJ, Kostuik JP: Evaluation of surgical treatment for burst fractures. *Spine* 15: 667–673, 1990.
4. Gaines RW Jr, Carson WL, Satterlee CC, et al.: Experimental evaluation of seven different spinal fracture internal fixation devices using nonfailure stability testing. The load-sharing and unstable-mechanism concepts. *Spine* 16: 902–909, 1991.
5. Ghanayem A, Zdeblick T: Anterior instrumentation in the management of thoracolumbar burst fractures. *Clin Orthop* 335: 89–99, 1997.
6. Hitchon PW, Torner JC, Haddad SF, et al.: Management options in thoracolumbar burst fractures. *Surg Neurol* 49: 619–626, 1998; discussion 626–627.
7. Kaneda K, Abumi K, Fujiya M: Burst fractures with neurologic deficits of the thoracolumbar-lumbar spine. Results of anterior decompression and stabilization with anterior instrumentation. *Spine* 9: 788–795, 1984.
8. Kaneda K, Taneichi H, Abumi K, et al.: Anterior decompression and stabilization with the Kaneda device for thoracolumbar burst fractures associated with neurologic deficits. *J Bone Joint Surg Am* 79: 69–83, 1997.
9. Okuyama K, Abe E, Chiba M, et al.: Outcome of anterior decompression and stabilization for thoracolumbar unstable burst fractures in the absence of neurologic deficits. *Spine* 21: 620–625, 1996.
10. Schnee CL, Ansell LV: Selection criteria and outcome of operative approaches for thoracolumbar burst fractures with and without neurological deficit. *J Neurosurg* 86: 48–55, 1997.

17 Anterior Thoracoscopic Discectomy

Thomas A. Zdeblick

INDICATIONS/CONTRAINDICATIONS

The primary indication for anterior thoracoscopic discectomy is disc herniation. The ideal indication for discectomy is myelopathy with cord compression caused by a central or lateral soft disc herniation. On occasion, discectomy is indicated for unremitting radicular or intercostal neuritic pain. The outcomes of discectomy, or discectomy plus fusion, for back pain alone are less certain. Hard discs, calcified discs, or lateral spurs may also cause myeloradiculopathy and may be amenable to anterior decompression (1,2,4,9). Other rare indications include débridement for disc space infection, vertebral body biopsy, and, on occasion, interbody fusion performed for pseudoarthrosis or degenerative disc disease (5,6). For conditions that necessitate corpectomy, I now perform a minithoracotomy with thoracoscopic assistance.

An absolute contraindication to thoracoscopic discectomy is the inability to tolerate single-lung ventilation (7). This may be present in older patients with interstitial lung disease or chronic obstructive pulmonary disease. Relative contraindications include previous thoracotomy, pleuritis, or pleurisy. Spinal levels that are amenable to thoracoscopic approach range from T3 to T11. However, this approach is more difficult at lower thoracic levels because retraction of the diaphragm and, on occasion, diaphragmatic division are required. Upper thoracic levels are difficult to reach if more than a simple release is required.

Technique

The side of pathology usually dictates whether the approach is right or left sided. With central herniations, I prefer a right-sided approach. The patient is positioned in the lateral decubitus position on a gel pad and beanbag. The ipsilateral arm is placed on an arm holder and extended superiorly (Fig. 17-1). Intubation with a double-lumen tube is a requirement. Bronchial blockers are usually not sufficient to maintain single-lung ventilation. To improve visualization, I usually roll the patient forward approximately 10 to 15 degrees (Fig. 17-2). This lets the lung fall slightly away from the vertebral column.

Fluoroscopy is utilized for initial portal placement. Three or four portals are typically utilized (Fig. 17-3). My preference is to use a posterior portal that is placed in the midaxillary line directly over the level of pathology and two anterior portals that are placed at the anterior axillary line (3,8). Usually, one of these is placed in line with the pathology, and the other is placed approximately two levels superiorly. This anterosuperior portal is typically placed first to avoid any chance of injuring the diaphragm. A 1-inch oblique skin incision is made just between the ribs, and sharp dissection is carried down to the intercostal muscle layer. Cautery is then utilized to make the initial division of the intercostal muscles. The ipsilateral lung is deflated, and the chest cavity is entered with a blunt clamp. A soft portal is placed in this anterior location. Thoracoscopic portals are typically 10 mm in diameter. Valves are not necessary. Each portal is placed using a blunt introducer. The remaining two or three portals can then be placed under direct vision, using the endoscope placed within the pleural cavity. After the skin incision, the approach to these portals is performed completely with cautery,

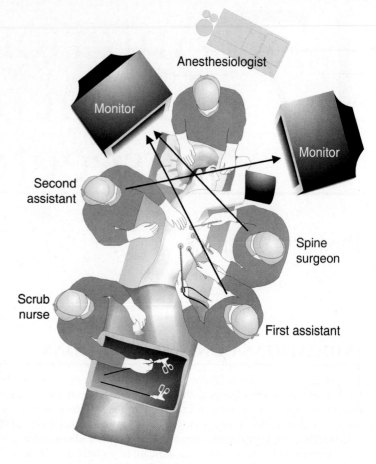

FIGURE 17-1

The patient is positioned in the lateral decubitus position. Care should be taken to pad both elbows well. Both the surgeon and the assistant stand at the abdominal side of the patient with the monitor directly across from them. This makes visualization and orientation easiest.

and I visualize the cautery coming through the pleura. Care should be taken that there is adequate space between the three portals in order to prevent "fencing." In general, each portal should be at least 2 to 3 inches from the next nearest portal.

Usually, the lung can be retracted anteriorly using a fan retractor. Often, it stays in this retracted position, and the fan can be removed. However, if the lung does not fully deflate or remains an obstruction, a fourth portal can be placed anteriorly and inferiorly for the use of the fan retractor.

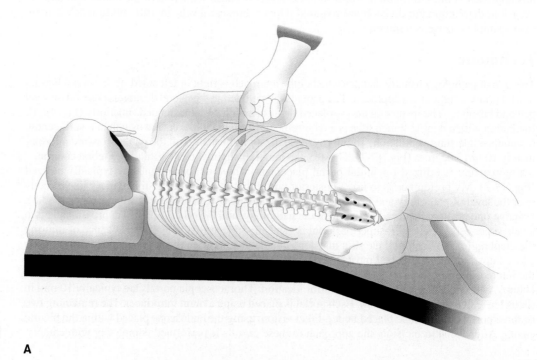

FIGURE 17-2

A,B: The table is usually tilted 20 to 30 degrees toward the surgeon. This allows the lung to fall forward away from the spine.

A

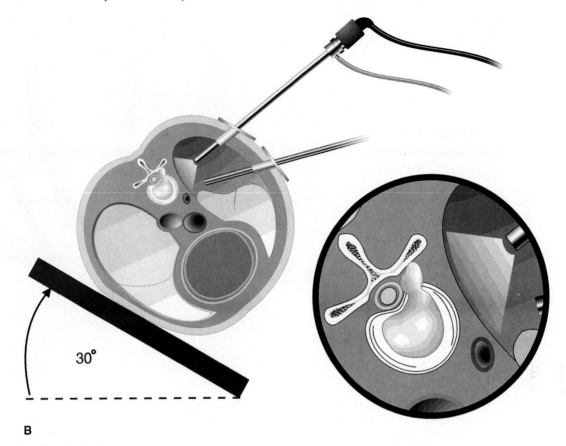

B

FIGURE 17-2 (*Continued*)

Both the surgeon and the assistant typically stand on the ventral aspect of the patient (Fig. 17-1). They can then look directly across at a monitor, which helps with orientation. The initial step is to palpate the involved disc space and confirm its level. Confirming the level of thoracic disc herniations is one of the most important aspects of this procedure. Of course, the pathologic level must first be accurately noted on a full sagittal magnetic resonance image, counted from C2. The intraoperative

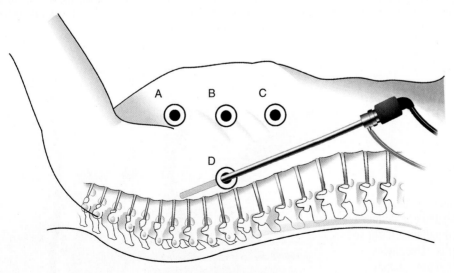

FIGURE 17-3

Three or four portholes are typically used for thoracoscopic discectomy. The central porthole (*B*) should be placed directly in line with the disc space to be operated upon and is usually placed under fluoroscopic guidance. If instrumentation is being performed, the more posterior porthole should also be placed centrally, directly above the operated disc space (*D*). Each porthole should be separated by 2 to 3 inches from the neck to avoid "fencing."

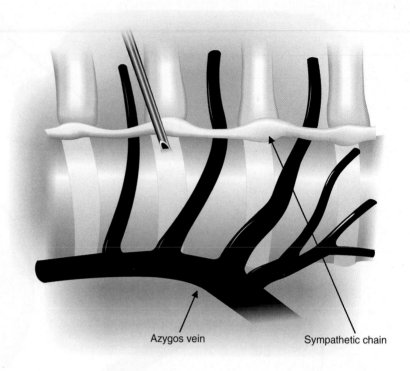

FIGURE 17-4

The surgeon should localize the disc space intraoperatively by placing a K-wire in the disc space through the central porthole. Fluoroscopy can then be utilized to count the space from both superiorly and inferiorly. Alternatively, the surgeon may, from inside the chest cavity, count the ribs.

Azygos vein

Sympathetic chain

level can be counted in three ways. A long K-wire is placed through the posterior portal into the disc space (Fig. 17-4). Anteroposterior (AP) fluoroscopy is then used to count up from the 12th rib. Similarly, lateral fluoroscopy can be used to count up from the 12th rib. In addition, the surgeon can count from within the thoracic cavity, beginning from the first rib and counting down. The first rib is usually partially covered by the subclavian artery. It should be remembered that the disc space is covered by the head of the rib just below (e.g., the eighth rib head covers the T7–T8 disc space).

Once the appropriate rib space has been localized, a hook cautery is utilized to make a vertical incision in the pleura overlying the vertebral bodies above and below the disc space. This pleural incision is then extended in a T-shaped manner posteriorly over the head of the rib. Approximately 2 to 3 cm of the proximal rib is then exposed subperiosteally by means of cautery. Cautery is also utilized to expose the vertebral bodies just above and below the disc space. For a discectomy, I do not typically ligate the segmental vessels above or below the disc space. However, with a small vertebral body or large segmental vessels, ligation may be necessary (Fig. 17-5). This would be carried out with right-angled Ligaclips (Ethicon, Inc., Somerville, NJ).

Segmental vessels

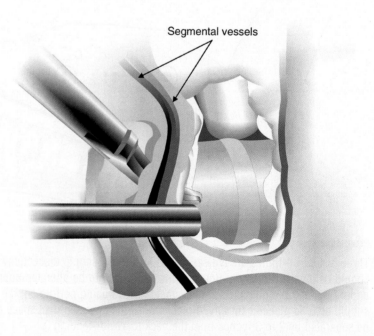

FIGURE 17-5

On occasion, the segmental vessels need to be ligated and divided. In small patients, in those with large osteophytes, or when more extensive decompression is required, segmental ligation is necessary. This is done with a fine right-angled clamp, Ligaclips, and bipolar cautery.

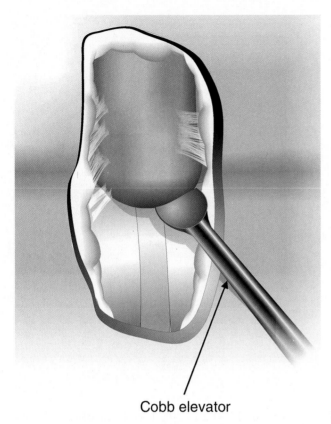

Cobb elevator

FIGURE 17-6

The proximal 1 to 2 cm of the rib needs to be isolated by cautery and sharp curettage. The costovertebral ligaments are strong and need to be sharply divided. The head of the rib overlies the disc space.

A hook cautery and a thoracoscopic Cobb elevator are then utilized to expose the rib head and divide the costovertebral ligaments (Fig. 17-6). The rib is then divided approximately 2 cm from its proximal end using a long Kerrison-style rib cutter. Alternatively, the rib can be divided with a high-speed bur. This proximal piece of rib is then removed (Fig. 17-7). Often there are tenacious ligamentous attachments between the rib head and the vertebral body. These must be sectioned sharply, typically with cautery or an angled curette. This portion of the rib is saved for later use as bone graft.

Once the rib head is removed, the posterior margins of the vertebral body are exposed using cautery and an elevator. For difficult cases, the exposure can be extended further posteriorly along the lateral aspect of the pedicle of both the upper and lower vertebral bodies (Fig. 17-8). If needed, a Kerrison rongeur can be used to resect the pedicle of the superior vertebra, exposing the exiting nerve root and orienting the surgeon to the location of the spinal canal. However, some epidural

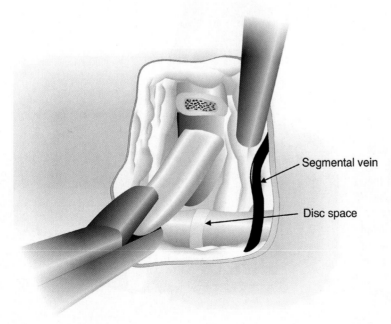

Segmental vein

Disc space

FIGURE 17-7

Once exposed, this proximal 1 to 2 cm of rib head is removed. The rib can be divided using either a Kerrison punch or a high-speed bur. This bone can be saved for later use as bone graft if a fusion procedure is being performed. Bleeding beneath the rib head can be controlled with bipolar cautery.

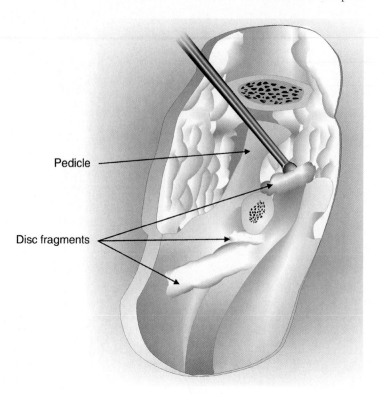

FIGURE 17-8

Once the rib head is removed, the disc space is entered with a no. 15 blade, a central discectomy is performed, and the posterior margin of the endplates of the vertebral bodies is resected using a high-speed bur. For orientation, the posterior corners of the endplates and the superior margin of the pedicle should be isolated.

bleeding should be expected after this maneuver (Fig. 17-9). Bleeding is typically controlled with thrombin-soaked sponges. Once the disc space is delineated with cautery, it is incised with a no. 15 blade. An initial discectomy of the central portion of the disc can be performed using pituitary rongeurs. I then use a high-speed bur to resect bone on either side of the endplate, on both sides of the disc space. This is performed approximately 3 to 4 mm on either side of the disc space and deepened to approximately 20 mm. The exact depth of this trough can be determined preoperatively from the computed tomography scan and/or magnetic resonance imaging scan. It should be deep enough to decompress the spinal canal for the entire width of the pathology. Once this trough is deepened in the central portion of the vertebra, the endplates can be resected with rongeurs or curettes, leaving only the posterior margin of the disc and the posterior endplate above and below the disc.

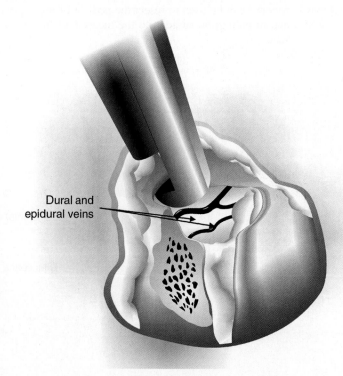

FIGURE 17-9

The dura can be visualized with partial resection of the superior aspect of the pedicle of the level below. This entails some epidural bleeding that can be controlled with thrombin-soaked sponges. The posterior corner of the vertebral bodies can then be visualized, or, typically, herniated fragments or osteophytes are located.

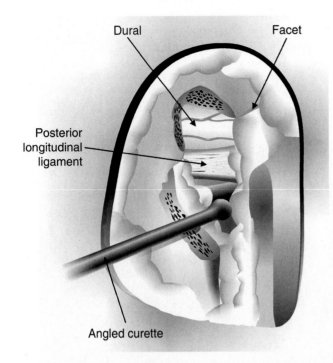

Dural   Facet

Posterior
longitudinal
ligament

Angled curette

FIGURE 17-10

The posterior endplates, osteophytes, and herniated disc fragments can then be safely removed
using fine-angled 3-0 curettes.
These fragments should be pulled
away from the dura with the curette,
which should land in the trough
created by the discectomy.

A high-speed bur is then used to carefully thin the posterior wall of the vertebral bodies above and below the disc space until only a thin shell of cortical bone remains. Curettes are used to peel this posterior cortex, as well as the posterior annulus of the disc, into the previously created trough. Fine curettes are utilized to remove the remaining aspects of the posterior longitudinal ligament, posterior annulus, and herniated or calcified fragments (Fig. 17-10). An angled curette or a long nerve hook can be utilized to continue to probe to retrieve any extruded fragments. The dura is then usually visualized, bulging into the decompression trough (Fig. 17-11). Most thoracoscopic instruments are marked with depth measurements so that the surgeon knows how far across the spinal canal the decompression has proceeded.

For lateral disc herniations, fusion is not usually required. However, if a large trough has been created or for central decompressions, a fusion is indicated. I typically utilize a titanium mesh or PEEK

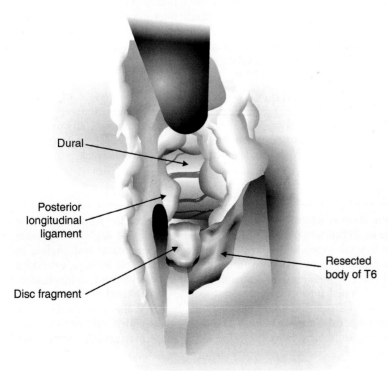

Dural

Posterior
longitudinal
ligament

Disc fragment

Resected
body of T6

FIGURE 17-11

After decompression, the
dura should be well visualized. Whether a fusion
needs to be performed is
dependent on how much
of the bony endplates was
resected. When more than
one-third of the endplates
are resected, I prefer to
perform a simple inter-
body fusion.

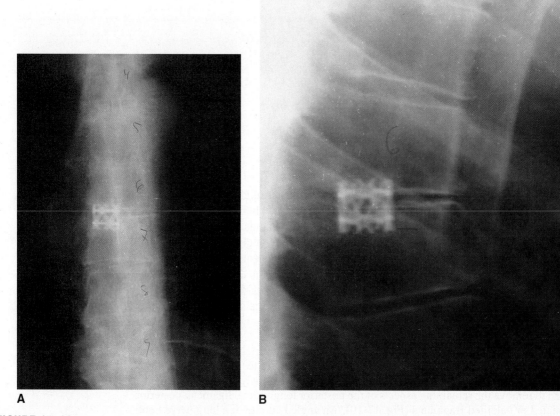

A   B

FIGURE 17-12

AP **(A)** and lateral radiographs **(B)** after thoracoscopic discectomy for myelopathy. Extensive bone resection was required, and a simple cage interbody fusion was therefore performed. The patient made a full recovery, and this radiograph was taken 6 months after surgery.

cage. This cage is filled with bone from the rib head and then impacted into the disc space. There should be a snug fit both superiorly and inferiorly into the vertebral bodies (Fig. 17-12). Remaining bone can then be packed anterior to the cage. Finally, AP and lateral fluoroscopic views are obtained to ensure acceptable cage placement. A chest tube is then placed through the most posterior portal site and secured. Each of the portals is then removed, and each incision is closed with a nonabsorbable suture in the intercostal muscle layer and with a subcutaneous suture.

POSTOPERATIVE MANAGEMENT

The chest tube is left to suction for 36 to 48 hours. Chest radiographs are obtained daily to ensure that there is no pneumothorax. If a fusion was performed, the patient is placed in a Jewett extension brace. Hospital discharge is usually on the 3rd or 4th day. The brace is used for 6 weeks.

COMPLICATIONS

The most devastating complication is neurologic deficit from contusion of the spinal cord. The surgeon must take great care at all times to remain oriented to the location and angle of the spinal canal. All motions with curettes must entail a pulling away from the spinal canal and landing in the previously made trough. Other potential complications include spinal fluid leakage, excessive bleeding, or chyle leakage. Recurrent hemothorax or pneumothorax is possible, and, as mentioned, chest radiographs should be obtained postoperatively. Postoperative intercostal neuritis is more prevalent when hard portals are utilized. Even with soft portals, however, this complication can occur from contusion of the intercostal nerve. Length of surgery may play a role in this complication. A postoperative intercostal block using lidocaine (Xylocaine) may greatly increase the patient's comfort.

RECOMMENDED READING

1. Bohlman H, Zdeblick T: Anterior excision of herniated thoracic discs. *J Bone Joint Surg (Am)* 70: 1038–1047, 1988.
2. Carson J, Gumpert J, Jefferson A: Diagnosis and treatment of thoracic intervertebral disc protrusion. *J Neurol Neurosurg Psychiatry* 34: 68–77, 1971.
3. Dickman CA: Commentary: thoracic discectomy and fusion. In: Regan JJ, McAfee PC, Mack MF, eds. *Atlas of endoscopic spine surgery*. St. Louis, MO: Quality Medical Publishing, 1995: 186–187.
4. Love JG, Schom VG: Thoracic disc protrusions. *JAMA* 191: 627–631, 1965.
5. Patterson R, Arbit E: A surgical approach through the pedicle to protruded thoracic discs. *J Neurosurg* 48: 768–772, 1978.
6. Ransohoff J, Spencer F, Slew F, et al.: Case reports and technical notes: transthoracic removal of thoracic disc. Report of three cases. *J Neurosurg* 31: 459–461, 1969.
7. Regan JJ, Mack MJ, Picetti GD III, et al.: A comparison of video-assisted thoracoscopic surgery (VATS) with open thoracotomy in thoracic spinal surgery. *Today's Ther Trends* 11: 203–218, 1994.
8. Rosenthal D, Rosenthal R, De Simone A: Removal of a protruded thoracic disc using microsurgical endoscopy. *Spine* 19: 1087–1091, 1994.
9. Williams MP, Cherryman GR, Husband IE: Significance of thoracic disc herniation demonstrated by MR imaging. *J Comput Assist Tomogr* 13: 211–213, 1989.

18 Posterior Spinal Fixation for Thoracolumbar Spinal Trauma

Kris Radcliff, C. Chambliss Harrod, Sapan D. Gandhi,
Christopher K. Kepler, and Alexander R. Vaccaro

INDICATIONS/CONTRAINDICATIONS

The goals of thoracolumbar fracture care are prevention of neurologic injury, restoration of sagittal alignment, and facilitation of early mobilization. Anatomically, several factors predispose the thoracolumbar junction to trauma and spinal cord injury. Forces across the thoracolumbar region are amplified by the rigid, long lever arm of the thoracic spine. There is also a transition of neurologic elements from spinal cord to the conus medullaris and a relatively small spinal cord to canal ratio as one moves distally. The mean normal thoracolumbar sagittal alignment is 0 to 3 degrees of lordosis (9). Mean normal lumbar lordosis is approximately 60 degrees (9) although the majority of lordosis is at L4–L5 and L5–S1. Mean thoracic kyphosis is 40 degrees (9).

Treatment decision making of thoracolumbar fractures includes assessment of fracture morphology, posterior ligamentous complex integrity, and neurologic status. The thoracolumbar injury classification system (TLICS) (17,21) is a classification algorithm to support decision making in thoracolumbar fractures (Fig. 18-1). Burst fractures are characterized by bony failure of the vertebral body (Fig. 18-2A). Isolated, neurologically intact thoracolumbar burst fractures without posterior ligamentous injury may be managed nonsurgically in the majority of circumstances. Distraction injuries, including flexion-distraction injuries (Fig. 18-2B) and extension distraction injuries (Fig. 18-2C), are often unstable and in the vast majority of cases benefit from surgical stabilization due to distraction failure of the vertebral elements and ligamentous injury. Translation-rotation injuries (Fig. 18-2D) are also unstable and are typically managed surgically. Relative indications for surgical stabilization include associated injuries (spinal, abdominal, or extremity) that would complicate compliance with bracing, inability to brace due to body habitus, or high risk of failure of nonsurgical treatment.

A posterior surgical approach is the most commonly used approach for thoracolumbar fractures as it is extensile, allows biomechanically rigid instrumentation, is more familiar to spinal surgeons, does not require the assistance of an approach surgeon, and allows fixation of multiple spinal segments.

The anterior approach is selected for direct decompression from anterior retropulsion of bony fragments at the conus and spinal cord injury level. An anterior approach may allow shorter fusion constructs and sparing of fusion levels.

Relative contraindications to posterior spinal fixation of thoracolumbar fractures include open wounds or compromised posterior soft tissues including skin or subcutaneous tissues, medical instability or Morel-Lavelle lesions. Other relative contraindications include significant retropulsion at the spinal cord level, which may be better addressed with an anterior approach.

FIGURE 18-1

Thoracolumbar injury classification system. The TLICS includes three elements: fracture morphology, posterior ligamentous complex injury, and neurologic injury. Fractures with a TLIC score greater than 5 are considered to be candidates for surgical intervention. (Adapted from Vaccaro AR, et al.: A new classification of thoracolumbar injuries: the importance of injury morphology, the integrity of the posterior ligamentous complex, and neurologic status. *Spine* 30(20): 2325, 2005.)

Thoracolumbar injury classification system		
Injury morphology	Compression	1
	Burst component	1
	Translation rotation	3
	Distraction	4
PLC integrity	Intact	0
	Indeterminate	2
	Disrupted	3
Neurological status	Intact	0
	Nerve root injury	2
	Complete	2
	Incomplete (cord or cauda equina)	3

PREOPERATIVE PREPARATION

Careful clinical assessment with a detailed physical and neurologic examination is essential. Mechanism of injury, associated spinal and nonspinal injuries, and precise physical examination are important in understanding the injury "character" and extent. Furthermore, patients should be queried about coagulopathy (either pharmacologic or pathologic) and history of previous spinal surgery or spondyloarthropathy.

Imaging Assessment

High-resolution computed tomography (CT) is a common trauma screening study in many centers. Sagittal and axial reconstructions are essential to appreciate translation and sagittal fracture lines.

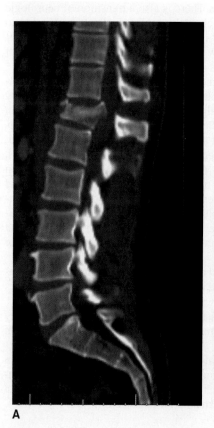
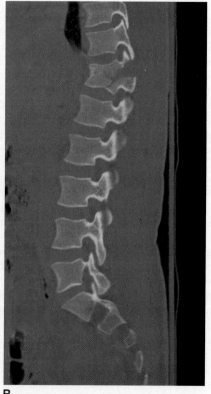

A   B

FIGURE 18-2

A: Midsagittal CT thoracolumbar burst fracture is characterized by involvement of the anterior vertebral body. **B:** Flexion-distraction injury.

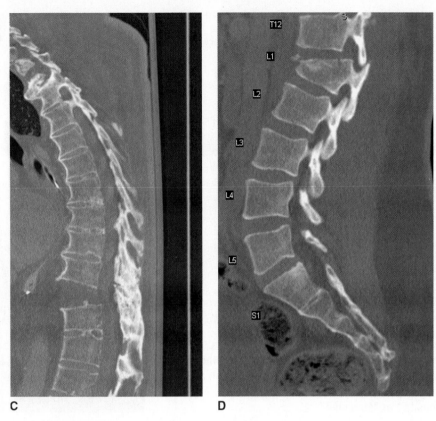

FIGURE 18-2 (*Continued*)

C: Extension distraction injury. **D:** Translation-rotation injury.

MRI is performed for evaluation of posterior ligamentous complex injury (10,16) (Fig. 18-3) and neurologic compression. Imaging studies, particularly in the thoracic spine, should include a scout or scanning view to enable the surgeon to directly count vertebrae from the sacrum to ensure correct-level surgery is performed (Fig. 18-4).

Prior to commencement of the procedure, the surgeon should inspect the preoperative CT scan for the fracture morphology, translation, and evaluation of the adequacy of the pedicles for instrumentation including length, axial convergence, axial vertebral body rotation, scoliosis, and pedicle diameter. Also inspect for location of the great vessels, rib fractures, and facet or pedicle fractures, which may obscure starting points.

Associated spinal and nonspinal injuries should be identified. Approximately 10% to 20% of patients have noncontiguous spinal fractures. Attention should be directed to the cervical spine and the necessity for immobilization or removal of a cervical collar prior to posterior spinal fixation for thoracolumbar trauma. Additionally, the surgeon should discuss with the trauma physicians about the possibility of hollow viscus organ injury particularly after flexion-distraction injuries.

Selection of Fusion Levels

Traditional posterior instrumentation for thoracolumbar fractures differs according to the patients' pathology. Burst fractures are unstable in axial loading, and traditionally, "long-segment" instrumentation (pedicular) is often considered two and sometimes three levels above and below the fractured level to resist compressive loads (14). Other fracture morphologies, including translation-rotation injuries, extension distraction injuries, and flexion-distraction injuries (2) (including "Chance" fractures), may be more stable to axial loading. Short-segment instrumentation, including one to two levels above and below the level of injury, may be more appropriate for selected fractures. The load-sharing score is a decision-making tool to enable surgeons to identify which fractures are most amenable to short-segment instrumentation (15). The load-sharing score assigns 0 to 3 points to fracture comminution, local kyphosis between 15 and 30 degrees, and axial fragment diastasis, and the total score is calculated 0 to 9 (13). Fractures that score 7 or more are considered to be poor candidates for short-segment fixation.

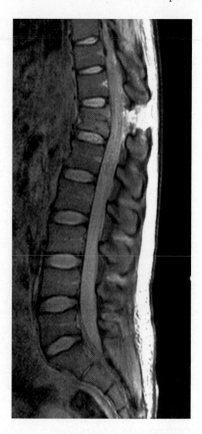

FIGURE 18-3

Posterior ligamentous complex spinal injuries. The posterior ligamentous complex of the spine includes supraspinous ligament, interspinous ligament, ligamentum flavum, and facet joint capsules. The capsules may be scored as "intact," "indeterminate," or "disrupted."

PERIOPERATIVE CONSIDERATIONS

Patients undergoing posterior spinal fixation for thoracolumbar fractures should undergo preoperative medical evaluation and risk stratification and optimization prior to surgery. Progressive neurologic deficit is considered a surgical emergency. Incomplete neurologic deficit is an urgent but not emergent condition best addressed with early surgery when medically cleared. There is no definitive high-level

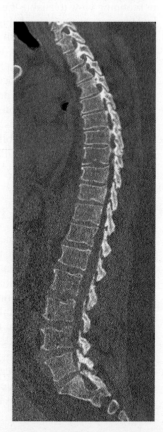

FIGURE 18-4

"Scout" view demonstrating T8 Chance fracture relative to the sacral endplate.

evidence supporting early surgery for thoracolumbar trauma at this time in the literature (20). Several studies have shown a benefit to early surgery in terms of reduction of medical complications (1,11). Consideration should also be given to the possibility of spinal shock and the possibility that an incomplete spinal cord injury may present as a complete injury due to spinal shock (4).

As part of perioperative management, the surgeon should inform the anesthetic team about special requirements including special positioning or intubation requirements, cervical spine clearance or stabilization, presence of other spinal injuries, blood pressure support, steroid dosing, need for one-lung ventilation if necessary, and expected blood loss. The authors' preference in the setting of a neurologic deficit is to maintain mean arterial pressure greater than 85 mm Hg during the procedure using continuous arterial blood pressure monitoring. The authors' preference is also for early involvement of plastic surgery if there is concern about adequate soft tissue for closure. Spinal cord injury is a major risk factor for deep venous thrombosis, increasing the risk eightfold over other isolated thoracolumbar trauma (8). Consideration should be given to deep venous thrombosis chemoprophylaxis to reduce the risk of pulmonary embolism. In cases where a prolonged period before thromboprophylaxis is considered and chemoprophylaxis is contraindicated, consideration should be given to placement of an inferior vena cava filter.

Given the biomechanical demands of spinal cord injury, the instability due to loss of protective muscle function, and the high prevalence of smoking in the trauma population, the authors' preference is autogenous iliac crest for arthrodesis of most patients with thoracolumbar trauma. Preoperative intravenous antibiotic prophylaxis is recommended on all surgeries. Antibiotics should be redosed if the surgical procedure lasts more than 4 hours or if estimated blood loss is greater than 1,000 mL. We monitor somatosensory evoked potentials and motor evoked potential for all spinal cord surgeries. We also perform dynamic triggered electromyography (EMG) for pedicle screw stimulation.

Technique

Positioning   Positioning should be dependent upon the fracture morphology. The authors perform the posterior approach prone on a radiolucent Jackson table (Fig. 18-5). The position of the chest pad (normally at the sternal notch) may be manipulated distally to effect kyphosis in the case of an extension distraction injury or fracture dislocation. Similarly, the iliac crest pads, which normally are located at the level of the anterior superior iliac crest, may be manipulated more proximally to effect kyphosis and more distally to increase lordosis. If the iliac crest pads are too low, the patient can develop meralgia paresthetica or a femoral nerve palsy postoperatively if they are directly in the inguinal region. The abdomen should be free to reduce venous pressure and epidural venous bleeding.

Arms are abducted forward out of the operative field and are supported on arm boards and are positioned in a manner so as to not obscure x-ray visualization. Care should be taken to pad the brachial plexus and the ulnar nerves. The head may be supported on a pillow or, for long cases or cases involving the cervicothoracic junction, held in a Mayfield head holder supported from the top of the Jackson table. Care should be taken to ensure that the patient's eyes are free and arterial pressure is carefully monitored to reduce the risk of blindness. The perineal region should be inspected to ensure that (in the case of male patients) the testicles hang free. The Foley catheter should be taped to the bed so it does not get caught on the C-arm if it hangs unsupported. The patients' knees rest on a gel pad on the Jackson table and are gently flexed. The patient's shins rest on one or two pillows. Sequential compression devices are applied to the patient's shins prior to prone positioning. Localization of levels with intraoperative fluoroscopy may be performed prior to prepping. The authors in some cases confirm adequate radiographic visualization with intraoperative fluoroscopy prior to prepping and draping to confirm that there are no monitors or wires, which are preventing adequate visualization. All surgeries are performed with an intraoperative blood salvage system to reduce the need for nonautologous blood transfusions.

Exposure   For thoracic cases, the spine is draped from lower cervical spine to the pelvis. For lumbar fractures, the spine is draped from the apex of thoracic kyphosis to the sacrum. If iliac crest graft is going to be harvested, then the iliac crest is draped into the field as well.

A midline posterior exposure is a standard extensile approach. The authors' preference is exposure of the fascia bilaterally prior to deeper exposure to facilitate closure at the conclusion of the case. The author will dissect and identify the fascia and undermine the plane between the subcutaneous fat and the fascia bilaterally several millimeters. The incision is midline. After exposure of the fascial plane (prior to violating the fascia), we repalpate the spinous processes and ensure that the midline is again identified. A cerebellar self-retaining retractor may be helpful at this stage. Exposure may proceed subperiosteally elevating the multifidus muscles off of the underlying spinous processes and laminae. Exposure then proceeds lateral to the facet joints and the transverse processes (TPs). In the lumbar spine, Gelpi retractors are placed deep to the paraspinous muscles to hold the muscles back while remaining in an unobtrusive location to avoid interfering with lumbar instrumentation.

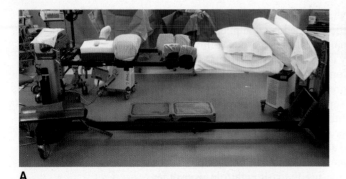

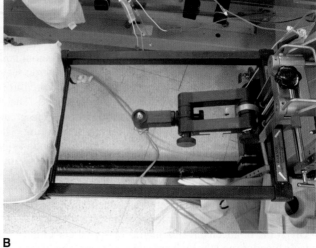

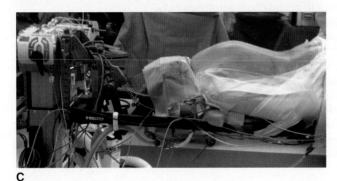

FIGURE 18-5

A: Positioning on a radiolucent Jackson table. The chest pads should be placed at the sternal notch. They may be moved distally to effect increased thoracic kyphosis. The iliac crest pads should rest on the anterior superior iliac spines. They may be moved more distally to increase lumbar lordosis. The abdomen should be free. The knees are gently bent on a gel pad. The feet supported on pillows. The arms should be supported on arm boards from the head of the table. **B:** Positioning a patient with a concomitant cervical and thoracic injuries with Mayfield attachment at the cephalad portion of the bed. The Mayfield attachment reduces pressure on the eyes and face. The Mayfield attachment also allows manipulation of the head and neck alignment. **C:** Example of positioning of patient with T6 flexion/compression injury. The patient was placed in a Mayfield head holder due to (a) her excessive thoracic kyphosis from the fracture and (b) a cervical fracture. The Mayfield attachment allowed direct control of the patient's cervical flexion/extension.

A midline, subperiosteal exposure of the spinous processes and laminae allows for the most efficient, bloodless exposure. The surgeon should avoid working into a hole or crevice as bleeding can quickly occur. Areas that are not being exposed should be packed with sterile sponges to tamponade venous bleeding. Care must be taken in areas of injury not to violate the spinal canal through defects in the laminae or tears in the ligamentum flavum that may have occurred as a result of the spinal fracture (Fig. 18-6). We expose several vertebral levels at once, first the spinous processes, then the laminae, then the pars interarticularis to avoid working in a hole. If necessary, exposure should also commence with identification of a normal anatomical area and then gentle dissection into unknown areas. Self-retaining retractors are helpful to maintain tension on the soft tissue structures during the exposure. Particular attention should be given to hemostasis over the lateral border of the pars interarticularis and the facet joints to avoid the parafacetal artery in that location. The surgeon should avoid violation of the cephalad facet joint of the levels to be fused to reduce the risk of adjacent segment disease. Other facet joints should be debrided of cartilage with electrocautery and/or a burr. Exposure is then carried to the tips of the TPs. In the lumbar spine, the TP is located in the caudal third of the facet joint. Care must be taken not to violate the intertransverse membrane to avoid excessive bleeding and possible iatrogenic nerve root injury.

Radiographic confirmation of levels is essential. The authors' preference for thoracic level identification in the absence of an obvious spinal abnormality is fluoroscopic localization of levels counting from the sacrum. Due to the caudal overhang of the spinous processes in the mid to lower thoracic spine, the tip of a spinous process can hang one or two vertebral levels below its corresponding pedicle. The authors' preference is marking a pedicle directly above and below the fractured segment. In the lumbar spine, a Kocher clamp or pedicle marker is sufficient. This informs the surgeon about the sagittal orientation of the pedicles relative to the floor.

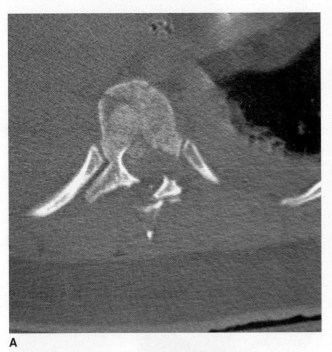

A

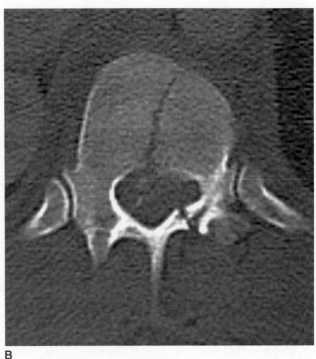

B

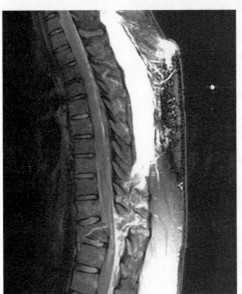

C

FIGURE 18-6

CT myelography demonstrating posterior lamina fracture in the axial view **(A and B)**, and the saggital view **(C)**. Care should be taken during exposure to avoid iatrogenic spinal cord injury by falling into the fracture site.

Instrumentation   Pedicle screw instrumentation is the authors' preference in the posterior approach for thoracolumbar fractures. Pedicle screw instrumentation allows segmental, anterior, and posterior spinal column fixation of multiple segments and the potential for manipulation of deformity. Pedicle screw instrumentation is a safe and effective procedure in the thoracolumbar spine (12,18,19,22).

There are two components to successful thoracolumbar pedicle screw instrumentation similar to other orthopedic instrumentation procedures: starting points and insertional angle. The pedicle is located at the junction of the TP and the superior articular process (SAP). Slight variations in the orientation of the TP to the pedicle (cephalad, same level, or caudal) distinguish spinal segments (Fig. 18-7A). The starting points of thoracic pedicle screws are approached based on two anatomical landmarks: the TP and the SAP. The smallest pedicles are at T4, T5, and T6. The most medially convergent thoracic pedicles are in the midthoracic spine.

The most important component of successful pedicle screw instrumentation is choosing correct starting points. It is difficult to salvage a poor starting point with screw trajectory. If difficulty is

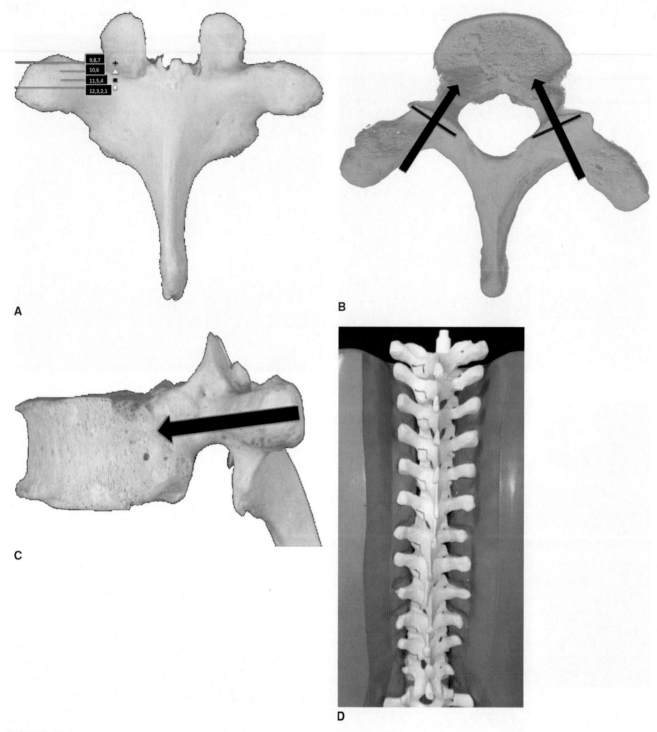

FIGURE 18-7

A: Thoracic pedicle screw starting points diagram. The medial-lateral position is located at the lateral edge of the SAP of the level to be instrumented. The vertebral level determines the proximal-distal position. Pedicle screw starting points are always in the cephalad half of the TP. The landmark is the bisector of a TP. The pedicle of T12, T3, T2, and T1 is located at the mid-point of the TP. The pedicles of T9, T8, and T7 are located at or above the cephalad border of the TP (on the superior facet). Two other points are defined between the top and midpoint of the TP. At the upper quadrant of the TP is the starting point of the T10 and T6 pedicles. At the lower quadrant is the starting point of the T11, T5, and T4. **B:** The axial orientation of the pedicles is perpendicular to a tangent line to the SAP. The trajectory of the pedicle screws are shown by the arrows. **C:** The sagittal orientation of the pedicles is often parallel to the TP. The trajectory of the pedicle screws are shown by the arrows. **D:** Model of thoracic pedicle screws/inferior facet osteotomy. On the left side, the inferior facet osteotomies have been marked. On the right side, inferior facet osteotomies have been performed to expose the superior articular facet. The pedicle screw starting points have been marked at every thoracic level on the right. Note how the inferior facet osteotomy improves visualization of the lateral aspect of the superior facet.

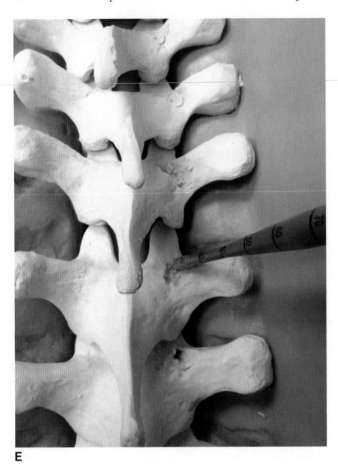

FIGURE 18-7 (*Continued*)

E: Example of cannulating right T7 pedicle with curved pointed gearshift. The instrument has been advanced 15 mm with the tip facing laterally. Now the tip has been redirected medially as it should have traversed the pedicle at this point and is entering the vertebral body. The depth markings on the gearshift enable to surgeon to determine the appropriate screw depth.

E

encountered in pedicle screw instrumentation, the surgeon should first reassess the pedicle screw starting point (Fig. 18-7A). The SAP is the medial-lateral thoracic pedicle screw starting point landmark. The ideal medial-lateral starting point is just lateral to the SAP. In the thoracic spine, the authors' preference is thinning or leveling the thoracic TP to expose the base of the SAP. This maneuver can be performed at all levels except the cephalad pedicle. A common error is failure to visualize the lateral edge of the SAP, resulting in a more medial starting point. The TP is the cephalad-caudal landmark for thoracic pedicle screw starting points. The surgeon should know the location of the TP relative to the pedicle starting point at every level.

The axial trajectory of the thoracic pedicles is perpendicular to the SAP (Fig. 18-7B). Accurate identification of the SAP is critical to successful screw placement. Sagittal trajectory of thoracic screws is often parallel to the TPs depending if a straightforward rather than an anatomic sagittal direction is chosen for improved pullout strength (Fig. 18-7C). After removal of the dorsal cortex of the TP with a Leksell rongeur, the pedicle screw starting point is identified with a high-speed bur and then cannulated. After creation of a starting point, the authors use either a curved, pointed pedicle finding gearshift or a straight 3-0 cervical curette for thoracic pedicle screw insertion. If a curved probe is used, the author advances the instrument 15 mm with the tip pointing laterally. At this point, the tip of the instrument should have traversed the pedicle. Then the author rotates and points the gearshift tip medially for 15 mm because at this point the instrument should be in the vertebral body. The author will advance the awl to 35 to 40 mm total, and then the hole is palpated. Five surfaces (medial, lateral, superior, inferior, and a floor) should be palpated. Our preference is undertapping by 1 mm or not tapping at all to optimize screw purchase while creating a bony path for the screw. The pedicle hole is palpated gently again with a ball tip probe. Pedicle screw trajectories can be checked with a pedicle marker or drill bit on anteroposterior (AP) or just lateral fluoroscopic views or plain x-ray to determine the correct trajectory prior to screw implantation.

In the case of difficulty with pedicle screw implantation, the author performs a laminoforaminotomy (Fig. 18-8) to palpate the medial, superior, and inferior pedicle wall. The initial step is resection of the inferior edge of the lamina of the cephalad level. The second step is resection of the cephalad edge of the level to be instrumented. Finally, we take a Kerrison rongeur and bite caudally-laterally at a 45-degree angle to identify the medial pedicle border and undercut the lamina/facet junction. The surgeon should then be able to palpate the medial border of the pedicle with a micro nerve hook.

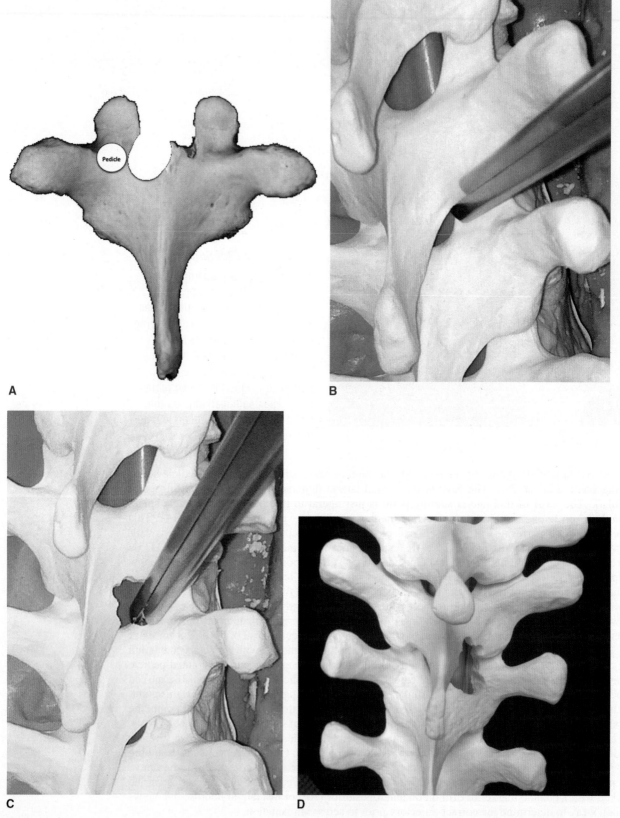

FIGURE 18-8

A: Diagram of laminoforaminotomy with pedicle projection marked. **B:** Start laminoforaminotomy with removal of the inferior edge of the cephalad lamina. **C:** Once adequate room is achieved, remove the bone medial to the pedicle with a high-speed burr or 1- or 2-mm Kerrison rongeur. Take care not to allow the back end of the instrument to contact the spinal cord. **D:** Completed laminoforaminotomy. The surgeon should be able to palpate the media, superior, and inferior borders of the pedicle with the Kerrison rongeur or a nerve hook after laminoforaminotomy is completed.

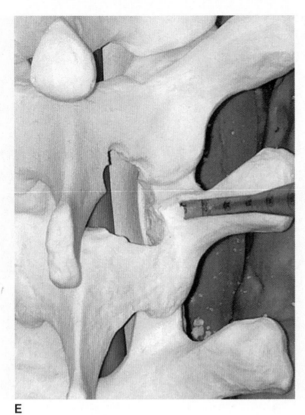
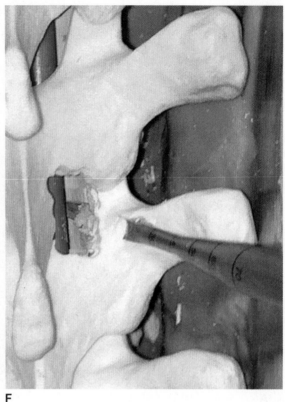

E   F

FIGURE 18-8 (*Continued*)

E: The surgeon may now cannulate the pedicle with direct knowledge of the location of the spinal canal. **F:** If an instrument breaches the medial pedicle border, the surgeon should be able to appreciate the defect either visually or with palpation.

Special pearls are that there is usually a rudimentary TP at L1 with a large mammillary process at that level. At L1, the pedicle has very little medial convergence, if any, and can occasionally diverge depending on starting point. Therefore, the surgeon has to be careful to avoid a medial breach at the L1 level. Fortunately, the L1 pedicles are usually large and therefore more amenable to pedicle fixation.

The axial trajectory of lumbar screws is fairly straightforward (Fig. 18-9). L1 screws have 5-degree medial convergence in most cases. There is 5 degrees of additional convergence per level below L1. Therefore, L2 screws 10 degrees, L3 screws 15 degrees, etc. The sagittal trajectory of lumbar screws is referenced around orientation to L3 in most cases. L3 screws are usually perpendicular to the floor in most cases as L3 is the apex of lumbar lordosis. The authors use the sagittal orientation of the radiographic marker as a guide.

Decompression   There are several options for decompression from a posterior approach in thoracolumbar trauma. We prefer decompression after instrumentation is placed (Fig. 18-10). For thoracic laminectomy, we first remove the spinous processes of the end levels with a Leksell rongeur to remove the distal overhanging portion of the spinous process to expose the ligamentum flavum above and below the laminectomy level. We then use a high-speed burr to create two troughs lateral to the dura. The thinned lamina is then lifted with a nerve hook and removed with a Kerrison or pituitary. Care should be taken to ensure that the bone fragment (lamina) does not rebound onto the spinal cord.

Depending on the pathology, a surgeon may choose unilateral transpedicular decompression (Fig. 18-11), bilateral transpedicular decompression, or costotransversectomy to address pathology ventral to the thecal sac. Transpedicular decompression is a technique to achieve ventral decompression of the thecal sac from a posterior approach. The authors cannulate the pedicle to be decompressed. The authors enlarge the pedicle channel with serial curette dilation and, ultimately, a high-speed burr to decancellate the entire pedicle and posterior lateral vertebral body. A tamp or reverse curette is used to breach the medial pedicle cortex, and a trough is created in the vertebral body. Then a reverse curette or angled bone tamp is used to reduce posterolateral bone fragments into the vertebral body. Transpedicular decompression does not violate the lateral pedicle wall and does

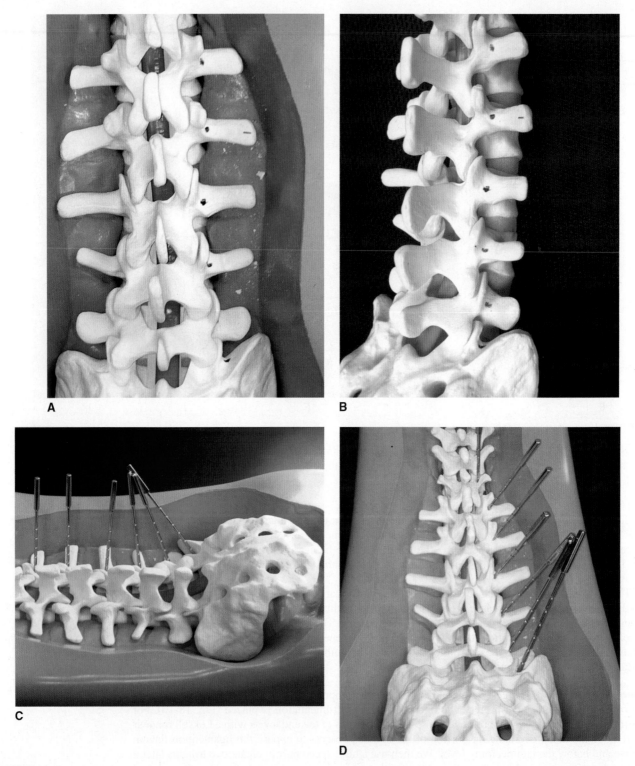

FIGURE 18-9

Lumbar pedicle screws (sawbones). **A:** Identification of starting from dorsal points (upslope of TP). **B:** Oblique view demonstrating the lumbar screw starting points at the junction of the TP and SAP. **C:** Sagittal angle of lumbar pedicle screws. Note the progressive caudal angulation most extreme in S1. **D:** Axial angulation of lumbar pedicle screws. Note that S1 has the most medial angulation.

not require disruption of the costovertebral junction. Transpedicular decompression is indicated for posterolateral pathology. Midline pathology or contralateral pathology may not be accessible via transpedicular decompression.

Costotransversectomy is a more lateral approach similar to transpedicular decompression. The surgeon dissects the lateral vertebral body wall free by osteotomizing the TP. The costovertebral

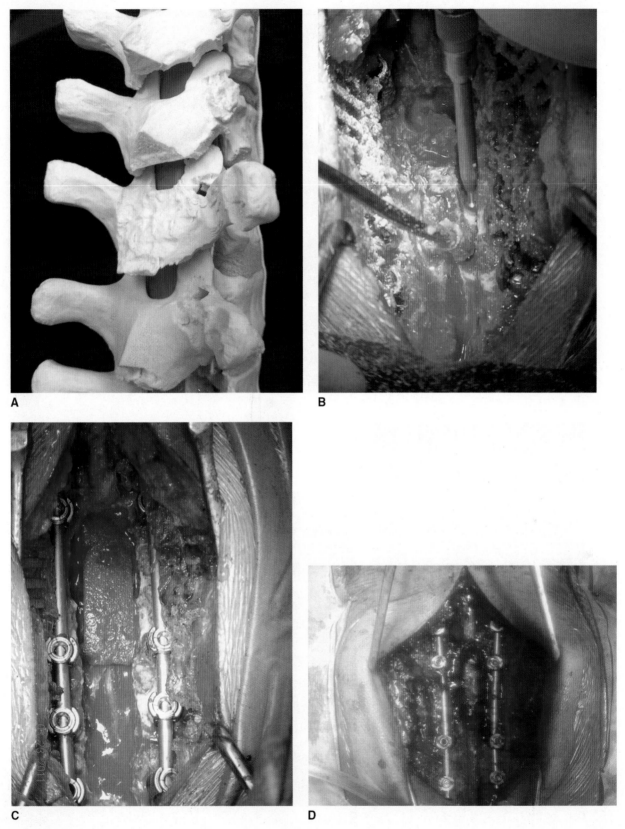

FIGURE 18-10

Thoracic laminectomy. **A:** The spinous processes have been removed, and dorsal cortex of the lamina has been removed. This enables easy identification of the cephalad and caudal border of the lamina. It is extremely difficult to do thoracic laminectomy without spinous process removal due to the overhang of cephalad levels obscuring the cephalad border of the lamina to the removed. The lamina has also been thinned to the ventral cortex. **B:** Drilling bilateral troughs. The thin lamina facilitates easy identification of ligamentum flavum and dura. The authors start at the caudal border since flavum protects the dura at this level. **C:** Example of thoracic laminectomy. **D:** Subdural/intramedullary spinal cord hemorrhage evident on thoracic laminectomy.

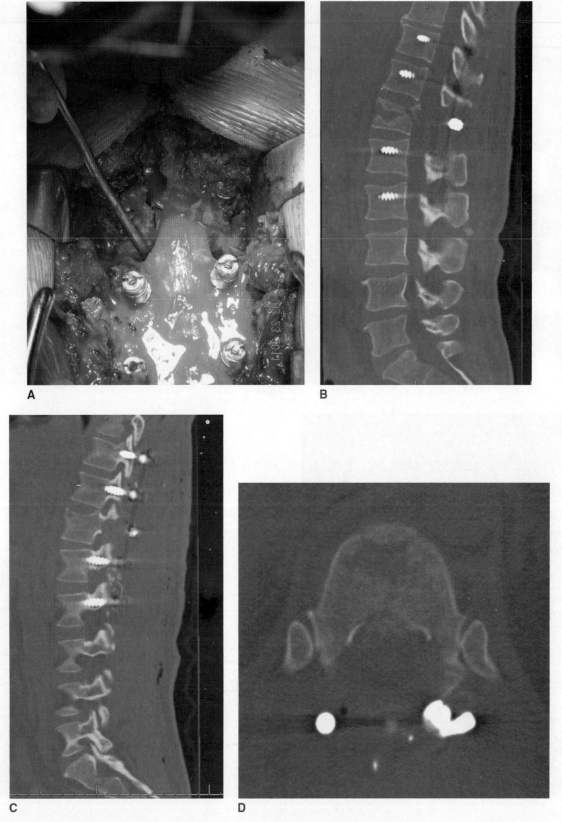

FIGURE 18-11

Transpedicular decompression/costotransversectomy. **A:** Bilateral transpedicular decompression. The surgeon is reaching into the vertebral body through the left pedicle, which has been removed. Note that the right pedicle has also been removed and bilateral nerve roots have been sacrificed. **B:** Example of transpedicular decompression for thoracolumbar burst fracture with incomplete spinal cord injury. Preoperative sagittal view demonstrates significant bony retropulsion. **C:** Postoperative sagittal view demonstrates reduction of fracture and resection of bony fragment. **D:** Axial view demonstrates bilateral transpedicular decompression.

junction is identified, and the rib head is osteotomized. The lateral and medial pedicle walls are taken down, which allows the surgeon to reach more medially across the thecal sac. Costotransversectomy may allow the surgeon to access midline and bilateral anterior pathology for a complete vertebrectomy. A cage or interbody graft may be placed anteriorly once the costotransversectomy is completed (Fig. 18-11C).

Traumatic durotomies may occur, particularly in the presence of a vertical laminar fracture, in thoracolumbar trauma. When possible, direct repair of the durotomy is the best possible outcome. The authors repair the durotomy with Castroviejo forceps with a 6-0 Gore-Tex suture on a CV6 needle. After a knot is tied in the suture, the authors in some cases bring the suture needles through a Duragen patch and/or a fascia or fat graft to augment the repair. The repair is then further supported with fibrin glue. If unable to repair, the authors recommend reduction of any herniated nerve rootlets then augmentation with a dural patch followed by prolonged bed rest of a day or 2. Consideration may also be given to subarachnoid drainage.

Deformity Reduction Maneuvers   The choice of reduction maneuvers depends on the specific pathology and direction of instability. Burst fractures usually require a combination of lordosis and distraction for reduction to correct kyphosis (Fig. 18-12). We recommend effecting lordosis initially with a cantilever maneuver or in situ bending and then distracting across the fractured segments. The distraction is a kyphosing maneuver. The rod should be contoured into an exaggerated lordosis prior to the reduction as some lordosis will be lost during the reduction. If the reverse maneuver is performed (distraction prior to lordosis), then the ligament tension may be maximized by kyphosis and may not be as effective in creating lordosis. In the case of fracture/dislocations, there is a shear mechanism that results in anterolisthesis of the proximal segment relative to the distal segment. If necessary, in the case of a fracture dislocation, the SAPs may be osteotomized bilaterally using a high-speed burr or osteotome to facilitate direct reduction. After instrumentation has been placed and decompression completed, we perform reduction of the proximal screws to the rods bilaterally using persuader instrumentation to reduce translation. A cantilever maneuver may also be employed by anchoring a contoured, corrected rod to one end of the construct and using a rod gripper to bring the opposite end of the rods anteriorly enough to capture the screws (Fig. 18-13). We recommend working bilaterally simultaneously while performing this maneuver to avoid unilateral screw failure. Extension distraction injuries must be reduced in kyphosis. In situ bending in kyphosis or distraction across the fracture segment will reduce these injuries.

Closure   All bony elements should be decorticated. Local bone from the decompression or spinous processes, debrided of soft tissue and morcellized, plus bone graft extender may be added to the decorticated posterior elements. The authors recommend autogenous iliac crest bone graft on trauma patients. There are some reports of the use of recombinant human bone morphogenic protein 2 (BMP2) in a capacity that is "off-label" by the FDA in thoracolumbar trauma cases. However, we recommend caution with use of BMP2 posterolaterally in the thoracolumbar spine due to basic science data that recombinant human BMP2 may penetrate the thecal sac and induce a signalling cascade (5) possibly causing gliosis (7).

After irrigation and bone grafting, closure should be performed in a layered fashion over a subfascial drain. Care should be taken to close all dead space, particularly in the subcutaneous fat over the thoracolumbar fascia.

Minimally Invasive Surgery   Although at this time controversial, selected patients may be candidates for percutaneous instrumentation with or without facet arthrodesis as an "internal brace" for selected fractures. Such percutaneous instrumentation may be a good choice in patients who are high risk for failure of nonsurgical treatment. Early studies have demonstrated no significant loss of radiographic alignment or high rate of early failures with application of such techniques, although long-term studies are still under way.

The technique of percutaneous instrumentation and fusion of thoracolumbar fractures involves insertion of pedicle screws under fluoroscopic guidance. The first step of percutaneous pedicle insertion is careful setup and radiographic mapping to identify the appropriate pedicle landmarks. Prior to instrumentation, the C-arm should be brought to be parallel to the vertebral body to be instrumented. The authors first confirm a perfect AP view (Fig. 18-14A). Left and right rotation should be used to ensure that the spinous process projection is equidistant from the pedicles bilaterally. This will ensure that the C-arm is not axially rotated relative to the vertebral body. Cephalad and caudal angulation should be used to move the C-arm parallel to the vertebral body endplates. It is important to accurately align the endplates so they are superimposed on one another.

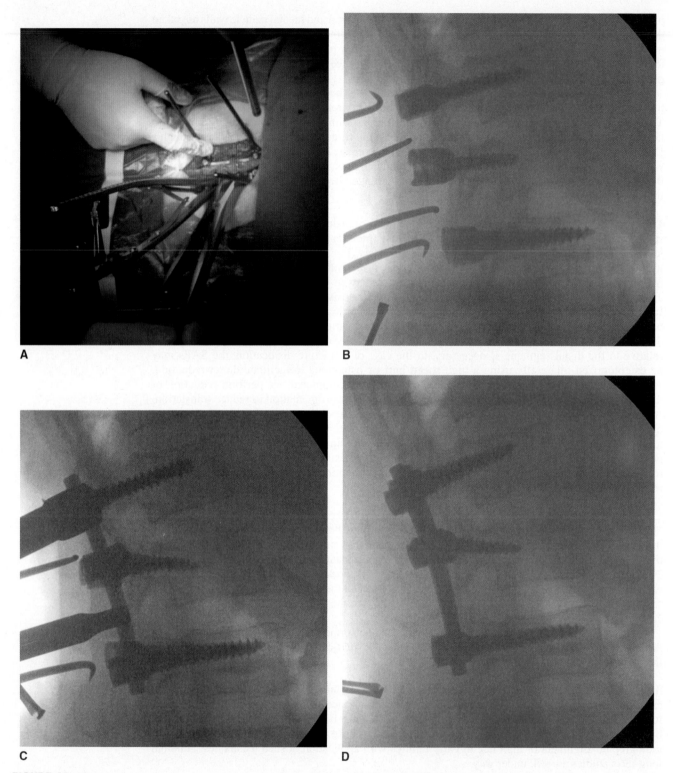

FIGURE 18-12

Distraction/lordosis reduction maneuver burst fracture. **A:** Intraoperative photo of distractor apparatus attached to rod gripper to effect distraction across thoracolumbar burst fracture. **B:** Example of thoracolumbar burst fracture reduction with distraction. Pedicle screws have been placed at L4, L3, and L2 for a burst fracture. **C:** Distractor applied intraoperatively to a fusion construct. The fracture has been reduced from kyphosis. **D:** Final construct showing reduction of the fracture with short-segment instrumentation and a screw in the fracture site as a fulcrum.

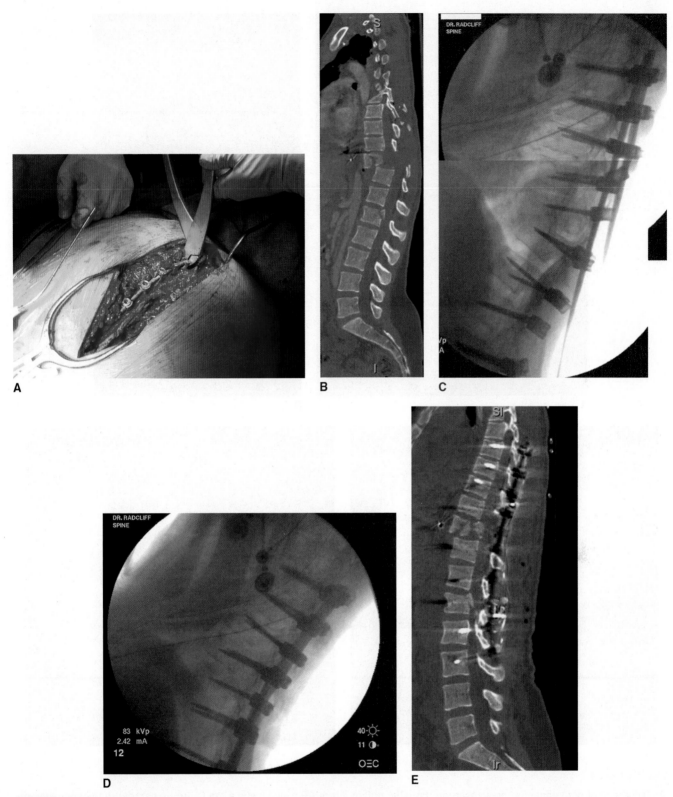

FIGURE 18-13

A: Intraoperative photo of a rod gripper applied to the cephalad end of a rod to effect a cantilever reduction. Instead of using a persuader to reduce the screws to the rod, a cantilever maneuver reduces the rod and distally attached screws to the remaining screw. **B:** Preoperative midsagittal CT scan of a T10 translation-rotation injury with complete spinal cord injury. Also note an L1 burst fracture. **C:** Intraoperative radiograph obtained prior to reduction maneuver displays persistent kyphosis and translation. Pedicle screws have been placed and long, contoured rods anchored at the cephalad aspect of the construct (T6 to T10). The rods have not been anchored distal to the fracture site. **D:** After bilateral cantilever reduction, the translation and kyphosis have been corrected. The rods were cut to appropriate length. **E:** Postoperative CT displays restoration of alignment.

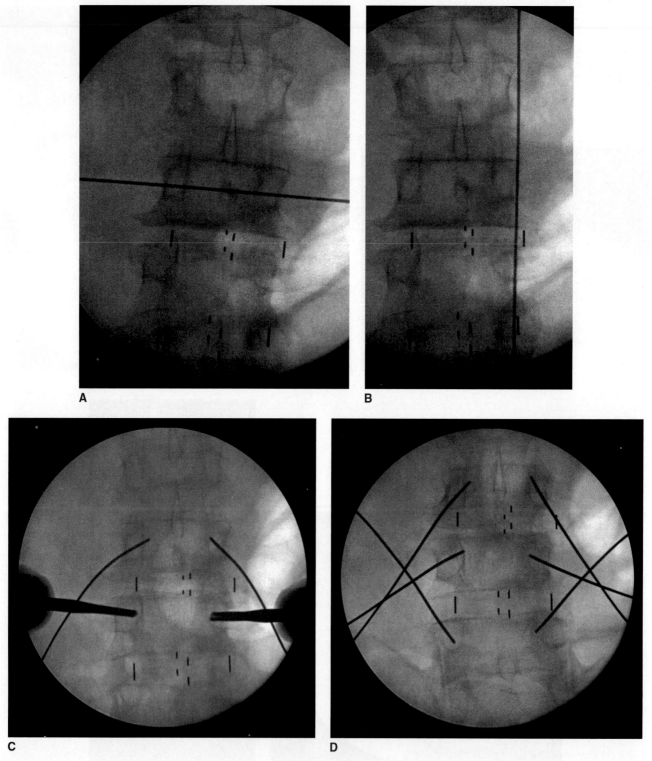

FIGURE 18-14

A: Technique of percutaneous screw insertion. Initially, obtain a true AP view in which the C-arm is parallel to the endplates of the vertebral body to be instrumented, and the spinous process is midline. After this is performed, the location of the pedicles can be marked on the skin by laying a guidewire across the skin parallel to the midpoint of the pedicles. **B:** Mark the skin at the location of the lateral pedicle boundary with a guidewire. The skin incision should be at least 2 cm lateral to the lateral pedicle border to medialize. **C:** Example of cannulating L4 pedicles. The Jim-Sheedy needles have been advanced exactly 15 mm. The tips are located at the midpedicle on an AP view and have not touched the medial L4 pedicle border. This is the correct position, and it implies appropriate medicalization. At this point on a lateral view, the Jim-Sheedy needles should be at the pedicle-vertebral body border. **D:** AP fluoroscopic image after guidewires are inserted at L3, L4, and L5. Notice that the C-arm is now orthogonal to L5 superior endplate and is no longer orthogonal to L3 vertebral endplates.

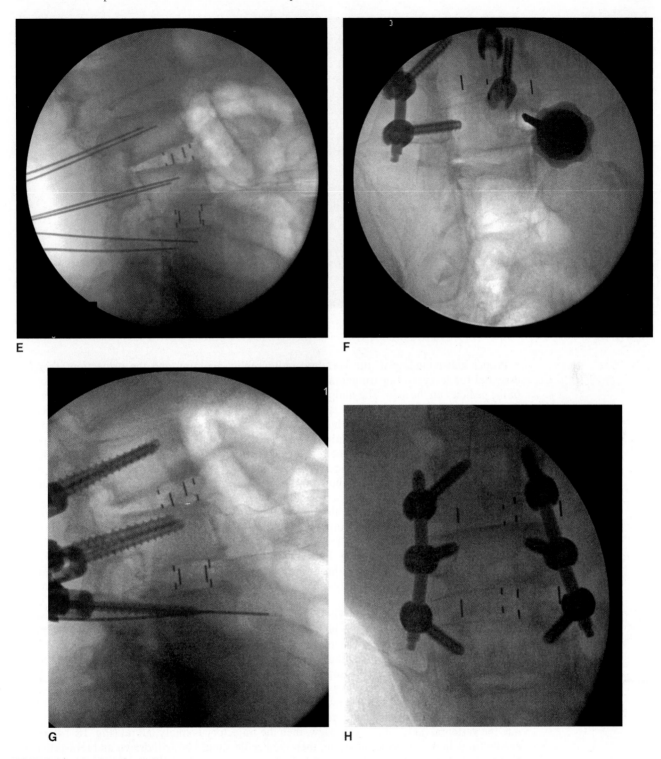

FIGURE 18-14 (*Continued*)

E: Lateral fluoroscopic view after guidewires is inserted. The left L5 guidewire is at the mid–vertebral body projection on the lateral view but is only at the medial pedicle wall on an AP view. This implies a lateral guidewire placement as the guidewire has traveled farther in the AP plane than the medial-lateral direction. **F:** "Owl's eye" or transpedicular oblique view may be obtained to directly visualize a pedicle in the case of difficulty with screw insertion on AP view. In this example, the gearshift is now in perfect position as it is midpedicle. **G:** Care should be taken to avoid guidewire migration with screw insertion. **H:** AP radiograph after the L5 screw was repositioned demonstrates final construct.

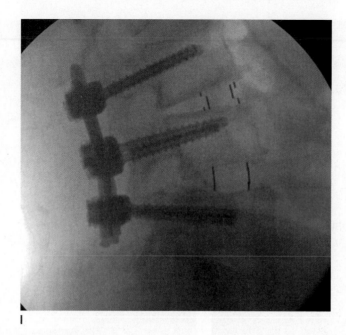

FIGURE 18-14
(*Continued*)

I: Lateral radiograph of final construct.

I

Proper understanding of the vertebral radiographic anatomy and the projections therein is essential for successful instrumentation. The authors carefully identify the anatomical location of the pedicles on the skin. The midpoint of the pedicle proximal-distal is identified (Fig. 18-14A). The lateral border of the pedicles is identified (Fig. 18-14B). A skin incision is performed 2 to 3 cm lateral to the lateral pedicle border. Lateral fascia should be incised generously to prevent difficulty with instrument angulation. If difficulty is encountered with percutaneous pedicle screw insertion, the authors lengthen the fascial incision longitudinally. The author bluntly dissects down to the TP with his finger and palpates the TP/facet junction. A Jim-Sheedy needle is carefully introduced directly onto the upslope of the TP having just palpated it manually followed by radiographic confirmation. Percutaneous pedicle screws should start at the 3 or 9 o'clock position on a true AP fluoroscopic image. The correct starting point anatomically is at the facet/TP junction. The surgeon should take care that he/she is starting ventral enough that the instrument does not become entrapped in the facet joint. A common error with percutaneous pedicle screws is starting the screw on the inferior articular process (too dorsal). This mistake is more likely if the skin incision is too medial. The pedicle is then cannulated with a Jim-Sheedy needle aiming medially. The Jim-Sheedy needle should be marked at a length of 15 mm from the skin. The needle is advanced approximately 15 mm at which point it should have traversed the pedicle (Fig. 18-14C). On the AP radiograph, the tip of the needle should have reached the midpoint of the pedicle. On a lateral view, the Jim-Sheedy needle should be at the pedicle-vertebral body junction if in the correct position. The ideal position after the Jim-Sheedy needle has traversed the pedicle (prior to entering the vertebral body) is on the midpoint of the pedicle on an AP radiographic view and at the posterior vertebral body on a lateral view. If the needle is located at the medial wall of the pedicle after insertion 15 mm but is still within the pedicle on a lateral view, then the trajectory is too medial and the screw will likely be medial. If the needle is at the midpoint of the pedicle on an AP view (Fig. 18-14D) but is into the vertebral body on a lateral view, then the trajectory is likely lateral (Fig. 18-14E). If the needle tip is in the incorrect position, then the needle should be withdrawn and reinserted. The best result is obtained if an entirely new trajectory is selected. In the case of difficulty with screw insertion, an oblique transpedicular view ("owl's eye," "Scotty dog") may be obtained. On this view, the Jim-Sheedy should be inserted 15 mm and should remain within the outline of the pedicle (Fig. 18-14F). After successful cannulation, a guidewire is advanced through the needle to engage the vertebral body. The Jim-Sheedy needle is then removed carefully to ensure that the guidewire is not also simultaneously removed. A cannulated tap is then introduced over the guidewire. Care should be taken to monitor the guidewire to ensure that the tip is not advanced with the advancing tap or screw insertion (Fig. 18-14G). Then the tap is removed, and the screw is introduced over the guidewire. Then a sleeve may be introduced over the screw, and the screw can be tested with dynamic triggered EMG. Final AP (Fig. 18-14H) and lateral views should be obtained (Fig. 18-14I).

POSTOPERATIVE MANAGEMENT

The authors recommend postoperative immobilization in a brace for 10 to 12 weeks depending on the injury and the patient's risk factors. Spinal cord injury, smoking, and burst fracture comminution are relative risk factors for late kyphosis.

Spinal cord injury patients require careful consideration for prophylaxis for soft tissue decubiti, pulmonary complications, gastrointestinal ulcers, and deep venous thrombosis. In particular, deep vein thrombosis (DVT) is particularly common in spinal cord injury patients, and therefore, we begin chemoprophylaxis on patients for DVT either immediately or on postoperative day 3 depending if a decompression is performed.

COMPLICATIONS

Complications may be grouped into the following categories: local and general.

Local complications include screw malplacement, traumatic durotomy, spinal cord injury, nerve root injury, wound infection, and hematoma. Wrong-level surgery is most common in the thoracic spine. Common causes of wrong-level surgery include open S1–S2 interspace (Fig. 18-14), inadequate C-arm penetration due to patient body habitus, arm boards overlying the spine, fractured posterior elements, or misinterpretation of landmarks in the wound. Complications can occur during positioning. Patients who had significant baseline kyphosis due to spondyloarthropathy (Fig. 18-15) should be supported in their position of kyphosis throughout the surgery. Chest pads and iliac crest pads should be manipulated to maintain kyphosis. Neurologic monitoring after positioning is helpful to determine if there are any complications due to the positioning. Laminectomy alone is inadequate to treat thoracolumbar trauma as patients will develop late kyphosis and instability (Fig. 18-16). Instrumentation can be malpositioned. Lateral malpositioned instrumentation in the thoracic spine generally endangers the great vessels. For this reason, the authors place screws 5 mm shorter on the left side to reduce the danger to great vessels in the event of lateral screw malpositioning. The natural history of instrumentation adjacent to the great vessels has not been well defined. Several case reports have been described of intravascular migration (3). However, at least one retrospective case series described no cases of vascular injury during a 5-year postoperative follow-up period (6) (Fig. 18-17). Medial screw malpositioning endangers the spinal cord. Infection can occur after any spinal surgery but is particularly increased after spinal trauma.

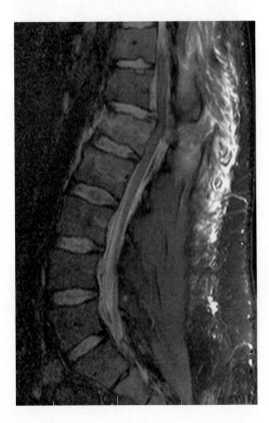

FIGURE 18-15

Patient with open S1–S2 interspace, which can confound identification of correct levels with intraoperative localization.

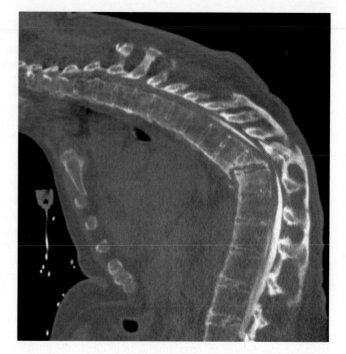

FIGURE 18-16

Patient with significant pre-operative kyphosis due to spondyloarthropathy. Care should be taken during positioning to avoid iatrogenic displacement. This patient will be highly unstable in extension. Positioning this patient into excessive extension may result in translation or instability and ultimately spinal cord injury.

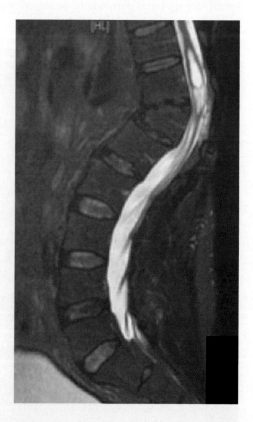

FIGURE 18-17

Patient with postlaminectomy kyphosis after treatment of a thoracolumbar burst fracture.

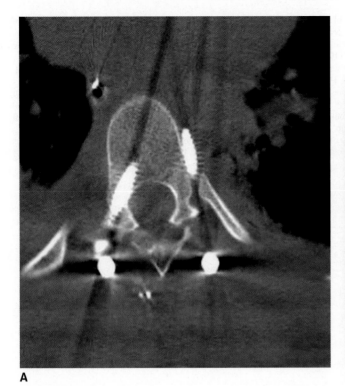

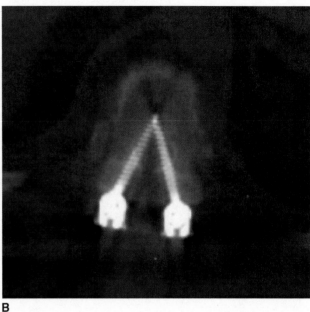

A   B

FIGURE 18-18

A: Lateral thoracic pedicle screw at T6 is near the aorta. **B:** Bilateral medial pedicle screw breaches at T11 in the impinged distal spinal cord.

General complications include thromboembolic disease (8), ileus, decubiti, pneumonia, and other unanticipated medical complications (Fig. 18-18).

RECOMMENDED READING

1. Cengiz L, et al.: Timing of thoracolomber spine stabilization in trauma patients; impact on neurological outcome and clinical course. A real prospective (rct) randomized controlled study. *Arch Orthop Trauma Surg* 128(9): 959–966, 2008.
2. Chapman JR, et al.: Thoracolumbar flexion-distraction injuries: associated morbidity and neurological outcomes. *Spine* 33(6): 648, 2008.
3. Clarke MJ, et al.: Combined endovascular and neurosurgical approach to the removal of an intraaortic pedicle screw. *J Neurosurg Spine* 15(5): 550–554, 2011.
4. Ditunno J, et al.: Spinal shock revisited: a four-phase model. *Spinal Cord* 42(7): 383–395, 2004.
5. Dmitriev AE, et al.: Bone morphogenetic protein-2 used in spinal fusion with spinal cord injury penetrates intrathecally and elicits a functional signaling cascade. *Spine J* 10(1): 16–25, 2010.
6. Foxx KC, et al.: A retrospective analysis of pedicle screws in contact with the great vessels. *J Neurosurg Spine* 13(3): 403–406, 2010.
7. Fuller ML, et al.: Bone morphogenetic proteins promote gliosis in demyelinating spinal cord lesions. *Ann Neurol* 62(3): 288–300, 2007.
8. Geerts WH, et al.: A prospective study of venous thromboembolism after major trauma. *N Engl J Med* 331(24): 1601–1606, 1994.
9. Gelb DE, et al.: An analysis of sagittal spinal alignment in 100 asymptomatic middle and older aged volunteers. *Spine* 20(12): 1351, 1995.
10. Haba H, et al.: Diagnostic accuracy of magnetic resonance imaging for detecting posterior ligamentous complex injury associated with thoracic and lumbar fractures. *J Neurosurg* 99(1): 20–26, 2003.
11. Kerwin AJ, et al.: The effect of early surgical treatment of traumatic spine injuries on patient mortality. *J Trauma* 63(6): 1308, 2007.
12. Kim YJ, et al.: Free hand pedicle screw placement in the thoracic spine: is it safe? *Spine* 29(3): 333–342, 2004; discussion 342.
13. McCormack T, Karaikovic E, Gaines RW: The load sharing classification of spine fractures. *Spine* 19(15): 1741, 1994.
14. McLain R, Sparling E, Benson D: Early failure of short-segment pedicle instrumentation for thoracolumbar fractures. A preliminary report. *J Bone Joint Surg Am* 75(2): 162, 1993.
15. Parker JW, et al.: Successful short-segment instrumentation and fusion for thoracolumbar spine fractures: a consecutive 41/2-year series. *Spine* 25(9): 1157, 2000.
16. Rihn JA, et al.: Using magnetic resonance imaging to accurately assess injury to the posterior ligamentous complex of the spine: a prospective comparison of the surgeon and radiologist. *J Neurosurg Spine* 12(4): 391–396, 2010.

17. Vaccaro AR, et al.: A new classification of thoracolumbar injuries: the importance of injury morphology, the integrity of the posterior ligamentous complex, and neurologic status. *Spine* 30(20): 2325, 2005.
18. Vaccaro AR, et al.: Placement of pedicle screws in the thoracic spine. Part I: morphometric analysis of the thoracic vertebrae. *J Bone Joint Surg Am* 77(8): 1193–1199, 1995.
19. Vaccaro AR, et al.: Placement of pedicle screws in the thoracic spine. Part II: an anatomical and radiographic assessment. *J Bone Joint Surg Am* 77(8): 1200-1206, 1995.
20. Vaccaro AR, et al.: Neurologic outcome of early versus late surgery for cervical spinal cord injury. *Spine* 22(22): 2609–2613, 1997.
21. Vaccaro AR, et al.: Surgical decision making for unstable thoracolumbar spine injuries: results of a consensus panel review by the Spine Trauma Study Group. *J Spinal Disord Tech* 19(1): 1, 2006.
22. Zindrick MR, et al.: Pedicle morphology of the immature thoracolumbar spine. *Spine* 25(21): 2726–2735, 2000.

19 Posterior Spinal Instrumentation Techniques for Spinal Deformity

Han Jo Kim, Lawrence G. Lenke, Yongjung J. Kim, and Anthony S. Rinella

Pedicle screw instrumentation has improved rigid fixation of the spine, lessening the need for anterior procedures while providing improved corrections. At our institution, spinal deformities are rarely approached with a combined anterior/posterior approach. We routinely use only the posterior approach for the vast majority of deformities. There are many benefits to using pedicle screws compared to hooks or sublaminar wires. Three-column fixation provided by the pedicle screw has shown biomechanical superiority and greater pullout strength (1,6). In addition, the ability to address the anterior column provides a greater ability to control for spinal deformity correction in the coronal, sagittal, and axial planes. In addition, fewer vertebral motion segments may need to be instrumented while obviating the need for any postoperative bracing. Other benefits include secure fixation during revision surgery settings where the posterior elements might be distorted or nonexistent (i.e., laminectomy) as well as to adequately stabilize the spine after three-column osteotomies. In patients with spinal deformity, pedicle screw fixation has demonstrated greater three-dimensional correction with decreased rates of curve progression and higher fusion rates (2,7–10). This has allowed for improved chest wall correction and improved pulmonary function particularly in adolescent idiopathic scoliosis (AIS) by obviating the need for thoracoplasty.

The majority of this chapter concentrates on the advantages and techniques of using pedicle screws in the thoracic and lumbar regions of the spine, with an emphasis on deformity analysis, surgical planning, and techniques for instrumentation and correction. For the purposes of simplicity and clarity, we will focus on adolescent idiopathic deformities. However, these techniques can be applied to adult deformities as well.

INDICATIONS/CONTRAINDICATIONS

The indications for surgery in adolescent idiopathic deformities (scoliosis and Scheuermann kyphosis) are consistent in the literature. Long-term studies have demonstrated that larger curves (greater than 45 degrees) in the coronal plane tend to progress into adulthood, and surgical stabilization should be considered. Additional considerations are patients who have pain, which is refractory to physical therapy and other conservative methods for management. It is not advisable to manage adolescent back pain with narcotic use. Typically, patients may have pain along the convexity of the curve after activity or with muscle spasms along the concavity. However, in patients with Scheuermann kyphosis, pain along the lower thoracic spine or distal to the kyphosis is typical due to compensatory lumbar hyperlordosis. In either case, the pain should resolve when lying down, and this is a good indication of whether surgery would be helpful. However, back pain alone is not a good indication for surgery and provides less predictable surgical outcomes.

Surgery is indicated in patients with progressive scoliotic curves greater than 45 degrees, with or without back pain, that have not obtained relief from physical therapy and for patients with a significant amount of distress from the appearance of their deformity (rib hump, gibbus).

PREOPERATIVE PREPARATION

Deformity Analysis

The selection of appropriate fusion levels, aiming to maximize correction while fusing the least levels as possible, is an important consideration in spinal deformity surgery. For AIS, the Lenke et al. (7) classification simplified and clarified the decision-making process by including all curve types and sagittal plane measurements in addition to the flexibility theories postulated by King et al. (4). Proximal thoracic (PT), main thoracic (MT), and thoracolumbar/lumbar (TL/L) curves are analyzed, in addition to thoracic sagittal measurements (T5–T12), with special attention given to the thoracolumbar junction (T10–L2). Structural and compensatory curves must be differentiated. Briefly, all major curves (largest Cobb measurement) greater than 40 degrees are considered "structural," whether the curve decreases to less than 25 degrees on side-bending radiographs or not. For all other minor curves, those that decrease to less than 25 degrees are considered "compensatory" and nonstructural, which generally do not need to be fused. Correspondingly, those that side bend greater than 25 degrees are considered structural minor curves, which generally do need to be fused. Sagittal measurements of the thoracolumbar junction must be considered, because a kyphotic angle that is greater than or equal to 20 degrees in this region (T10–L2) implies a double major curve, regardless of coronal flexibility measurements. Specific measurement ratios must be taken into account with flexibility measurements close to the 25-degree threshold. The initial goal of these ratios was to help distinguish true and false double major curves within the King et al. (4) system; however, they apply today to threshold values in the Lenke et al. (7) system as well.

In analyzing scoliosis, the relative Cobb angles, apical vertebral translation (AVT), apical vertebral rotation (AVR), sagittal plane measurements, as well as shoulder balance and pelvic obliquity should be considered. The thoracic AVT is the distance from the center of the vertebral body at the thoracic apex to the C7 plumb line (C7PL). Similarly, the TL/L AVT is measured from the center of the lumbar apical vertebral body to the center sacral vertical line (CSVL). When the patient is perfectly balanced, the C7PL and CSVL are the same. The AVR is assessed using the Nash-Moe rotation index, which is graded on a scale from 0 to 4 where 0 is neutral or no rotation to grade 4, which is the most severely rotated (one pedicle is invisible, and the contralateral pedicle crosses the midline).

In analyzing kyphosis, the normal sagittal plane parameters are measured including the thoracic kyphosis from T2–T5 to T5–T12, the thoracolumbar kyphosis from T10 to L2, and the lumbar lordosis, which is measured from L1 to S1. In addition, we also consider the maximum kyphosis, which is measured from the vertebral endpoints showing the maximum deformity. Then, to consider sagittal balance, the sagittal sacral vertical line is used. Recently, occipitocervical parameters have been introduced (3). They provide guidelines for the orientation and position of the skull in relation to the cervical spine as well as the thoracic spine in relation to the maintenance of forward gaze and global sagittal balance.

Clinical assessment of the deformity is also an important aspect of deformity analysis. It is not unusual for curves with lower magnitudes to demonstrate large clinical deformities, or vice versa, where curves with larger magnitude only have smaller amounts of clinical deformity. This information is important for the surgical decision-making process with regard to the selection of fusion levels. For example, large clinical deformities might make selective fusions a less likely option in selecting fusion levels. This clinical impression should be correlated with standing, supine, and push-prone radiographs. Frequently, analysis of the relative heights of the clavicles, coracoid processes, and the T1 rib angle in relation to horizontal line can help predict postoperative shoulder position. These images can help determine rigid curves, which might require osteotomies for correction. During the clinical exam, it is important to note which shoulder is higher as supine or push-prone radiographs may indicate the contralateral shoulder to be higher. This is usually due to the flexibility of the lumbar or MT curve, or the rigidity of the PT curve, which is important to consider when determining fusion levels and the amount of correction desired as to not overcorrect the MT curve, thus resulting in shoulder imbalance.

Selection of Fusion Levels

To determine endpoints of the fusion, radiographic considerations are based on the Harrington stable zone and the neutral vertebra in addition to the aforementioned assessment of the clinical deformity present. The stable vertebra is the most proximal TL/L vertebra bisected by the CSVL. This lower endpoint is considered to be the most safe, but frequently we can stop one to two levels short of the stable vertebra, depending on rotation, curve magnitude, flexibility, coronal and sagittal balance, as well as other factors. Review of supine, push-prone, and lateral bending radiographs provides a sense of the postoperative balance. As a rule, the lowest instrumented vertebra (LIV) can be chosen as the most cephalad TL/L vertebra "touched" by the CSVL (Fig. 19-1) unless a significant amount of rotation exists at this level.

To determine the proximal endpoint of the fusion, shoulder position as well as flexibility and size of the PT curve must be taken into consideration. Under conditions where the PT curve is inflexible, where the supine or push-prone radiographs demonstrate contralateral shoulder elevation, or the upright clinical position of the contralateral shoulder is high, we usually extend the fusion proximally to T2. By "contralateral shoulder," we mean the shoulder opposite the main curve: that is, the left shoulder for a right thoracic curve or the right shoulder for a left lumbar curve. When the PT curve is somewhat flexible or the shoulders are in neutral position, we consider fusing to T3, whereas with flexible PT curves or a low contralateral shoulder, we typically fuse to T4.

When performing selective fusions, the degree to which the compensatory curves must accommodate must be considered. For thoracic major curves, ratios for all three variables of AVT, AVR, and curve magnitude between the MT and TL-L are used to determine curves, which may be able to undergo a selective fusion. Ratios that are close to 1.0 imply similar deformity characteristics to both curves; therefore, both curves should be fused. Ratios greater than 1.2 imply a false double major pattern, and selective fusion should be strongly considered. For TL/L major curves, the ratio is inverted (TL/L-MT), and a threshold of 1.25 is used. These are rough guidelines, which can provide some insight into how the compensatory curve will behave under the setting of a selective fusion.

The LIV should be tilted to allow for smooth transition into the compensatory curves. For type A coronal lumbar modifiers in the Lenke et al. (7) classification, the distal endplate of the LIV can often be corrected to horizontal. Mild tilt is allowed for the LIV of type B modifiers (CSVL touches the apical concave pedicle or medial vertebral body). For type C modifiers (CSVL lies medial to the apical lumbar vertebral body), an appropriate degree of tilt must be allowed. Intraoperative radiographs can aid in determining the remaining tilt of the LIV; however, supine and bending radiographs can help in the estimation.

In kyphotic deformities, sagittal plane considerations govern the fusion levels. We use the sagittal stable vertebra (SSV) concept to assess the correct distal level for fusion. The SSV is the vertebra touched by the posterior sacral vertical line. In some cases, this line might barely touch the anteroinferior corner of the vertebrae making the decision for selecting the distal fusion level ambiguous. If so, attention is turned toward the orientation of the adjacent disc space. If the proximal

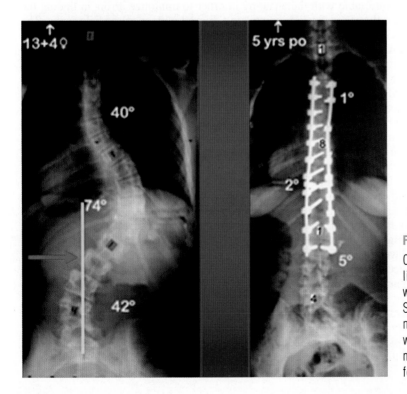

FIGURE 19-1

Center sacral vertebral line touching L2, which was selected as the LIV. Successful posterior spinal fusion was performed with good alignment maintained at 5-year follow-up radiographs.

disc space is lordotic, this vertebra is usually safe to choose as the distal fusion level. The next step is to locate the apex of the kyphosis on upright x-rays, which helps to determine the proximal level for fusion. For example, if an apex of the kyphosis is at T8 and the SSV was L2, we will usually maintain symmetry of the construct and extend the fusion roughly the same extent proximally (in this example, to T2).

Osteotomy Selection

Osteotomies can be excellent corrective tools for spinal deformities in the coronal and/or sagittal plane. The selection of the type of osteotomy will depend on the type, character, flexibility, and location of deformity. This information can be obtained from the radiographs as well as advanced imaging such as computer tomography (CT scans) and magnetic resonance imaging (MRI). Radiographs can be used to assess the rigidity of the curve, and CT scans and MRI can be used to assess the posterior elements and the anterior discs to assess flexible versus fixed segments. Generally speaking, if there is an area with prior anterior and posterior column fusions, a three-column osteotomy (pedicle subtraction, vertebral column resections) will be the only method capable of achieving correction. On the other hand, if the anterior column is not fused, posterior column osteotomies (Smith-Petersen or Ponté) may be sufficient. In addition, the magnitude and angularity of the deformity is important to consider. For example, smaller sagittal plane deformities may benefit from posterior column osteotomies alone, while those with a larger sagittal imbalance may need a three-column osteotomy (pedicle subtraction) to obtain sufficient correction. We usually perform pedicle subtraction osteotomies in the lumbar spine for fixed sagittal imbalance greater than 15 cm.

It is important to remember the general concept that posterior column-based osteotomies lengthen the anterior column, while three-column osteotomies shorten it. Therefore, MRI is useful for assessing anterior column structures. For example, in cases of kyphosis, it is essential to evaluate the quality of the thoracic discs when planning osteotomies. When there are significant disc bulges, posterior column osteotomies can result in stress load transfer to the disc space, thereby resulting in intraoperative disc herniation that can impinge on the spinal cord. In addition, MRI will show the amount of space available in order to determine whether a posterior column osteotomy can be performed without inadvertent risk to the spinal cord. In such cases, it may be safer to perform a three-column osteotomy, and the decision to proceed will rely on surgeon preference and comfort with performing them.

TECHNIQUE

Pedicle Screw Placement

It is essential to become comfortable with the anatomy in order to minimize errors in finding the pedicles as well as to ensure that good fixation points are achieved with every pedicle screw. The starting points for all thoracic screws are slightly variable and based on the posterior element anatomy visualized intraoperatively. This anatomy includes the transverse process, the lateral portion of the pars interarticularis, and the base of the superior articular process. Usually the supine preoperative film is very helpful for localizing the ideal starting point because of prone positioning during surgery. It is also beneficial to place each screw in a position parallel to the superior endplate of the thoracic spine as to maximize the strength of the fixation. We aim perpendicular to the lamina in the lower thoracic spine, where the facet joints are moving from a horizontal/coronally oriented position proximally to a vertical/sagittally oriented position in the lumbar spine. In the midthoracic spine, we aim perpendicular to the starting points at the junction of the transverse process, the facet, and the lamina.

In general, the surgeon should visualize the starting point based on as much anatomic information as possible and should always start from the neutrally rotated and distal vertebra. In starting distal at T12, there is a trend toward using a more medial and cephalad pedicle starting point on the posterior elements as the surgeon proceeds toward the apical midthoracic region (T7–T9). Proximal to this, the starting point tends to be more lateral and caudal as the surgeon proceeds more proximal to the T1 level. It is advantageous for the surgeon to note these trends when placing a screw at each level in succession, working in a distal-to-proximal direction in the thoracic spine, and to make fine adjustments to the trajectory of the previous level's screw or contralateral screw. It is also important to have smooth transitions between each screw for easy rod placement. When performing a selective thoracic or lumbar fusion, the surgeon must remember that the pedicles may be smaller in the concavity of the upper or lower compensatory curves. If hooks are used during the procedure, they are typically placed at the level of the uppermost thoracic vertebra because of the small pedicle size on the PT concavity. We routinely implement the free-hand pedicle screw placement technique.

In order to do this, however, the facet joints must be thoroughly cleaned and partially osteotomized to enhance visualization and fusion (Fig. 19-1). The inferior 3 to 5 mm of the inferior facet and the articular cartilage on the superior facet are removed except for at the most distal and most proximal levels. Adequate visualization of the superior articular process for imaginary localization of the ventral pedicle is essential for finding the correct starting point. This method provides consistent and correct localization of the starting points and obviates or minimizes the need for intraoperative radiography, fluoroscopy, or computer-guided systems.

First, a 5.5- or 3-mm bur (depending on patient size) is utilized to create a posterior cortical breach to a depth of approximately 5 mm until the pedicle "blush" should be visualized; this suggests entrance into the cancellous bone within the pedicle. This may not be seen in smaller, apical concave pedicles because of the limited intrapedicular cancellous bone. If so, the funnel technique can be used to find the cancellous track.

The blunt-tipped gearshift is placed in the pedicle and used to search for a cancellous bone indicating entrance to the pedicle (Fig. 19-2). The gearshift is initially pointed lateral as a safety measure to avoid medial wall perforation. The inner diameter of the pedicle can be quite small; thus, the gearshift should be allowed to "fall" into the pedicle. After the gearshift is inserted 20 to 25 mm, the gearshift is removed and the tip is turned to face medially and then advanced. The path down the pedicle is then continued medially into the body; use of the thoracic gearshift should proceed in a smooth and consistent manner with a snug feel. Any sudden advancement of the gearshift suggests a violation of a pedicle wall or vertebral body and should be investigated immediately in order to possibly salvage the pedicle and avoid complications. Usually, the ultimate depth averages 35 to 45 mm for the lower thoracic region, 30 to 40 mm for the midthoracic region, and 25 to 35 mm for the PT region in adolescents and adults. The surgeon rotates the gearshift 180 degrees, making room for the screw after advancing the finder to the approximate length of the desired screw. In addition, it allows the wider tip of the ball-tipped probe to extend the length that the gearshift has been inserted. This allows for accurate assessment of tract length and, ultimately, screw length. When using the ball-tipped pedicle probe, bone should be felt along the entire length of the pedicle (Fig. 19-3).

Once the ball-tipped pedicle probe confirms the five intraosseous borders (medial, lateral, superior, inferior, and anterior cortex of the vertebral body), the surgeon marks the length of the tract with a clamp. If the tract appears too shallow, consideration should be given to replacing the gearshift and advancing it to the appropriate length. The pedicle tract is undertapped with a tap 0.5 to 1.0 mm less in diameter than the intended screw (e.g., 4.5- or 5.0-mm tap for a 5.5-mm-diameter screw). If there is difficulty passing the tap, the surgeon should use the next smaller tap and retap the pedicle. If the pedicle is quite small or when more than one pass has to be made into a pedicle with the thoracic gearshift, a K-wire is placed down the pedicle tunnel into the body, and cannulated tapping can occur over that. It is mandatory that a bone floor exist when K-wire is used so as not to advance the K-wire beyond the anterior or lateral cortex. If there is any question of whether the anterior wall is intact, a K-wire must not be used.

Once the pedicle probe is removed, the tract is visualized to ensure a slow steady bleed from the pedicle tract. If excessive bleeding occurs, it might be an indication of an epidural vein secondary to a medial pedicle breach, and the screw may need to be redirected. Rarely, cerebrospinal fluid (CSF) may leak from the tract in which case the leak should not be explored. Placing bone wax over the defect will suffice and help prevent further CSF leakage.

We select the screw diameter based on preoperative assessment as well as how the pedicle "feels" with the pedicle finder. Pedicle diameter transitions occur gradually; therefore, segmental fixation allows the surgeon to note the fine variations between levels, with the goal of maximum fit and fill of the screw within the pedicle.

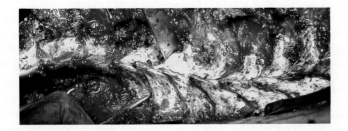

FIGURE 19-2

Complete exposure and partial facetectomy. The spine is systematically exposed to the edge of the transverse process bilaterally. The inferior facets are removed with a 0.5-inch straight osteotome (down to T10) or a rongeur (below T10). A small curette is used to remove articular cartilage from the superior facet of the inferior vertebrae.

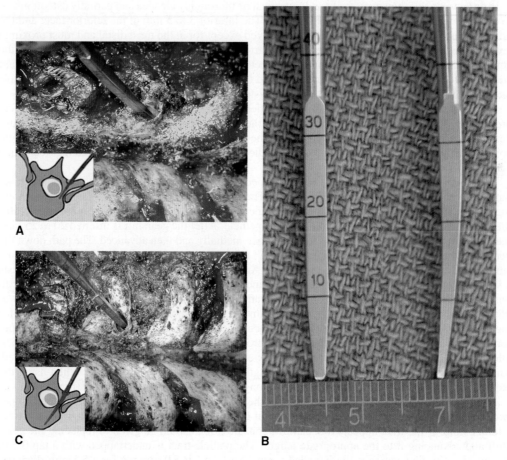

FIGURE 19-3

Creating the pedicle tract. **A:** After establishing the starting point, the 2-mm curved gearshift is inserted. The gearshift is initially directed laterally to the depth of 20 mm (the approximate depth of the pedicle) to diminish the likelihood of medial pedicle perforation. **B:** Two views of the thoracic gearshift with millimeter-depth markings. **C:** The gearshift is then removed and redirected medially. It is important to make sure the gearshift is inserted completely to the 20-mm depth before advancing. The surgeon should use the nondominant hand to brace the gearshift against sudden movement.

Although the ideal screw diameter is 80% of the pedicle diameter, screws up to 115% of the pedicle diameter may be inserted without causing a significant decrease in the screw's holding power, because of plasticity of the pedicular cortex in pediatric patients (8). We have determined the screw diameter by using the internal diameter of the neutrally rotated spine as a reference diameter and the tightness of the tap. We can insert screws if the internal diameter of the pedicle is more than 3 mm. After tapping, the pedicle tract is palpated again to make sure the five osseous borders are intact. This second palpation often allows palpation of distinct bone ridges, which helps confirm intraosseous position, and the tract length is remeasured with a clamp.

"Hubbing" the screws have been shown in biomechanical studies to reduce the pullout strength of the pedicle screw and are not routinely performed unless there is insufficient soft tissue coverage where screw profile prominence is an issue. This is rarely the case in AIS, although under adult revision settings for the thoracic spine, it might be more pertinent.

Correction Maneuvers

The correction maneuver is the most surgeon-dependent aspect of deformity surgery and typically follows a distinct sequence. In performing correction maneuvers, general concepts must also be remembered. Specifically, we must keep in mind that posterior compression is a lordosis-generating maneuver, and posterior distraction is a kyphosis generator. With this in mind, the concave rod is usually placed first for scoliosis, which is typically lordotic at the apex. While in kyphoscoliosis, the convex rod is usually placed first because corrective maneuvers of convex compression tend to remove kyphosis. In purely kyphotic deformities, the sequence of rod placement can occur from top-down or bottom-up.

Following pedicle screw insertion, the rods are measured and contoured into the sagittal and coronal plane alignment. It is often helpful to orient the cut end of the rod in a vertical direction while contouring to serve as a reference point. We typically secure the rod with two clamps and hold the rod over the wound to allow visualization during contouring. The rod tends to rotate with three-dimensional contouring; therefore, the use of two clamps and rod-reference orientation is helpful.

For scoliosis correction employing multiple apical concave reduction screws, after the rod is contoured, the concave rod is placed first and provisionally into the proximal fixation points. Usually, the proximal three to four fixation points are engaged, and set screws are placed temporarily into position to keep the rod engaged. Distally, the rod will be far from the pedicle screws. Then, with a combination of derotation and cantilever bending, the contoured rod is engaged into the pedicle screws distally along the apex of the curve, and set screws are placed to keep them engaged. The distal set screws are then tightened resulting in reduction of the deformity. Once the distal three to four fixation points are tightened down, it will be evident that the rod is not completely seated along the periapical segments. Attention is then turned toward tightening the reduction set screws down along the apical region. As the reduction set screws are gradually tightened, the spine is posterior laterally translated resulting in the apical correction. Care is taken to move up and down the periapical region in tightening the set screws as well as to not place too much force on one fixation point. This will distribute the forces evenly and will minimize the occurrence of screw pullout. Vigilant visualization of the screw/bone interface is essential at this point so that the correction maneuver can be modified or stopped if there is evidence of screw pullout. Once the rod is closer to fully engaging the rod along the apical region, distractors are used along the apex of the curve to fine-tune the correction and enhance apical kyphosis. Care is taken to proceed very slowly as to not exceed three to five clicks with the distractor over any given fixation point at one time. Once this is completed, the set screws are provisionally tightened, and attention is turned toward placement of the contralateral rod. The contralateral rod is contoured and placed allowing for apical compression along the convexity that can also help to fine-tune the reduction. Compression is performed slowly as to not exceed three to five clicks over any one level. In situ benders are then used to fine-tune the reduction further to ensure adequate sagittal plane parameters are contoured into the correction. This is done with the set screws loosely placed as to not compromise fixation points by placing too much stress on the screw with the bending moments caused by rod contouring. Finally, once the set screws are provisionally tightened, an assessment of the coronal balance is roughly assessed intraoperatively. Long-cassette radiographs are then taken to assess overall balance.

In cases of kyphosis correction, the sequence of rod placement is less important. Usually, we will place both rods before the correction maneuver is initiated. Once the rods are secured at the apex of the kyphosis, a series of compression maneuvers are performed above and below the apex bilaterally and simultaneously toward the apex to achieve correction. Several passes may be necessary to allow viscoelastic relaxation to occur and to ensure the bone-screw interface is not weakened or compromised. Long-cassette AP and lateral radiographs are taken to assess the instrumentation, correction, and overall balance.

We routinely perform periapical posterior column osteotomies for the majority of scoliosis or kyphosis deformities. This allows for a thorough release of the ligamentous and bony attachments along the apical regions, which allows us to achieve a better correction and, more importantly, "frees" up the spinal segments to allow us to perform our corrective maneuvers with less resistance, resulting in less stress on the pedicle screw/bone interface. Three-column osteotomies are reserved for more severe and/or angular deformities or under revision settings where there maybe fused or rigid segments.

POSTOPERATIVE MANAGEMENT

Pediatric patients are typically observed in a pediatric intensive care unit setting overnight and then transferred to the pediatric orthopedic floor. They are placed on a patient-controlled analgesia regimen and then oral narcotic medications once they are tolerating fluids and passing flatus. Physical therapy begins on postoperative day 1 with the patient sitting and then briefly standing with assistance on the 1st day. This is gradually progressed to ambulation independently on subsequent days. The Foley catheter is removed when a patient is ambulating well. Prophylactic antibiotics are discontinued after the drains, and Foley catheter is removed, typically on postoperative day 3 or 4. Standing long-cassette AP and lateral radiographs are obtained when the patient is able to walk in the halls without difficulty. We do not routinely implement postoperative bracing. The patient may shower after discharge from the hospital at 2 weeks postoperative, if the wound is healing well. The patient also begins mild trunk range-of-motion exercises according to the comfort level.

COMPLICATIONS/RESULTS

We studied the results of these techniques in 114 consecutive patients with AIS treated by the senior author at our institution with a minimum of 3-year follow-up (5). The average preoperative Cobb angle of the major curve was 65 degrees (range, 42 to 149 degrees). The postoperative Cobb angle of the major curve averaged 18.8 degrees (average correction, 71.8% ± 15.2%). The correction rates according to the Lenke et al. (7,9) curve classification system were 72.8% in type 1 scoliosis (41 patients), 70.4% in type 2 (18 patients), 65.4% in type 3 (18 patients), 65.3% in type 4 (8 patients), 77.8% in type 5 (5 patients), and 83.6% in type 6 (10 patients). No complications from screw insertion, such as neurologic injury, were noted with our techniques.

CONCLUSION

Thoracic and lumbar pedicle screw instrumentation minimizes complications resulting from implant failure or dislodgment while providing three-column fixation of the spine. Using our techniques, we have not seen neurologic complications related to pedicle screw placement to date. The tremendous three-dimensional correcting power of pedicle screws has allowed us to obviate the need for anterior surgery, and in the last 7 years, we have not needed to perform AIS surgery with an anterior and posterior combined approach regardless of curve magnitude. This has clearly redefined how scoliosis is operatively managed at our institution.

RECOMMENDED READING

1. Cinotti G, Gumina S, Ripani M, et al.: Pedicle instrumentation in the thoracic spine. A morphometric and cadaveric study for placement of screws. *Spine* 24: 114–119, 1999.
2. Hamill CL, Lenke LG, Bridwell KH, et al.: The use of pedicle screw fixation to improve correction in the lumbar spine of patients with idiopathic scoliosis. Is it warranted? *Spine* 21: 1241–1249, 1996.
3. Kim HJ MD, Lenke LG MD, et al.: Occipital Incidence—a Novel Morphometric Parameter for Understanding Occipitocervical Spinal Alignment. Presented at the International Meeting in Advanced Spinal Techniques, Istanbul, Turkey, 2012—Whitecloud Award Nominee.
4. King HA, Moe JH, Bradford DS, et al.: The selection of fusion levels in thoracic idiopathic scoliosis. *J Bone Joint Surg Am* 65: 1302–1313, 1983.
5. Lehman RA Jr, Lenke LG, et al.: Operative treatment of adolescent idiopathic scoliosis with posterior pedicle screw-only constructs: minimum three-year follow-up of one hundred fourteen cases. *Spine* 33: 1598–1604, 2008.
6. Lehman RA Jr, Polly DW Jr, Kuklo TR, et al.: Straight-forward versus anatomic trajectory technique of thoracic pedicle screw fixation: a biomechanical analysis. *Spine (Phila Pa 1976)* 28(18): 2058–2065, 2003.
7. Lenke LG, Betz RR, Harms J, et al.: Adolescent idiopathic scoliosis: a new classification to determine extent of spinal arthrodesis. *J Bone Joint Surg Am* 83: 1169–1181, 2001.
8. O'Brien MF, Lenke LG, Mardjetko S, et al.: Pedicle morphology in thoracic adolescent idiopathic scoliosis: is pedicle fixation an anatomically viable technique? *Spine* 25: 2285–2293, 2000.
9. Suk SI, Kim WJ, Lee SM, et al.: Thoracic pedicle screw fixation in spinal deformities: are they really safe? *Spine* 26: 2049–2057, 2001.
10. Suk SI, Lee CK, Kim WJ, et al.: Segmental pedicle screw fixation in the treatment of thoracic idiopathic scoliosis. *Spine* 20: 1399–1405, 1995.

20 Lumbar Pedicle Subtraction Osteotomy

Sigurd H. Berven and Praveen Mummaneni

INDICATIONS/CONTRAINDICATIONS

Posterior-based osteotomies contraction (PSO) in the lumbar spine encompass a spectrum of techniques that are intended to realign the spine through resection of posterior elements with variable resection of the anterior column of the spine. The spectrum of posterior-based osteotomies is listed in Table 20-1. The spectrum of osteotomies is a continuum, and the osteotomy techniques share steps including resection of the facet joints, decancellation, and partial or complete corpectomy from a posterior approach. The spectrum of osteotomies begins with a resection of the facet joints alone and realignment of the spine with an axis of rotation at the anterior longitudinal ligament in a mobile spine (type 1) or anterior column osteoclasis through a rigid spine (type 2). Decancellation of the vertebral body through the pedicle permits a controlled fracture of the anterior column and may be useful in realigning the spine in the coronal and sagittal plane, as described by Heinig in the "eggshell osteotomy" (type 3). The lumbar pedicle subtraction osteotomy is a wedge resection of the vertebral body from below the pedicle to the anterior cortex of the vertebra, and the wedge resection may be entirely intraosseous with a hinge on the superior third of the vertebral body (type 5) or at the supraadjacent disc (type 6). Finally, a posterior resection of one or more vertebra and discs may be useful in treating more complex deformity including translation of the trunk. The purpose of this chapter is to describe the technique of the lumbar pedicle subtraction osteotomy.

The lumbar pedicle subtraction osteotomy (transpedicular vertebral wedge resection) is a useful technique for the operative correction of both sagittal and coronal plane deformity (4). The clinical impact of deformity is determined and predicted primarily by the sagittal plane (12,18). The primary indication for the technique is correction of sagittal plane deformity in the patient who has had a previous circumferential fusion of the spine. The transpedicular wedge resection technique was first described by Thomasen (27) in 1989 for the management of fixed sagittal plane deformity in ankylosing spondylitis. Common etiologies of fixed sagittal plane deformity include ankylosing spondylitis, or iatrogenic causes of fixed sagittal plane deformity including flatback syndrome (8) and kyphotic decompensation syndrome (10). More generally, lumbar spine kyphosis with variable degrees of rigidity may be the result of degenerative change, congenital anomaly, trauma, neoplastic disease with pathologic fracture, or infection. The rigidity of lumbar kyphosis and the apex of the deformity are important determinants of the surgical approach. In a spine with a mobile anterior column, or a flexible deformity, posterior-based osteotomies with facet resection and deformity correction through the disc space or osteoclasis of the anterior column may be useful. In a spine with an apex of deformity at L4 or L5, a combined anterior and posterior approach to the spine may be useful in recreating lordosis at the lumbosacral segments and correcting a rigid coronal obliquity of a fractional curve from L4 to S1. The lumbar pedicle subtraction osteotomy may be used at any level of the lumbar spine and is most useful for rigid

257

TABLE 20-1 Spectrum of Posterior-Based Osteotomies

Type	Description	Diagram	Reference
1	Resection of posterior elements from mid-pars above to pedicle below with realignment of the spine through hinging through a mobile disc anteriorly		Ponte
2	Resection of posterior elements from mid-pars above to pedicle below with realignment of the spine through hinging through the anterior column of the spine which is ankylosed. The opening involves osteoclasis rather than movement through a mobile intervertebral disc		Smith-Peterson
3	Posterior-based transpedicular decancellation of the vertebral body with realignment through controlled fracture of the anterior column		Heinig
4	Posterior-based intraosseous wedge resection of the vertebral body with realignment through osteoclasis of the proximal third of the anterior vertebral body		Thomasen
5	Posterior-based wedge resection with extension of the osteotomy into the supraadjacent disc and realignment hinging on the anterior column at the intervertebral space		Modified Thomasen
6	Posterior-based vertebral column resection including one or more vertebra with adjacent discs		Suk

deformity, which requires resection of bone including a portion of the anterior column for mobilization and realignment. The technique may also be used above the level of the conus including the cervical and thoracic spine.

The lumbar pedicle subtraction osteotomy fits best in the spectrum or posterior-based osteotomies as an option for patients with a sagittal deformity that is correctable with an apical resection of approximately 30 degrees and coronal imbalance less than 8 cm (1). Although the lumbar pedicle subtraction osteotomy may be used in the patient with open disc spaces and mobility of the anterior column of the spine, the authors prefer to use a combined anterior and posterior approach (5), or posterior-based osteotomies as described by Ponte for the patient with a mobile anterior column as these techniques permit a more gradual and harmonious realignment of the spine through the creation of trapezoidal intervertebral disc spaces (11). If osteoclasis is possible for the anterior column, the Smith-Peterson osteotomy may be useful to create segmental realignment (23). In the patient with a severe lumbar kyphosis that requires more than 40 degrees of correction, or trunk translation and coronal imbalance greater than 8 cm, a vertebral column resection may prove more advantageous (6,26).

PREOPERATIVE PREPARATION

Patient Assessment

The patient with a fixed sagittal plane imbalance presents with an inability to maintain horizontal gaze, fatigue to the thighs and hips, and back pain that is often intractable. Normal sagittal alignment of the spine follows a vertical axis from the center of C2, in front of T7, behind L3, and to the posterior margin of the sacrum (Fig. 20-1). Forward displacement of C7 relative to the pelvis may be due to regional malalignment in the lumbar, thoracic, and cervical spine. Extraaxial causes of global sagittal malalignment may commonly be caused by hip flexion contracture, especially in older patients, patients with neuromuscular scoliosis, and patients with ankylosing spondylitis. A differentiation of the anatomic source of sagittal plane deformity may be gleaned from a thorough physical examination. On standing, the patient's deformity is best appreciated with the knees fully extended. On sitting, if sagittal balance corrects or if the trunk appears with good balance relative to the pelvis, then a hip flexion contracture may be the cause of sagittal plane malalignment. A hip flexion contracture can be demonstrated using the Thomas test. If the patient remains

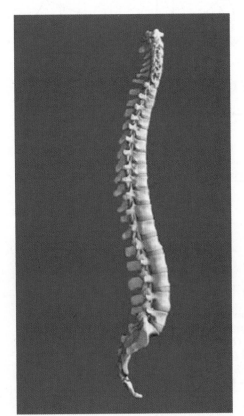

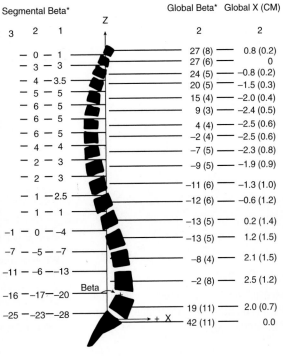

FIGURE 20-1

Normal sagittal alignment of the spine.

with forward displacement of the occiput relative to the pelvis on sitting, then the patient should be evaluated in the supine position. In the patient with deformity localized to the lumbar spine, the patient will be able to lie with shoulders on the table in the supine position with flexion of the knees and extension of the hips. In contrast, if the patient remains with head and upper thoracic spine elevated from the table in the supine position, fixed deformity in the cervical and/or thoracic spine is likely.

The patient with fixed sagittal imbalance will present with a characteristic stance and gait pattern. Patients extend at the hips and flex at the knees in order to maintain sagittal balance. This compensatory mechanism leads to significant fatigue of the quadriceps and limited standing and walking tolerance. Patients typically walk with short steps and may require a walker for support in cases of more severe imbalance. The patient with a wide-based gait or ataxia should be evaluated for myelopathy and possible spinal cord pathology. Hip extension may be quantified by measuring the pelvic tilt radiographically. On clinical exam, extension of the hips is identifiable by inspection of the position of the anterior superior iliac spine compared with the posterior superior iliac spine and by an apparent flattening of the buttocks. The cervical spine may also be affected by global deformity in the thoracic and lumbar spine, and neck pain is a common clinical complaint of patients with sagittal deformity due to hyperextension of the cervical spine to maintain horizontal gaze.

Radiographic Evaluation

Standing 14 × 36 inch radiographs in the posteroanterior and lateral projections are most useful for an assessment of the global and regional alignment of the spine. The lateral radiograph represents the spinal deformity most accurately with the knees fully extended and the shoulders at 30- to 60-degree forward flexion (28). Placing the proximal interphalangeal joints in the clavicular fossa may result in a more accurate radiographic assessment of sagittal alignment and less radiographically apparent sagittal malalignment than having the arms in 60 degrees of forward flexion (13). Inclusion of the proximal femur in the lateral view permits an assessment of the femoropelvic contribution to sagittal deformity and measurement of pelvic tilt and pelvic incidence (Fig. 20-2). Normal lumbar

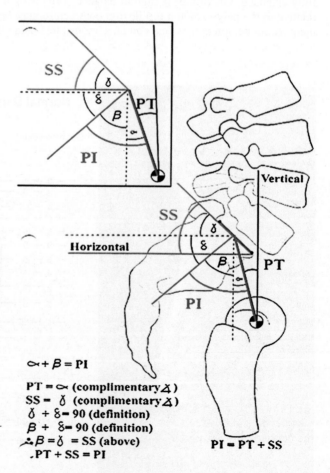

$\alpha + \beta = PI$

$PT = \alpha$ (complimentary $\angle$)

$SS = \delta$ (complimentary $\angle$)

$\delta + \epsilon = 90$ (definition)

$\beta + \epsilon = 90$ (definition)

$\therefore \beta = \delta = SS$ (above)

$\therefore PT + SS = PI$

$PI = PT + SS$

FIGURE 20-2

Measurement of lumbopelvic parameters. PT, Pelvic tilt; PI, Pelvic incidence; SS, Sacral scope.

lordosis is closely correlated to the pelvic incidence. Realignment of the spine should aim to match lumbar lordosis to within 10 degrees of pelvic incidence (1). Patients with a high pelvic incidence may require significantly more than 40 degrees of lumbar lordosis for optimal sagittal alignment of the spine. Even small losses of segmental lordosis in the lower lumbar spine may translate to large changes in global alignment between C7 and the sacrum. Flexion and extension radiographs, including imaging over a bolster, are useful to determine the flexibility of the deformity above and below the planned osteotomy.

Magnetic resonance imaging is most useful in assessing the space available for the neural elements, especially in the region of the planned osteotomy. In the presence of spinal instrumentation, a computerized tomogram with myelography can provide accurate imaging of the spinal canal. Computerized tomography may also be useful in measuring ankylosis of motion segments and rigidity of the spine. An assessment of spinal stenosis is particularly important in the patient in whom an anterior first stage may be considered for deformity correction because introduction of lordosis in a stenotic lumbar spine may lead to significant loss of space for the neural elements and neurologic deficit. If significant stenosis is present on preoperative imaging of the spinal canal, special care must be taken to first decompress and then to mobilize the posterior portion of the intervertebral space with parallel distraction of the disc space to avoid hinging of the intact posterior longitudinal ligament and worsening the stenosis.

Measurement of Wedge Resection and Prediction of Correction

Sagittal alignment of the spine may be considered at the segmental, regional, and global levels. The goal of segmental alignment of the spine is the creation of trapezoidal intervertebral disc spaces, either through segmental lordosis across the disc space or through lordosis over an interbody implant. The goal of regional alignment of the spine is thoracic kyphosis in the physiologic range of 30 to 40 degrees (29). There is significant variability in normal lumbar lordosis, and matching lumbar lordosis to the pelvic incidence is an important goal of regional realignment of the spine (19). At the cervicothoracic junction, restoration of a chin-brow angle to neutral is an important goal (25). An accurate assessment of the amount of correction to expect from a single-level transpedicular wedge resection may be made using the 36-inch preoperative lateral image and basic trigonometry. The amount of global realignment of the spine from a transpedicular wedge resection osteotomy is a function of the level of the osteotomy, with more correction at lower levels, and by the size of the wedge resected. Ondra et al. described a mathematical model for the prediction of sagittal plane realignment after pedicle subtraction osteotomy (PSO) (30). The transpedicular wedge resection will leave the height of the anterior column intact, but the posterior column will be compressed as a wedge, the height of which equals the height of the planned resection. An important limitation of this technique is that the sagittal offset of the C7 plumb line from the sacrum may underestimate the actual global sagittal plane deformity. Pelvic tilt is an important component of sagittal plane alignment. Unintended reciprocal changes of the uninstrumented thoracic spine and the femoropelvic junction may be difficult to predict and may compromise overall sagittal plane realignment (15).

TECHNIQUE

Positioning

Patient positioning is an important portion of the correction of deformity (24). In the patient with a mobile spine, prone positioning on a Jackson frame may directly result in significant improvement in sagittal alignment and may influence the decision to perform a PSO compared with an osteotomy of the posterior facet joints only. Intraoperatively, resection of the facet joints with the patient extended over a chest and pelvic frame may also lead to significant spontaneous sagittal plane correction during the early stages of the osteotomy and may influence the type of osteotomy to pursue. The patient with a fixed sagittal plane deformity presents a challenge for positioning in both the supine and the prone position. In the supine position for intubation, the patient will require head support and elevation because the shoulders may be elevated from the table. Fiberoptic nasotracheal intubation facilitates visualization of the true vocal cords in the patient with significant deformity and rigidity in the cervicothoracic region.

In the prone position, the patient with a fixed sagittal plane deformity in the lumbar spine may not fit well on a standard four poster, with incongruity between the pelvis and the hip pads, and the ribs and the chest pad that may lead to point loading of the skin and skin breakdown. We prefer to use a technique with two separate posts each for the chest and the pelvis. In separating the posts, we may flex the operating room table to accommodate the preoperative deformity and permit the chest and pelvis to be congruent with the contour of the post. The hips are positioned in full extension, with care to keep pressure off of the patella and other bony prominences including the elbows and periorbital region. After the osteotomy is complete, reversal of the flexion of the table permits and facilitates a controlled closure of the wedge resection.

Surgical Approach

The posterior approach to the spine is a standard midline open approach. A subperiosteal dissection is completed to the level of the transverse process tips of the segments to be fused. The spine is exposed at least from a level at least two segments above the planned osteotomy to at least two segments below, because stable internal fixation requires instrumentation to two of three segments above and below the osteotomy at a minimum. Pedicle screws are placed at the levels above and below the osteotomy. In order to include three segments below the osteotomy, the instrumentation may extend to include the ilium using one or two iliac screws (Galveston technique).

At the level of the planned lumbar pedicle subtraction osteotomy, the transverse processes are removed and saved for local bone graft. Using a Penfield elevator followed by a small osteotome, an interval between the lateral walls of the vertebra and the psoas muscle is developed, just lateral to the pedicle. The exiting nerve root from the level above the osteotomy is protected within the psoas muscle. By remaining at the level of the pedicle, the segmental vessels are avoided. A sponge or retractor is useful to preserve the exposure of the lateral cortex. Adequate exposure and subsequent wedge resection of the lateral cortex is critical for an effective, low-energy osteotomy closure. Decompression of the spinal canal begins at the lamina of the vertebra to be osteotomized. The margins of the posterior resection are from the mid-pars of the vertebra above to the pedicle of the vertebra below. It is important to extend the decompression to at least one level above and one level below the pedicle subtraction, meaning a partial or complete laminectomy of L3 and L5 if the L4 pedicle is to be resected. If a wide decompression is not accomplished, the posterior elements may impinge upon the spinal canal with the wedge closure.

After a wide midline decompression, the remaining posterior elements (the superior facet, the inferior facet, and the pars) of the vertebra to be osteotomized are removed. The goal in this portion of the surgery is to skeletonize the pedicles such that there is no remaining attachment to the pedicles bilaterally. After removal of the posterior elements, the remaining pedicle is visible as are the nerve roots above and below (Fig. 20-3). Fat and perineurium should be left around the nerve roots during this exposure. Hemostasis is maintained by bipolar electrocautery and thrombin-soaked Gelfoam.

Excision of the pedicle effectively creates a single foramen shared by the nerve root above the osteotomy and the nerve root at the level of the osteotomy. Excision of the pedicle and partial corpectomy of the vertebra may be done with an osteotome and a direct wedge resection, or may be done with decancellation of the vertebra through the pedicle. In the process of decancellating the pedicle and vertebral body, the pedicle is thinned with a pedicle probe to the point of breaking spontaneously, to be removed with a pituitary rongeur. The technique of decancellation is especially effective in patients with osteoporosis and limits blood loss. In patients with more rigid or dense bone, use of an osteotomy to directly cut a wedge from the posterior elements is useful. The orientation of the wedge resection is important. The nerve root exiting below the pedicle defines the inferior margin of the resection. The superior margin is defined by the superior endplate of the osteotomized vertebra (type 4 posterior osteotomy) or by the disc above (type 5 posterior osteotomy). If the disc above the osteotomy is to be included in the osteotomy, then a complete discectomy including meticulous endplate resection should be performed prior to starting the pedicle excision and partial corpectomy. Meticulous endplate preparation facilitates bone healing across the osteotomy when the disc is removed.

Resection of the pedicles should proceed to one side at a time. Placing a temporary short rod from the pedicle screw above to the screw below will prevent translation of the spine and preserve the space for working ventral to the neural elements. On the side where the first pedicle is resected, extending the medial margin of the resection beyond the midline facilitates resection

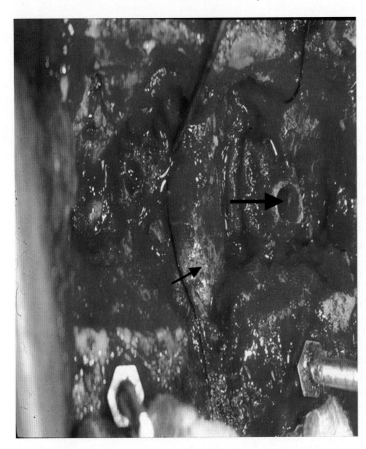

FIGURE 20-3

Isolation of the pedicles bilaterally after midline decompression with resection of the superior facet above, the pars interarticularis, and the inferior facet below. *Large arrow*—L3 pedicle; *small arrow*—thecal sac.

of the residual posterior vertebral wall with excision of the second pedicle. Decancellation of the vertebra ventral to the posterior wall is achieved with a reverse angle curette and permits a simple resection of the thin posterior wall by ventral displacement using little force. Any posterior vertebral wall that may remain after resection of the pedicles may be removed with a reverse angle curette pushing the posterior cortex ventral from the protected neural elements. A Penfield 3 is useful to protect the neural elements during resection of the posterior cortex of the vertebra. Wedge resection of the vertebral body is systematic, and the posterior height of the resection extends across two-thirds or more of the vertebral body, while anteriorly the wedge ends just posterior to the anterior cortex of the vertebral body. It is easier to remove bone that is well anterior to the neural elements, and a tendency to resect bone from the anterior portion of the vertebra should be avoided as this will create a gap anteriorly that will remain after closure of the wedge. Asymmetric resection of bone from the right and left sides of the vertebra permits significant coronal plane realignment with osteotomy closure. The last portion of the vertebra to remove is the lateral cortex. The lateral cortex is easily visualized medial to the sponge or retractor that separated the vertebra from the psoas muscle. A wedge resection of the lateral cortex may be accomplished with a narrow rongeur or an osteotome. The anterior extent of the wedge should be near the anterior cortex of the vertebral body.

Closure of the osteotomy is guided over temporary rods to prevent translation of the spine and compression of the neural elements. Loosening the set screws on the temporary rod that was used to maintain intervertebral height during the osteotomy will permit some spontaneous closure of the osteotomy after resection of the lateral wall. Temporary rods bent to 70 degrees may be placed two levels above the osteotomy and one level below to use a gentle cantilever technique to close the osteotomy. Gentle compression between the screw above and below will facilitate complete closure of the osteotomy. At the time of osteotomy closure, a Penfield may be used to confirm that the osteotomy is closed congruently. Temporary rods may be replaced by long permanent rods that span all of the instrumented segments of the spine. An alternative is to leave short rods across the osteotomy spanning one level above and below, and long rods spanning over the osteotomy level across the entire instrumented spine. The latter technique results in four rods across the osteotomy, which increases rigidity of fixation across the osteotomy site (17).

PEARLS AND PITFALLS

Potential pitfalls of the lumbar pedicle subtraction osteotomy include neural injury, excessive blood loss, and nonunion. Removal of the pedicle, decancellation of the vertebral body, and closure of the osteotomy are portions of the procedure in which the neural elements are at risk and bleeding may be quite brisk. Meticulous exposure of the osseous elements is useful in avoiding excessive bleeding. Use of a bipolar electrocautery on the epidural vessels and thrombin-soaked Gelfoam is useful to control bleeding prior to the osteotomy. A sharp periosteal elevator is used to dissect the soft tissue laterally to the base of the pedicle and anteriorly along the outer wall of the vertebral body, taking great care to avoid injury to the segmental vessels and exiting nerve roots. If there is a tear of the segmental vessel, bipolar electrocautery will control ventral bleeding. Blunt dissection with a surgical sponge in the subperiosteal plane avoids sharp injury to the segmental vessels. The use of cell saver intraoperatively and autogenous blood donation preoperatively reduces the need for allogenic blood product. Anticipation of coagulopathy with blood loss over 1 L or 4 hours of surgical time, and early transfusion of cell saver or fresh frozen plasma will prevent exponential rates of blood loss associated with coagulopathy. Bleeding may also be limited by the use of antifibrinolytic drugs during surgery (3).

In order to protect the neural elements during resection of the vertebral body, we use two handheld dural retractors positioned for each pedicle. A Woodson elevator and a Penfield 3 to mobilize the ventral aspect of the dura from the posterior longitudinal ligament will help prevent a ventral dural tear. The neural elements are also at risk from possible translation of the spine at the level of the osteotomy. Placement of a temporary rod to span the osteotomy on one side while working on the opposite side will protect against uncontrolled closure of the osteotomy or translation of the spine across the osteotomy. The neural elements are at risk at the time of closure of the osteotomy. The fracture through the anterior cortex is a greenstick fracture (torus type) and does not involve a complete disruption of the anterior cortex. The anterior cortex serves as a hinge and prevents translation of the spinal column. In the case of ankylosing spondylitis, or prior circumferential fusion of the spine, special care is necessary to ensure that the anterior cortex remains a hinge and is not completely disrupted by translation. Forceful fracture reduction should be avoided as this can lead to loosening of the screws adjacent to the osteotomy, and translation and uncontrolled closure of the osteotomy. The osteotomy should close spontaneously over temporary rods with minimal posterior compression. If the wedge is not closing easily with posterior compression, the lateral wedges and the anterior cortex should be reevaluated. Distraction across the osteotomy will permit further resection of bone from the lateral wall and from the anterior one-third of the vertebral body. The osteotomy shortens the spinal canal and may lead to infolding of dura, especially in revision cases with significant dural scarring. Shortening of the spinal canal is protective for neural blood flow and nerve function. Dural infolding is rarely symptomatic. Transient neurologic deficits have been reported in up to 20% of transpedicular wedge resection osteotomies, and an adequate decompression is important in reducing the incidence of this complication (7). Motor evoked potentials with multiple myotomes are sensitive techniques for monitoring neurologic function and are followed closely during the wedge closure. If there is a change in motor evoked potentials, then immediate reversal of the osteotomy closure will usually result in a prompt return of signals. Exploration of the epidural space for sources of compression, and extension of the decompression cephalad, caudad, and laterally, is important prior to reclosure of the osteotomy. If infolding of dura is determined to be the cause of neural compression, then an anterior cage may be used as a fulcrum to lengthen the anterior column of the spine and permit similar angular closure with less posterior shortening. An excision of epidural scar or even a resection of a posterior segment of dura may rarely be required if infolding is significant and symptomatic.

Pseudarthrosis is an important late complication of the lumbar pedicle subtraction osteotomy. Symptomatic pseudarthrosis has been reported in up to 30% of cases at 5-year follow-up (14). Symptomatic rod fracture has been identified in 16% of patients after PSO (21). Posterior arthrodesis is optimized by meticulous preparation of the transverse processes above and below the osteotomy for a posterolateral fusion. The midline decompression prevents a midline fusion. Approximation of the mid-pars above to the pedicle below may facilitate bridging bone across the posterior columns, but a gap between the pars and the pedicle may be useful to preserve space for the shared neural foramen for the nerves above and below the pedicle excision. The most reliable fusion is of the anterior column. The cancellous bone of the vertebral body will heal reliably. However, a mobile anterior column with open disc spaces above and below the osteotomy may lead to nonunion. In patients with open disc spaces anteriorly, a transforaminal interbody fusion at the level below the osteotomy, and an extension of the osteotomy to the disc space above the osteotomy, is useful to gain solid arthrodesis of the anterior column. Circumferential fusion of the discs above and below may also be accomplished with posterior or direct lateral interbody arthrodesis at the level above and below the osteotomy.

POSTOPERATIVE MANAGEMENT

We place subfascial drains at the end of the procedure, and these are removed when drainage is less than 30 mL per shift. Early mobilization of the patient minimizes postoperative complications including atelectasis, ileus, thromboembolic disease, and skin compromise. Most patients are transferred from the operating theater to a surgical floor after surgery. The patient may remain intubated overnight after this surgery depending upon the length of surgery, laryngeal edema, fluid shifts, and the difficulty of intubation. Postoperatively, the patient may transfer from a bed to the chair without a brace on day 1. We use a thoracolumbar sacral orthosis for patients with poor bone quality or patients who may be at significant risk of junctional kyphosis, specifically patients who have osteoporosis, thoracic kyphosis more than 30 degrees, and a kyphotic proximal junctional motion segment.

RESULTS

Pedicle subtraction osteotomy is a powerful tool to correct spinal imbalance. Realignment of sagittal balance can result in a significant improvement of patient-reported health status and high rates of patient satisfaction (1,4). The PSO compared favorable to alternative procedures including combined anterior and posterior surgery for sagittal deformity, including in cases of posttraumatic kyphosis (9). However, previous reports have documented significant morbidity in patients undergoing PSO, including neurologic deficits, infections, spinal fluid leakage, visual deficits, deep vein thrombosis, and pulmonary embolism. These complication rates are higher in revision cases (16,22). Inadequate correction of deformity may also be common in patients with larger preoperative sagittal plane deformities (20). In a recent publication reviewing the results of 87 PSO operations with 2 years of follow-up, Auerbach et al. reported a 38% rate of major surgical complications. These authors reported a nearly 2-L mean blood loss for their PSO cases (with a mean of ten levels of fusion). Risk factors for major complications included over 4 cm of sagittal imbalance, age over 60 years, and three or more medical comorbidities. In spite of these complication rates, the authors reported a significant improvement in the scoliosis research society subscores for pain and function for those who underwent PSOs for correction of global spinal balance (2). Rhin et al. reported complications in 62% of patients in the perioperative or late follow-up period. Despite complications, the majority of patient had a significant improvement of leg and back pain at long-term follow-up averaging over 6 years.

ILLUSTRATIVE CASE FOR TECHNIQUE

A 68-year-old male retired man underwent prior fusion for degenerative lumbar changes from L3 to S1. After surgery, the patient reported a significant increase in low back pain with difficulty standing upright. He reported standing intolerance of more than 10 minutes and inability to walk more than two blocks without support. He was treated with a PSO at the level of L3, with instrumented fusion from T11 to S1. A lateral interbody fusion was performed at L2–L3 to secure circumferential fusion of the spine around the osteotomy. At 2-year follow-up, the patient was able to walk unlimited distances and reported no significant back pain (Fig. 20-4).

Radiographic Measures

	Preop	Post-op	Change
C7 Plumb line	123	38	85
Lumbar lordosis	18	56	38
Thoracic kyphosis	18	46	28
Pelvic tilt	40	18	22
Sacral slope	10	32	22

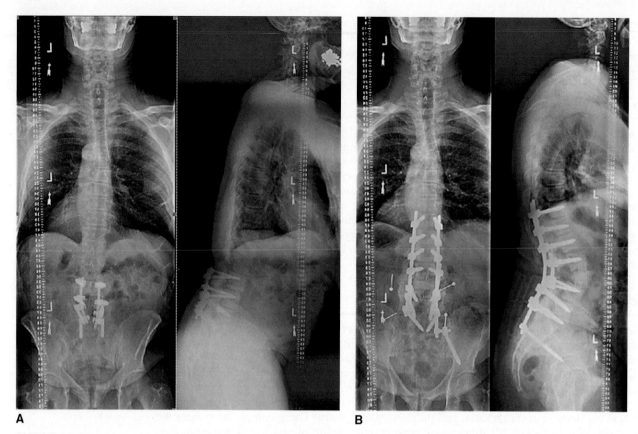

A   **B**

FIGURE 20-4

Preoperative **(A)** and postoperative **(B)** radiographs demonstrating the pedicle subtraction osteotomy.

RECOMMENDED READING

1. Ames CP, Smith JS, Scheer JK, et al.: Impact of spinopelvic alignment on decision making in deformity surgery in adults: a review. *J Neurosurg Spine* 16(6): 547–564, 2012.
2. Auerbach JD, Lenke LG, Bridwell KH, et al.: Major complications and comparison between 3-column osteotomy techniques in 105 consecutive spinal deformity procedure. *Spine (Phila Pa 1976)* 37(14): 1198–210, 2012.
3. Baldus CR, Bridwell KH, Lenke LG, et al.: Can we safely reduce blood loss during lumbar pedicle subtraction osteotomy procedures using tranexamic acid or aprotinin? A comparative study with controls. *Spine (Phila Pa 1976)* 35(2): 235–239, 2010.
4. Berven S, Deviren V, Smith J, et al.: Management of fixed sagittal plane deformity: results of the transpedicular wedge resection osteotomy. *Spine* 26(18): 2036–2043, 2001.
5. Berven SH, Deviren V, Smith JA, et al.: Management of fixed sagittal plane deformity: outcome of combined anterior and posterior surgery. *Spine (Phila Pa 1976)* 28(15): 1710–1715; discussion 1716.
6. Boachie-Adjei O, Bradford DS: Vertebral column resection and arthrodesis for complex spinal deformities. *J Spinal Disord* 4(2): 193–202, 1991.
7. Buchowski JM, Bridwell KH, Lenke LG, et al.: Neurologic complications of lumbar pedicle subtraction osteotomy: a 10-year assessment. *Spine (Phila Pa 1976)* 32(20): 2245–2252, 2007.
8. Doherty JH: Complications of fusion in lumbar scoliosis: proceedings of the Scoliosis Research Society. *J Bone Joint Surg Am* 55: 438, 1973.
9. El-Sharkawi MM, Koptan WM, El-Miligui YH, et al.: Comparison between pedicle subtraction osteotomy and anterior corpectomy and plating for correcting post-traumatic kyphosis: a multicenter study. *Eur Spine J* 20(9): 1434–1440, 2011.
10. Farcy JP, Schwab FJ: Management of flatback and related kyphotic decompensation syndromes. *Spine* 22: 2452–2459, 1997.
11. Geck MJ, Macagno A, Ponte A, et al.: The Ponte procedure: posterior only treatment of Scheuermann's kyphosis using segmental posterior shortening and pedicle screw instrumentation. *J Spinal Disord Tech* 20(8): 586–593, 2007.
12. Glassman SD, Bridwell K, Dimar JR, et al.: The impact of positive sagittal balance in adult spinal deformity. *Spine* 30(18): 2024–2029, 2005.
13. Horton WC, Brown CW, Bridwell KH, et al.: Is there an optimal patient stance for obtaining a lateral 36" radiograph? A critical comparison of three techniques. *Spine (Phila Pa 1976)* 30(4): 427–433, 2005.
14. Kim YJ, Bridwell KH, Lenke LG, et al.: Results of lumbar pedicle subtraction osteotomies for fixed sagittal imbalance: a minimum 5-year follow-up study. *Spine (Phila Pa 1976)* 32(20): 2189–2197, 2007.
15. Lafage V, Ames C, Schwab F, et al.; International Spine Study Group: Changes in thoracic kyphosis negatively impact sagittal alignment after lumbar pedicle subtraction osteotomy: a comprehensive radiographic analysis. *Spine (Phila Pa 1976)* 37(3): E180–E187, 2012.
16. Mummaneni PV, Dhall SS, Ondra SL, et al.: Pedicle subtraction osteotomy. *Neurosurgery* 63(3 Suppl): 171–176, 2008.

17. Scheer JK, Tang JA, Deviren V, et al.: Biomechanical analysis of revision strategies for rod fracture in pedicle subtraction osteotomy. *Neurosurgery* 69(1): 164–172, 2011.
18. Schwab F, Ungar B, Blondel B, et al.: Scoliosis Research Society-Schwab adult spinal deformity classification: a validation study. *Spine* 37(12): 1077–1082, 2012.
19. Schwab FJ et al.: Sagittal realignment failures following pso surgery. Are we doing enough? *J Neurosurg Spine* 16(6): 539–546, 2012.
20. Schwab FJ, Patel A, Shaffrey CI, et al.: Sagittal realignment failures following pedicle subtraction osteotomy surgery: are we doing enough?: clinical article. *J Neurosurg Spine* 16(6): 539–546, 2012.
21. Smith JS, Shaffrey CI, Ames CP, et al.; International Spine Study Group: Assessment of symptomatic rod fracture after posterior instrumented fusion for adult spinal deformity. *Neurosurgery* 71(4): 862–867, 2012.
22. Smith JS, Sansur CA, Donaldson WF III, et al.: Short-term morbidity and mortality associated with correction of thoracolumbar fixed sagittal plane deformity: a report from the Scoliosis Research Society Morbidity and Mortality Committee. *Spine (Phila Pa 1976)* 36(12): 958–964, 2011.
23. Smith-Peterson MN, Larson CB, Aufranc OE: Osteotomy of the spine for correction of flexion deformity in rheumatoid arthritis. *J Bone Joint Surg Am* 27: 1–11, 1945.
24. Stephens GC, Yoo JU, Wilbur G: Comparison of lumbar sagittal alignment produced by different operative positions. *Spine (Phila Pa 1976)* 21(15): 1802–1806, 1996.
25. Suk KS, Kim KT, Lee SH, et al.: Significance of chin-brow vertical angle in correction of kyphotic deformity of ankylosing spondylitis patients. *Spine (Phila Pa 1976)* 28(17): 2001–2005, 2003.
26. Suk SI, Kim JH, Kim WJ, et al.: Posterior vertebral column resection for severe spinal deformities. *Spine* 27(21): 2374–2382, 2002.
27. Thomasen E: Vertebral osteotomy for correction of kyphosis in ankylosing spondylitis. *Clin Orthop Relat Res* 194: 142–152, 1985.
28. Vedantam R, Lenke LR, Bridwell KH, et al.: The effect of variation in arm position on sagittal spinal alignment. *Spine* 25(17): 2204–2209, 2000.
29. Winter RB, Lonstein JE, Denis F: Sagittal spinal alignment: the true measurement, norms, and description of correction for thoracic kyphosis. *J Spinal Disord Tech* 22(5): 311–314, 2009.
30. Yang BP, Chen LA, Ondra SL: A novel mathematical model of the sagittal spine: application to pedicle subtraction osteotomy for correction of fixed sagittal deformity. *Spine J* 8(2): 359–366, 2008.

21 Vertebral Resection for the Correction of Fixed Coronal Deformity

Clifford B. Tribus

INDICATIONS/CONTRAINDICATIONS

The spine surgeon has several different options for reestablishing spinal balance in the patient with spinal deformity of the thoracolumbar spine. In patients with flexible deformity in the sagittal or coronal plane, a posterior, anterior, or combined anterior and posterior approach will typically suffice to correct the deformity and maintain spinal balance. When a fixed spinal deformity exists, particularly with spinal imbalance, spinal osteotomy is often necessary to reestablish spinal balance. A rare subset of patients exists who have a fixed spinal deformity in the coronal plane. In these patients, posterior osteotomy alone and even anterior/posterior osteotomy procedures are not sufficient to correct coronal deformities (3,5,7,9,12,13). In order to reestablish spinal balance safely in these patients, the spine must be shortened and translated. This requires vertebral body resection (VBR) (1,2,4,6).

The indication for VBR is loss of spinal balance in the coronal plane. As with other spinal deformity problems, the indications for surgery are pain, progression, neurologic deficit, and cosmesis. Additionally, the patients with coronal deformity will frequently have a substantial functional deficit.

The diagnosis leading to a fixed coronally decompensated spine is most commonly postsurgically treated idiopathic scoliosis. Congenital scoliosis or other postsurgical deformity patient may also lead to fixed coronal deformity.

Confirming the diagnosis of fixed coronal deformity is self-evident on physical exam and standing plane radiographs. Supine bending films will confirm the fixed nature of the deformity. Vertebral resection is not necessary, however, unless the shoulders are parallel or angled away from the coronal deformity. If the shoulders are positioned in this manner, resection is necessary to allow shortening and translation of the spine enabling the shoulders to be rebalanced and centered over the pelvis.

The wide utilization of the pedicle subtraction osteotomy (PSO) has allowed the expansion of the PSO technique to include dorsal vertebral column resection (VCR). This evolving technique allows a full three-column resection of the vertebral column from the posterior approach and is a viable alternative to the anterior and posterior VBR. The neural elements are more readily identified from the posterior side, while risk to the local vasculature is greater (10,11,14–16). The surgical technique for both will be presented.

PREOPERATIVE PLANNING

Patients indicated for VCR require extensive preoperative evaluation. A cursory review of posture and radiographs will establish the necessity of the procedure, but a careful physical exam and assessment of the patient's state of health is required to determine if the patient is a candidate for this extensive procedure.

These deformities are typically quite complex. Any neurologic deficit needs to be explained and the question of its reversibility answered. Preoperative cardiopulmonary and nutritional status should be assessed. In addition to being physically prepared to undergo extensive surgery, the patient should be emotionally prepared. A support system should be in place, and most importantly, the goals between physician and patient should be matched and realistic. If the patient is a candidate, he or she should donate autogenous blood.

Radiographic studies would include standing AP and lateral radiographs on long films, as well as supine bending films to assess flexible correction. MRI is useful to assess neurologic elements as well as discs of areas not to be included in the fusion. A CT scan with sagittal and coronal reconstructions is needed to assess previous fusions and to plan for hardware placement and resection. Consideration should be given to utilizing intraoperative computer-assisted technology for the placement of hardware and performance of VCR.

The surgeon should plan for neurologic monitoring depending on the level of the resection and proposed hardware placement. Both Tc motor evoked potentials and somatosensory evoked potentials should be utilized. The potential need for a wake-up test should be discussed with the patient preoperatively. The need for a monitored bed in an intensive care unit should be anticipated and prearranged.

SURGICAL TECHNIQUE

The Anterior Approach

In the case when an anterior/posterior resection is planned, the anterior spine is approached first. The typical scenario is a two-level resection at the apex of the deformity. For the purpose of discussion, a resection of T12 and L1 will be described. Neurologic monitoring should also be established prior to positioning.

The patient is positioned, well padded, on the operating table in the lateral position with the convexity of the deformity up. A double arm board, axillary roll, and pillows between the knees are useful adjuncts to a beanbag and three-inch cloth tape to secure the patient to the operating table. Take care to protect the peroneal nerve on the down leg. In planning the incision, be mindful of the rib/vertebral angle, as the ribs may be quite vertical, thus requiring the approach to be made through a more proximal rib. Additionally, if the approach is proximal to the ninth rib, a double-lumen endotracheal tube should be considered. A standard thoracic, thoracolumbar, or lumbar approach is performed, and the levels to be resected are exposed. To approach T12–L1, a thoracolumbar approach is performed.

The incision is created with a skin knife, and subcutaneous tissues and underlying muscle layers are incised with electrocautery. If the diaphragm needs to be mobilized, it may be peeled directly off of the chest wall with electrocautery either from above or below. I prefer the superior approach, applying traction on the diaphragm with a sponge stick and incising the diaphragm at its insertion on the chest wall. A cuff of diaphragm may be left on the chest wall to facilitate later closure or the diaphragm may be directly repaired to the chest wall. Particular care should be given to incising the crus of the diaphragm as large segmental vessels are often found just deep to the crus.

Ipsilateral segmental vessels are controlled and markers placed to confirm radiographically that the appropriate levels are exposed (Fig. 21-1). An osteoperiosteal flap is then elevated. The purpose of the flap is to later contain the morcelized graft placed in the vertebrectomy site, yet in adults, a true flap is difficult to develop.

In performing the resection, you need to recognize and utilize as many visual clues as to the location and orientation of the spinal cord as possible. Discectomies are performed proximal and distal to the levels to be resected. Often the patient has already had an anterior fusion ablating the discs. The CT scan with reconstructions should be scrutinized for residual landmarks in the fusion mass. The pedicles are a particularly reliable landmark for the initial localization of the cord. Given that these deformities are in three dimensions, however, once the cord is localized, its direction is still often not clear. At the start of the resection, a rongeur is used so that resected bone may be reused as bone graft. As the posterior cortex is approached, use a diamond-tip burr to reduce the risk of dural tear. The posterior cortex is thinned and then resected with small curettes and Kerrison rongeurs. The posterior longitudinal ligament (PLL) should be left intact as both a landmark and a biologic barrier (Figs. 21-2 and 21-3). However, all bone needs to be resected off

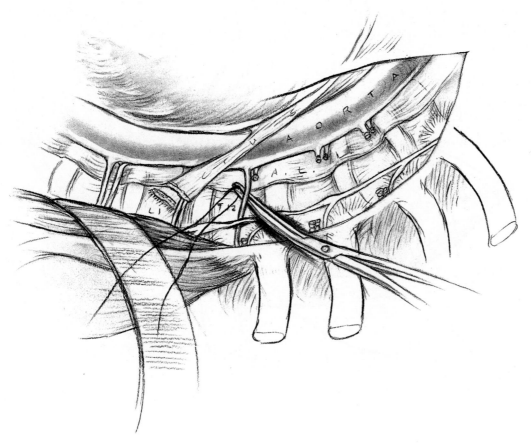

FIGURE 21-1
Anterior approach demonstrating ligation of segmental vessels.

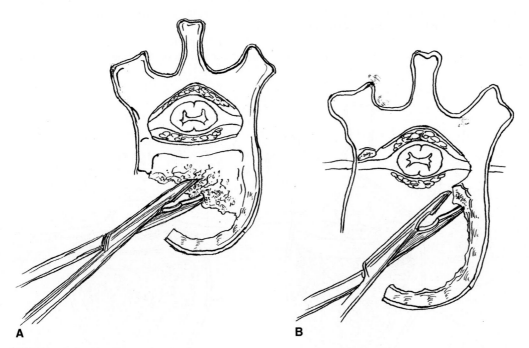

A   **B**

FIGURE 21-2
Axial views demonstrating the periosteum being elevated **(A)** and the vertebral body resected **(B)**.

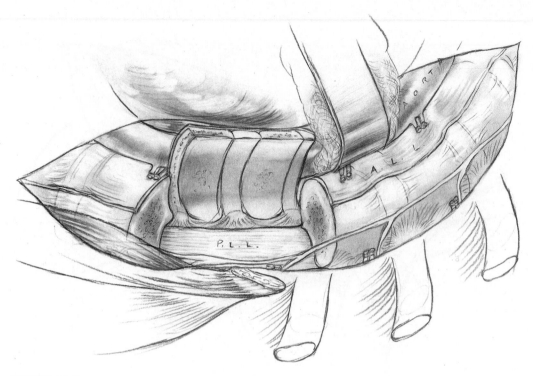

FIGURE 21-3

The periosteal flap is elevated, the vertebrectomy is complete, and the PLL is exposed.

of the PLL to prevent buckling into the cord at the time of posterior correction of the deformity. Complete resection of the concave pedicle is not often possible from the anterior approach, yet the base of the pedicle needs to be resected at this time to assure a safe posterior removal of the residual pedicle.

A small amount of Gelfoam is used to augment the PLL as a barrier between the cord and the bone graft, which is morcellized and loosely placed into the anterior vertebrectomy site. The osteoperiosteal flap is then secured over the vertebrectomy site preventing the graft from displacing (Figs. 21-4 and 21-5). A standard closure is performed.

At this point, you must decide whether to proceed with the posterior approach in one setting or to stage the procedure. If the decision is to stage the procedure, a central line for total parenteral

FIGURE 21-4

A: Axial view of Gelfoam (Ethicon, Somerville, NJ) in place, protecting the nerve; the bone graft in place; and the periosteum being repaired. **B:** Axial view showing subsequent posterior completion of the vertebral resection.

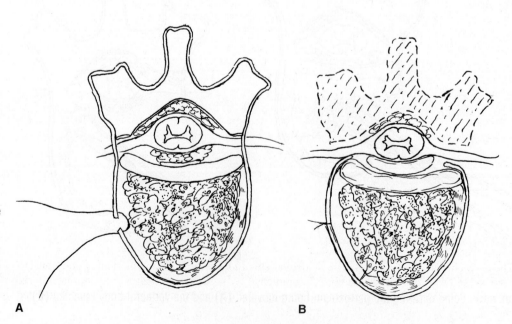

A   B

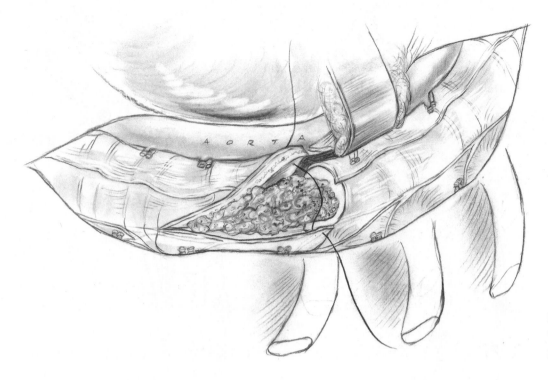

FIGURE 21-5
The periosteal flap
being closed.

nutrition should be placed on the same side as the chest tube while the patient is still under general anesthesia. The patient may be mobilized out of bed to a chair between stages.

The Posterior Approach

The patient is positioned prone for the posterior approach. A frame, which allows full extension of the hips and a freely dependent abdomen, is required. The spine is exposed through a midline approach. Generally, I complete the exposure, obtain bone graft, and place the screws and hooks to be utilized. Completing the resection prior to securing fixation is ill advised. The spine will be highly unstable when the resection is completed; you need to minimize the time of instability and the trauma inflicted when placing hooks and screws. Additionally, you need to be certain that good fixation proximal and distal to the planned resection is secured prior to committing the patient to a completed resection. Instrument at least three levels proximal and distal to the levels resected. I will generally reinstrument all previously fused levels and extend the fusion if the three-level rule is not met (Fig. 21-6).

The resection is then completed. The entire lamina and both pedicles of each level resected anteriorly are removed posteriorly.

In the case where the entire resection is being preformed via a posterior approach, the planned resection is marked through the fusion mass posterolaterally with a burr (Fig. 21-7). Generally, the resection will be pars to pars over one or more levels (Fig. 21-8). The laminectomy is extended proximally and distally to the planned resection to allow for dural buckling. The pedicles are then isolated and resected to their base (Fig. 21-9). Next, identify the proximal and distal end of the vertebral resection. The disc spaces may be utilized, but in the case where the anterior column is solidly fused, mid–vertebral body may also be used. The lateral cortex of the vertebral body can then be exposed by bluntly dissecting extraperiosteally in the waist of the vertebral body. The segmental vessels can be ligated or preserved but should be identified. The resection proceeds by alternating between decancellation, decortication, and discectomy (Fig. 21-10). The posterior cortex of the vertebral body is retained until the resection is almost complete. A temporary rod can be placed to stabilize the vertebral column while the resection is being performed. The anterior cortex is thinned and then resected with a curette or Kerrison. Just prior to correction, the posterior cortex is removed and morcelized bone graft is placed in the corpectomy site. Alternatively, the correction can be performed and then the anterior column rigidly reconstructed.

The correction is then effected. The maneuver should have the effect of shortening and translating the spine. Distraction is absolutely contraindicated. My preference is a two-rod approach to the convexity. A rod is placed proximally and distally. The deformity is then shortened and translated by manipulating the rods, and a domino device is used to connect the two rods. A/P and lateral

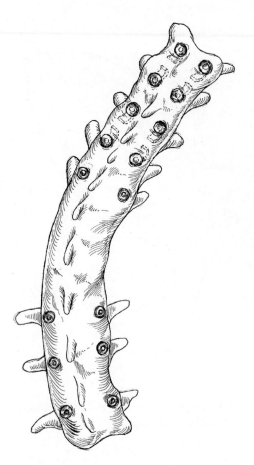

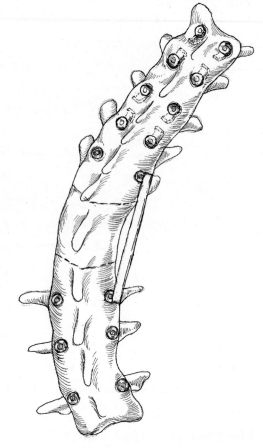

FIGURE 21-6

Anteroposterior view of the posterior fused spine exposed. Hardware is placed before the resection is completed. Screws are placed distally and around the proposed resection site. Hooks are placed directly into the fusion mass in a "claw" construct proximally.

FIGURE 21-7

Anteroposterior view of a temporary rod placed on the concavity, spanning the proposed resection.

radiographs on 36-inch films are then obtained to assure spinal balance, while a wake-up test is performed. A single concave rod is then placed neutrally, and cross-links complete the construct (Figs. 21-11 and 21-12). A small amount of Gelfoam is placed to protect the dura, and bone graft is placed spanning the resection gap (Figs. 21-13 and 21-14).

POSTOPERATIVE MANAGEMENT

As previously stated, if the patient's two procedures are staged, then total parental nutrition should be instituted between the two procedures. A monitored bed should be arranged for the first 1 to 2 postoperative days. Patient-controlled analgesia as well as ulcer and deep venous thrombosis (DVT) prophylaxis are instituted. I use only mechanical DVT prophylaxis given the relatively low thrombus risk and the neurologic risk of bleeding in the area of exposed spinal cord. The chest tube is placed to suction and typically remains for 48 to 72 hours. The Foley catheter should be removed at roughly the same time as the chest tube. After the chest tube has been removed, the patient is fitted for a custom thoracolumbosacral orthosis (TLSO). The TLSO is worn whenever the patient is out of bed, but it is not necessary to sleep in the brace. The patient is then mobilized in the TLSO. A walker is usually necessary with the start of gait training. Assistance is required in rising from bed.

Decisions as to placement in a skilled nursing facility can be made by the 3rd to 5th postoperative day as needs can be anticipated based on the patient's progress to this point. The diet is also slowly progressed according to bowel sounds and flatus. Standing AP and lateral radiographs are obtained prior to discharge. The typical hospital stay is 5 to 7 days post-op with some patients able

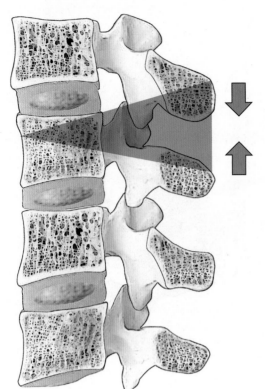

FIGURE 21-8

Schematic of lateral view demonstrating planned resection for PSO (darkened area) and VCR (darkened area plus single shaded area).

to go directly home at this point, while others require a more extended transitional time in a skilled nursing facility.

REHABILITATION

After discharge, patients are followed with serial exams and radiographs to assure that spinal balance is maintained and healing obtained. I do not generally continue formal physical therapy past discharge as long as independent ambulation has been obtained. Walking is the mainstay of

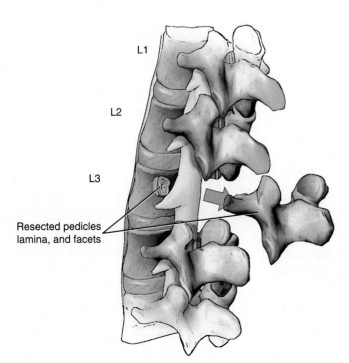

L1

L2

L3

Resected pedicles lamina, and facets

FIGURE 21-9

The posterior fusion mass, lamina, facets, and pedicles are resected.

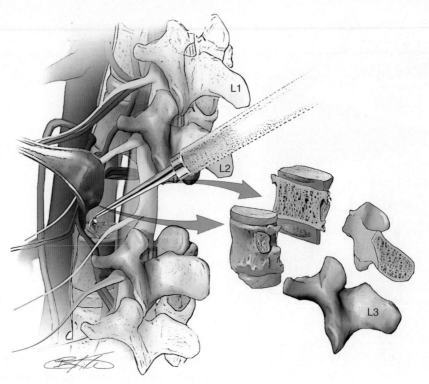

FIGURE 21-10

The vertebral body is resected with the proximal and distal disc.

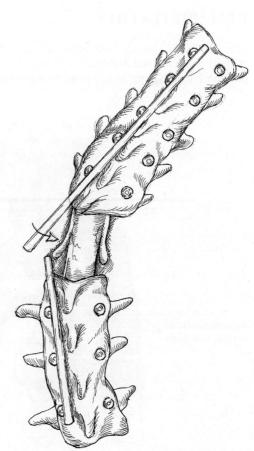

FIGURE 21-11

A proximal and distal rod are placed on the convexity of the deformity. The rods were previously bent, so that subsequently attaching them will affect correction of the deformity by shortening and translating the spine. The temporary rod is removed and correction performed as the two convex rods are attached to each other by a domino side-to-side connector.

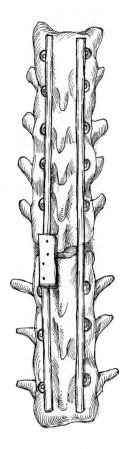

FIGURE 21-12

The alignment of the spine is improved. The single concave rod is placed, and the osteotomy site bone is grafted.

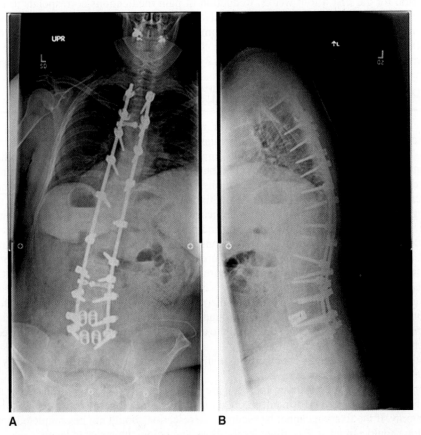

A   B

FIGURE 21-13

Preoperative anteroposterior **(A)** and lateral **(B)** radiographs demonstrating fixed coronal imbalance.

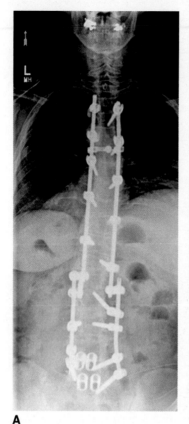

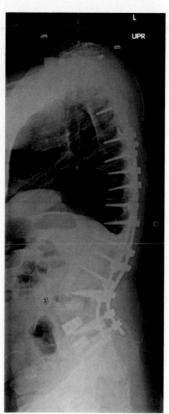

A   B

FIGURE 21-14

Postoperative antero-posterior **(A)** and lateral **(B)** radiographs demonstrating corrected coronal imbalance.

rehabilitation for the first 4 to 6 weeks. Reduction of pain medications corresponds to increasing activities. Generally, by 4 to 6 weeks postoperatively, the patient may drive a car, ride a stationary bicycle, and swim. Brace wear continues approximately 8 to 10 weeks. Lifting, bending, and twisting activities are limited until at least 3 months. Return to work full time should not be expected before 3 months. Visits are scheduled at 6 weeks, 3 and 6 months, and 1 and 2 years postoperatively.

COMPLICATIONS AND RESULTS

The anticipated complications of VBR mirror those of other extensive thoracolumbar spinal reconstructions (1,3,4,8,10,12–15). The most catastrophic complication, short of death, would be paralysis. The procedure is designed to allow correction of fixed spinal deformities with as much consideration for neurologic safety as possible, but it is technically demanding. Maintaining one's orientation is difficult and crucial. The time during which the correction is being performed posteriorly is critical. The cord is essentially free floating at this point. The corrective forces should be shortening and translation only, followed by efficacious and rigid fixation. The resection must be complete. Residual bone will inhibit correction and pose a neurologic risk.

The anterior approach exposes many vital organs including lung, diaphragm, vascular, renal, and intestinal organs, any one of which may be injured. Once the retroperitoneum has been entered, blunt dissection is the preferred mode of exposure. Control of segmental vessels without avulsing them will save greatly on blood loss.

Dural tears and neurologic injury during the anterior approach are typically due to loss of orientation. There is usually no scar tissue around the nerve, and the PLL is an excellent barrier. When I create an anterior dural tear, I do attempt to close the injury primarily. If this is not technically possible, fibrin glue can prove helpful.

Disruption of the sympathetic chain leading to mild ipsilateral autonomic dysfunction is common but frequently is mild and reverses itself.

The complications of the posterior approach are neurologic as previously discussed or related to fixation. Fixation may be very difficult to obtain due to multiple operations, osteoporosis, or distorted anatomy. If the fixation cannot be secured, the resection should not be completed posteriorly. The fixation should extend at least three levels above and below the resected levels.

Pseudoarthrosis may be a cause of late fixation problems. Rigid fixation, good bone grafting techniques, and postoperative bracing should minimize risk of pseudoarthrosis.

Prolonged surgery promotes positional risk, increased risk of infection, and coagulopathy. The surgeon must be decisive, efficacious, and cautious in the operating room.

The risk of complication for vertebral resection is between 25% and 40%. This substantial risk combined with the operative insult and extensive postoperative rehabilitation must be balanced with the patient's desires and preoperative dysfunction. Both surgeon and patient need to be committed to the idea of good communication, extended follow-up, and the aggressive treatment of complications. If these ideals are followed, successful patient outcomes and satisfaction rates should be 75% to 80% good to excellent, or similar to other large reconstructive spinal procedures.

RECOMMENDED READING

1. Boahchie-Adjei O, Bradford DS: Vertebral column resection and arthrodesis for complex spinal deformities. *J Spinal Disord* 4(2): 193–202, 1991.
2. Bradford DS, Boahchie-Adjei O: One-stage anterior and posterior hemivertebral resection and arthrodesis for congenital scoliosis. *J Bone Joint Surg Am* 72(4): 536–540, 1990.
3. Bradford DS, Tribus CB: Current concepts and management of patients with fixed decompensated spinal deformity. *Clin Orthop Relat Res* 306: 64–72, 1994.
4. Bradford DS, Tribus CB: Vertebral column resection for the treatment of rigid coronal decompensation. *Spine* 22(14): 1590–1599, 1997.
5. Bridwell KH: Decision making regarding Smith-Petersen vs. pedicle subtraction osteotomy vs. vertebral column resection for spinal deformity. *Spine* 31(19): S171–S178, 2006.
6. Fountain SS: A single-stage combined surgical approach for vertebral resections. *J Bone Joint Surg Am* 61(7): 1011–1017, 1979.
7. Gill JB, Levin A, Burd T, et al.: Corrective osteotomies in spine surgery. *J Bone Joint Surg Am* 90(11): 2509–2520, 2008.
8. Lü GH, Wang XB, Wang B, et al.: Complications of one stage posterior vertebral column resection for the treatment of severe rigid spinal deformities. *Zhonghua Wai Ke Za Zhi* 48(22): 1709–1713, 2010.
9. LaFage V, Schwab F, Vira S, et al.: Does vertebral level of pedicle subtraction osteotomy correlate with degree of spinopelvic parameter correction?" *J Neurosurgery Spine* 14(2): 184–191, 2011.
10. Lenke LG, O'Leary PT, Bridwell KH, et al.: Posterior vertebral column resection for severe pediatric deformity. *Spine* 34(20): 2213–2221, 2009.
11. Matsumoto M, Watanabe K, Tsuji T, et al.: Progressive kyphoscoliosis associated with tethered cord treated by posterior vertebral column resection. *Spine* 34(26): E965–E968, 2009.
12. Smith JS, Wang VY, Ames CP: Vertebral column resection for rigid spinal deformity. *Neurosurgery* 63(3): A177–A182, 2008.
13. Sucato DJ: Management of severe spinal deformity. *Spine* 35(25): 2186–2192, 2010.
14. Suk SI, Chung ER, Lee SM, et al.: Posterior vertebral column resection in fixed lumbosacral deformity. *Spine* 30(23): E703–E710, 2005.
15. Suk SI, Kim JH, Kim, WJ, et al.: Posterior vertebral column resection for severe spinal deformities. *Spine* 27(21): 2374–2382, 2002.
16. Xie J, Li T, Wang Y, et al.: Change in Cobb angle of each segment of the major curve after posterior vertebral column resection (PVCR): a preliminary discussion of correction mechanisms of PVCR. *Eur Spine J* 21(4): 705–710, 2012.

PART III
LUMBAR SPINE

22 Lumbar Microdiscectomy

C. Chambliss Harrod, Roman Trimba, and Alan S. Hilibrand

BACKGROUND/ANATOMY

The lumbosacral spine is the region of the skeleton that transitions from the appendicular to the axial skeleton. Ambulation is most functional when the head is centered over the pelvis in both the coronal and sagittal planes, which are typically balanced in adult patients with cervical and lumbar lordosis counteracting thoracic and sacral kyphosis. Walking places significant biomechanical loads across the lumbosacral junction. Approximately 80% of the weight is supported via the anterior column consisting of vertebral bodies and intervertebral discs, while the posterior bony and ligamentous structures including the neural arches and zygapophyseal (facet) joints accommodate approximately 20%. Typically, the lordotic lumbar spine consists of five nonrib-bearing, mobile osseous segments between the rigid thoracic and fused sacral vertebrae, which serve as a conduit for the cauda equina. Normal lordosis ranges from 40 to 60 degrees with over 50% stemming from L4–S1 as the lumbosacral intervertebral disc is often much taller ventrally than dorsally. Normal lower extremity function depends on mobile joints powered by musculotendinous units, which derive their neurologic innervation via nerve roots stemming from the spinal cord, conus medullaris, and cauda equina.

INDICATIONS/CONTRAINDICATIONS

Compression of the neurologic elements can be secondary to degenerative, neoplastic, congenital, infectious, or traumatic etiologies, although herniation of lumbar nucleus pulposus through the peripheral annulus is most common. Patients are often present with lower extremity radiculopathy (combination of pain, weakness, numbness, paresthesias, loss of function) though bowel, bladder, and autonomic nervous system abnormalities culminating in cauda equina syndrome are possible. Nonoperative management is effective in the vast majority of cases with activity modification, physical therapy, medication, and interventional pain management techniques. Absolute indications for surgical treatment include progressive neurologic deficit and cauda equina syndrome. Relative indications include recalcitrant pain after failed conservative management. Analysis of disc location, size, and extent and surgical goals allows the correct approach to achieve the surgical goal—decompression of neural elements while maintaining spinal stability. Disc herniations can be located centrally, paracentrally, foraminally, or extraforaminally. Removal of offending compressive lesions under direct vision has been the standard of care over thermal ablative techniques. Posterior-based approaches are utilized below the level of the conus medullaris and include midline, paramedian (Wiltse), or far lateral open, tubular, endoscopic, or arthroscopic techniques with laminectomy, hemilaminectomy, hemilaminotomy, or transforaminal (foraminoplasty) bony resections to perform the discectomy. Each of these techniques has its own unique advantages and disadvantages. Experience of the surgeon, cosurgeon availability, and familiarity with the approach and anatomy of the patient are of utmost importance when deciding on which approach to use. Additionally, most surgeons use loupe magnification or the operating microscope to improve visualization and safety. Studies have shown that results of lumbar microdiscectomy have been superior to traditional techniques (subtotal or complete discectomy). We have enjoyed a low complication profile with use of a 2- to 3-cm open midline or Wiltse paramedian approach to treat nearly all primary recalcitrant symptomatic lumbar disc herniations under loupe magnification. We discuss this approach in the following technique.

PREOPERATIVE PLANNING

Understanding of anatomy and radiographic data will facilitate preoperative planning, allowing a smaller incision, with less dissection, blood loss, and tissue trauma. A careful physical examination should inspect for any prior incisions, scars, skin lesions (i.e., psoriasis or acne), infection, or signs of spina bifida (dimpling, hairy tufts, and lack of spinous processes). Morbidly obese patients can increase the difficulty of the operation, necessitating increased radiation to identify one's level, larger incisions, longer instruments, and longer operating times.

Lumbar spine imaging must include plain radiography with anteroposterior and neutral, flexion, and extension lateral views to clearly identify the lumbosacral junction, the 12th (or most caudal) rib, the number of lumbar vertebrae, presence of transitional (or sacralized) vertebrae, and superimposed level of the iliac crest. Adequate plain radiographs aid in preventing wrong-level surgery. Flexion-extension views allow identification of instability, while oblique views are occasionally helpful in identifying pars interarticularis fractures. Computed tomography is of limited importance though can be helpful to quantify the amount of foraminal stenosis and osteophytic compression. In revision lumbar spine surgery with instrumentation and for patients who cannot undergo magnetic resonance imaging (MRI), addition of myelography is helpful to identify disc herniations and stenosis. MRI best assesses the extent of nerve root, thecal sac, conus medullaris, or spinal cord compression with or without intradural extension. Gadolinium administration with enhancement is useful with neoplasms, infections, revision microdiscectomy cases, and as an aid in diagnosing an early reherniation. T1 parasagittal images are vital in assessing the amount of foraminal root compression in far lateral disc herniations. Rarely, an anomalous or bifid nerve root may also be identified that will alter decompression tactics. In addition, engorged epidural plexi should be noted as occasionally large ventral epidural leashes will be encountered and can be difficult to control. Lastly, we typically require a recent MRI (within 3 months) prior to performing surgical decompression as lumbar disc herniations can resorb over that period of time.

In order to minimize incision length and bony removal, while still obtaining adequate decompression, one must understand the exact location of the disc herniation prior to surgery. Lesions can be characterized using the McCulloch "three-floor anatomic house," which provides a three-dimensional grid of the spinal canal. Vertically, the house is broken down into three floors (Fig. 22-1). The most inferior or caudal floor contains the disc level ("1"). The second floor extends from the inferior border of the pedicles to the inferior endplate and contains the foraminal level. The third or most cephalad is the pedicle level and spans from the superior endplate to the inferior border of the pedicle. One flaw in this vertical system is that it is designed for cranial migration of discs (i.e., an L4–L5 disc migrating toward the L4 pedicle). Caudal disc herniations are given the nomenclature of a "minus-one" (−1) level. An example would be an L3–L4 disc migrating to the level of the pedicle of L4. Disc pathology is further divided in the sagittal plane from medial to lateral into central, subarticular (lateral recess), foraminal, and extraforaminal (far lateral) zones (Fig. 22-2). Medially, the central zone is situated between the edges of the dura, while the subarticular (lateral recess zone) sits between the lateral edge of the dura and the medial borders of the pedicles. The foraminal zone lies from the medial to lateral border of the pedicle, and the extraforaminal zone is lateral to the pedicles. The seven posterior bony elements include the superior and inferior articular processes, spinous process, lamina, pedicle, transverse process, and pars. The pedicle and transverse process are the only ones that lie in a single floor, the third or pedicle level. All other structures straddle two floors.

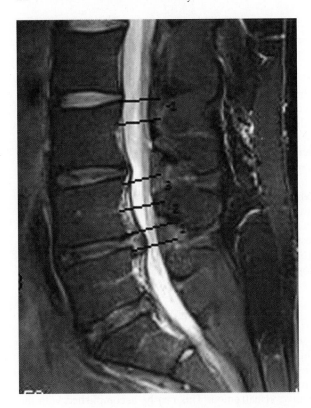

FIGURE 22-1

A T2-weighted midsagittal MRI image demonstrates the McCulloch 3-floor technique with an L4–L5 disc herniation at the level of the disc level (first floor). Labeled are the second and third floor corresponding to foraminal- or pedicle-level cranial herniations. Caudal herniations are given the nomenclature "–1" when at the level of the caudal pedicle.

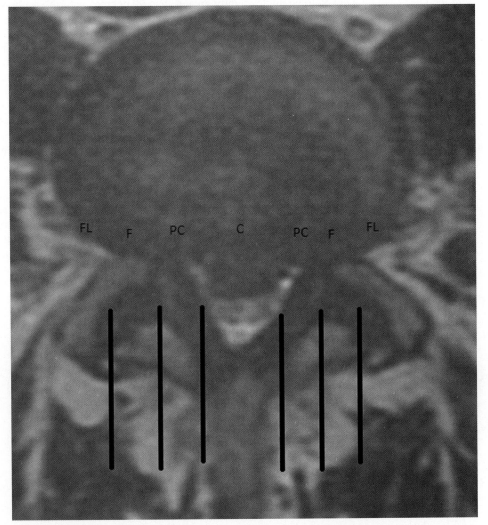

FIGURE 22-2

A T2-weighted axial MRI image at the L4–L5 disc level from Figure 22-1 demonstrates a central disc herniation with lateral recess stenosis with compression of the caudal equina. The patient clinically had left-sided radiculopathy, so a left-sided hemilaminotomy with microdiscectomy was planned with a low threshold to convert to either bilateral hemilaminotomy or laminectomy if the appropriate-sized fragment was not removed. The central (C), paracentral (PC), foraminal (F), and extraforaminal or far lateral (FL) zones are defined.

TECHNIQUE

Anesthesia

The majority of microdiscectomies are still performed under general anesthesia; however, some patients opt for spinal and/or epidural anesthesia. The degrees of sedation are determined according to the preference of the patient and/or surgeon. While a small percentage of patients chose to be awake and watching the procedure on the television monitor, the majority prefer to be unconscious. An epidural anesthetic dilates the vessels in the lower extremities, resulting in lower intraoperative bleeding. It is also associated with lower recovery room times, faster return to orientation and alertness, and general absence of postoperative nausea and vomiting compared to a general anesthetic. However, there are several disadvantages to using an epidural or local anesthetic. The peripheral vasodilation caused by the epidural may lead to general hypotension. Lack of general anesthesia and complete sedation may cause difficulty with patient positioning and moving during the procedure, as well as difficulty establishing an emergency airway in case of a complication. Increased incidence of urinary retention with epidural anesthetic may lead to an overnight stay during what would normally be an outpatient procedure. Neurologic complications may also result from the epidural anesthetic/procedure itself; the anesthesiologist may inadvertently cause a dural tear necessitating a repair.

Patient Positioning

Careful patient positioning can facilitate a successful lumbar microdiscectomy. The first is to minimize lumbar lordosis as much as possible. This will increase the interlaminar space allowing for easier access into the spinal canal and resulting in a smaller laminotomy to expose the disc. The second goal is to decrease abdominal compression to decrease venous pressure, which results in markedly reduced epidural blood loss and enhanced intraoperative visualization. This can be accomplished with the Andrews frame in a knee-chest position. The patient is placed with his/her back parallel to the floor with the knees and hips flexed to an angle slightly greater than 90 degrees with the frame kneeling angle increased to maximum. The patient should be positioned prone on an Andrews frame or table if the patient weighs less than 250 pounds; otherwise, a Jackson table with a sling is preferred to allow the abdomen to hang freely to decrease venous congestion and subsequent epidural venous bleeding (Fig. 22-3). The Andrews frame is secured to a regular operating room table with the legs flexed to the floor (the surgeon or assistant should test with his or her own weight that the frame is rigidly affixed prior to patient placement). The patient must be rolled prone onto the table, knees are secured initially with both feet strapped in place, a buttocks plate is placed at the appropriate height, and then the patient is translated caudally. A semifirm gel bolster is used as a chest or sternal roll and must be 2 cm caudal to the sternal notch to not impinge on the airway or cause cranial vascular engorgement. The arms are then gently rotated into a "90-90" position, and care must be taken to pad bony prominences and ensure the safety of the peripheral nerves and brachial plexus. The surgeon must then ensure that the patient's back is parallel to the floor by either raising or lowering the legs or more typically cranking the tibial tray up or down. Finally, lateral bolsters are squeezed on the midthighs to ensure patients are safely and securely fastened. Note that patients should be examined preoperatively for adhesive capsulitis (frozen shoulder) or shoulder pathology as those with such disorders will not be able to be positioned with the arms in the "90-90" position. They will require the arms to be at the side, which should be low enough not to block the marker radiograph. We typically drape out the operative field widely with 1,010 drapes and then mark the iliac crests transversely; the posterior superior iliac spines

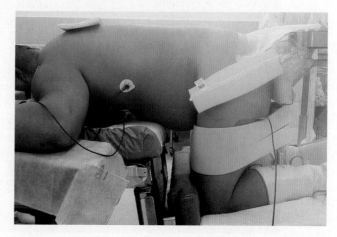

FIGURE 22-3

The patient is appropriately positioned on the Andrews frame.

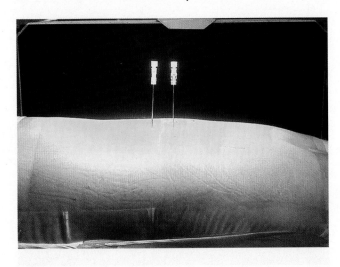

FIGURE 22-4

After prepping, two 18-guage spinal needles are inserted into spinous processes vertically, and a lateral marker radiograph is made.

are vertically marked bilaterally. After scrubbing skin and prepping with ChloraPrep, a World Health Organization (WHO) "time out" is performed to verify the details of the procedure and equipment and review major intraoperative risks with the anesthesia, surgical, and nursing teams.

Localization of the Level

Based on the relationship of the spinous processes to the iliac crest on preoperative lateral flexion, we then insert two 18-gauge spinal needles vertically into the appropriate spinous processes. Care must be taken to place the needle vertically to avoid an incision at the wrong disc space. The size of the incision is then determined by the location and size of the disc fragment and the laminotomy needed to remove it. If landmarks are difficult to palpate, needles may be placed shallower to avoid dural perforation. A lateral radiograph is taken to ensure the correct location for incision (Figs. 22-4 and 22-5). A 0.5 to 1 mL indigo carmine is then injected as the needle is withdrawn to mark the appropriate spinous process (Fig. 22-6).

The needles may then be removed, and the region prepped and draped. Indigo carmine dye may cause a greenish tint to the urine. Methylene blue dye is not recommended because it may cause neurotoxicity if inadvertently injected intradurally. Additional radiographs are then not necessary to localize the level. The distance between the two needles allows the surgeon to determine the exact location and size of the incision when comparing it to the magnified radiograph. We typically mark the caudal spinous process, as it is easier to stray a level cranial in the low lumbar spine. Once this is done, the incision is measured to be approximately 1 inch (2.5 cm) and placed approximately 5 mm paramedian to the midline for easier exposure past the spinous processes. We then reprep the skin with a second ChloraPrep solution and then drape the operative field.

Surgery

Exposure   Preoperative identification of abnormal anatomy is vital for this stage. Incision is made sharply with a knife. Depending on the size of the patient, dissection through the subcutaneous tissue is then done either with an electrocautery or with blunt dissection. The lumbodorsal fascia is

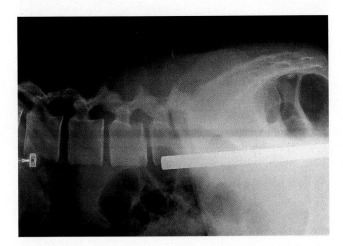

FIGURE 22-5

A lateral radiograph demonstrates that the spinal needles are correctly positioned on the L4 and L5 spinous processes.

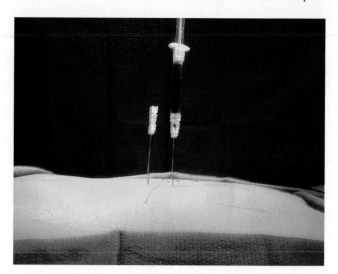

FIGURE 22-6

Indigo carmine is injected onto the L5 spinous process as the needle is removed creating a tract down to the spinous process.

then opened with the Bovie on cut with care not to cause the underlying muscle to bleed. A Weitlaner self-retaining retractor may now be inserted. The slightly paramedian flap provides a strong buttress for the medial hook of the retractor and allows for improved lateral excursion of the self-retaining retractor system. This results in easier retraction of muscles and allows the medial hook to rest on a flap of fascia as opposed to the interspinous-supraspinous ligament complex.

Deep Dissection/Muscle Elevation   Following the fascial incision, subperiosteal dissection of the multifidus muscle off the two laminae is then done up to the medial portion of facet joint. Care is taken not to injure the facet joint capsule. If there is any doubt regarding spinal levels, a Penfield 4 or Woodson elevator placed in the interlaminar interval can unambiguously verify the disc space on a lateral radiograph.

Muscle elevation is started on the leading edge of the caudal spinous process using a Cobb elevator. This is an avascular plane, inferior to the insertion of the multifidus tendon. The dissection continues down the slope of this lamina. Extensive cephalad dissection beyond the initial skin markings may lead to exposure of the proximal level. The muscle of the trailing edge of the cephalad lamina and spinous process is then dissected subperiosteally, and the lateral pars must be identified cranially to ensure its integrity through the procedure. Hook-blade combination self-retaining retractors can now be placed into the wound (Fig. 22-7). The hook portion is placed between the spinous processes superficial to the spinolaminar junction, while the blade is placed laterally to retract the paraspinal muscles superficial and lateral to the facet joint. Soft tissues are then cleared from the laminae and ligamentum flavum (Fig. 22-8).

Flavectomy and Entry into Spinal Canal   At this point, the surgeon has the option of utilizing loupes or the surgical microscope for entry into the spinal canal. Both have been affective in performing the surgery; however, there are several advantages to using the microscope. These include better lighting, better optics, and an identical field of vision for the surgeon and

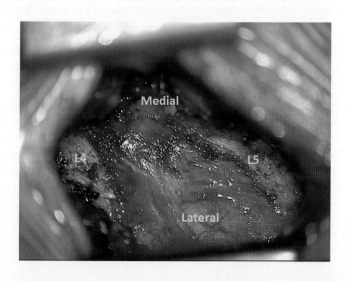

FIGURE 22-7

After dissection and elevation of the multifidus muscles, the L4 and L5 lamina, interspinous ligaments medially, ligamentum flavum, and facet capsules laterally are visualized.

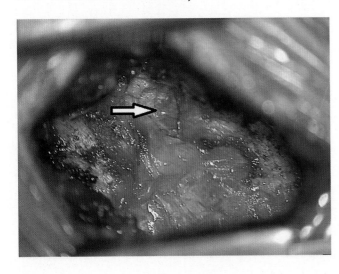

FIGURE 22-8

Ligamentum flavum release is released with L5 hemilaminotomy.

assistant. The microscope coaxial optics also allow for a smaller incision due to direct downward vision.

Although some surgeons advocate for a ligamentum flavum sparing or flap approach, we typically perform flavectomy. The ligamentum flavum can be detached from the inferior portion of the superior lamina or the superior portion of the inferior lamina. We prefer the latter at L5–S1 since the ligamentum flavum detaches more easily at the leading edge of the inferior lamina laterally to the facet joint. This is done with a no. 2 straight or curved curette in a lateral-to-medial direction with no downward-directed force to avoid inadvertent plunging into the canal. The surgeon must be aware of a possible dorsally displaced root that may become injured during this procedure.

Inferior Laminotomy/Laminectomy   After passing a Woodson elevator or Penfield dissector under the free edge of flavum, the margins can be gently inspected for any adhesions to the underlying dural sac. The ligamentum flavum can then be thinned using a pituitary rongeur and the lateral 5 to 10 mm removed using a Kerrison rongeur though we typically leave a small amount underneath the trailing edge of the cranial lamina at this time to protect for our inferior hemilaminotomy. A small portion of the caudal lamina may be resected for better exposure of the lateral dural sac and the exiting nerve root at this caudal level (Figs. 22-9 and 22-10).

After the ligamentum flavum is detached from the inferior lamina, the cranial inferior hemilaminotomy may be performed. The amount of lamina to be removed depends on the size of the interlaminar interval as well as its relation to the disc space. At the lower lumbar levels (L4–L5 and L5–S1), the interlaminar interval is usually close to the disc space; thus, a smaller amount of lamina needs to be removed. At more cephalad levels, the disc space lies more caudal to the interlaminar interval necessitating the creation of a larger bony window (occasionally requiring complete hemilaminectomies). We prefer to use a high-speed burr with a 3-mm matchstick tip to thin the superior hemilamina with the remaining flavum protecting the thecal sac. A Kerrison punch can then perform final bony and flavum removal. Partial medial facetectomy can be performed for any lateral recess stenosis secondary to flavum and facet capsule and bony hypertrophy. Note that in the case

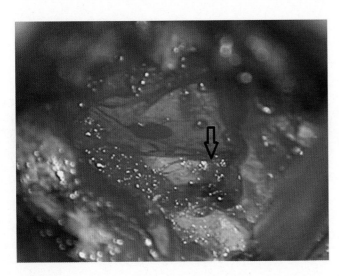

FIGURE 22-9

The traversing L5 (*arrow*) is exposed.

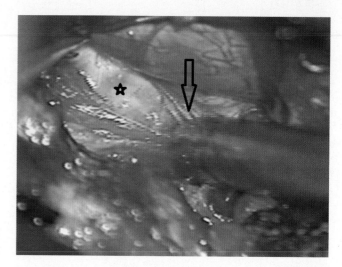

FIGURE 22-10

Mobilizing L5 nerve (*arrow*) off disc herniation (*star*).

of a trefoil canal, more medial facetectomy may be required if the root is tucked away laterally as opposed to normally laying in line with the medial edge of the facet. During the hemilaminotomy, excessive bony resection can lead to an iatrogenic fracture of the lateral pars interarticularis. An iatrogenic pars fracture is more likely during discectomy at more proximal levels due to the more medial location and smaller pars width. This may also lead to iatrogenic inferior articular process fracture with potential instability. It is important to leave at least 7 mm of lateral pars to prevent an iatrogenic pars fracture.

Pedicle and Traversing Nerve Root Identification   After adequate bony resection, attention is turned to identification of the traversing nerve root. The lateral border can typically be found with a Penfield 4 elevator. Once found and gently retracted, we use the bipolar cautery to cauterize the lateral longitudinal epidural leash, which lies on the dorsal vertebral bodies and disc. We like to use a Woodson elevator to palpate the caudal pedicle, directly visualize the traversing root exiting medial to it and out the subjacent foramen. We then typically gently pack a thrombin-soaked 0.5×0.5-cm pledget patty caudally to mobilize the traversing root medially. This facilitates mobilization of the thecal sac with a Love nerve root retractor, allowing visualization of the herniated disc from the disc space (Fig. 22-11). In addition to hemostasis, using pledgelets allows a cushion and dissipation of focal forces that a nerve root retractor alone places on the neural elements. Great care must still be taken not to overretract the root to minimize postoperative neuralgia.

Discectomy   The disc herniation should be clearly visible and must be correlated with preoperative MRI findings. If there are major discrepancies, repeat radiograph must be obtained with a marker to verify correct-level surgery. If the herniation is readily visible, the surgeon can now excise the ruptured fragment of disc with a pituitary rongeur. If an annular defect already exists, the surgeon may choose to work within it or extend it as necessary. An attempt can be made to remove the disc fragment without extending the annulotomy as clinical findings show that patients with smaller

FIGURE 22-11

Exposure of the herniation. A Love retractor gently retracts the thecal sac and traversing nerve root while the disc herniation and annulus are visualized while patties are used gently to provide hemostatic control of epidural bleeding.

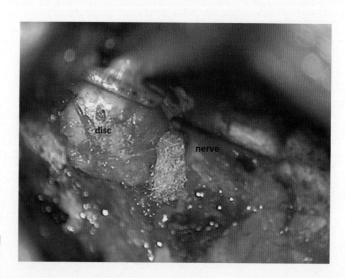

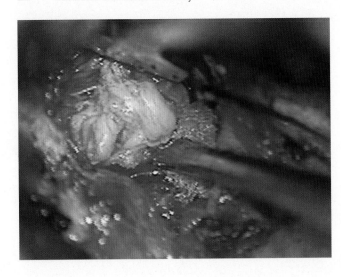

FIGURE 22-12

Peeling of the membrane over the disc material with Penfield dissector.

annular defects tend to have fewer recurrences. In the absence of an annular defect, annulotomy can be performed with a no. 15 blade. The surgeon may chose a box, slit, or cruciate approach leaving as small an annular defect as possible, taking care to cut away from the nerve roots. The disc fragments are removed with a Penfield no. 4 and a pituitary rongeur (Figs. 22-12 to 22-15). If a hard disc or posterior vertebral body osteophytes are prominent, we use a reverse-angled curette to impact away from the thecal sac and roots and remove with a pituitary. We then perform disc space lavage with Frasier sucker tips and large syringes to flush any additional lose fragments as well as ensure removal of offending chemical cytokines and irritants. If there are any major discrepancies between operative findings and MRI, a repeat radiograph should be obtained with a marker to verify correct-level surgery.

Confirmation of decompression is then performed by probing the ventral surface of the canal and dural sac both proximal and distal to the disc space for extraligamentous and subligamentous disc fragments or osteophytic ridges. We typically explore the floor of the canal with a Murphy probe to ensure there are no sequestered fragments. The contralateral ventral surface, lateral subarticular recess, and foramen are also inspected. If the foramen is found to be stenotic, it should be decompressed. The traversing nerve root should be freely mobile at the end of the procedure.

Closure   Meticulous hemostasis is obtained with the temporary use of thrombin-soaked Gelfoam, bone wax, and pledgets. We irrigate profusely and then remove all sponges or pledgelets including Gelfoam to ensure no space-occupying lesions exist. Bone wax is used to control any bleeding from exposed cancellous bone. The retractors are then removed and the paraspinal muscles inspected for bleeding. We apply 0.5 mL of dexamethasone locally over the nerve roots and then close watertight in layers the muscle, fascial, subdermal, and subcuticular layers with no. 1 Vicryl, 2-0 Vicryl, 3-0 Vicryl, and 4-0 Monocryl followed by application of a tension-free dressing (Fig. 22-16). We typically do not need a closed suction drain and let our patients go home the day of surgery after ambulating and voiding with pain controlled.

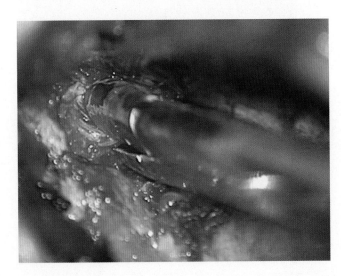

FIGURE 22-13

A pituitary now easily removes the large herniation.

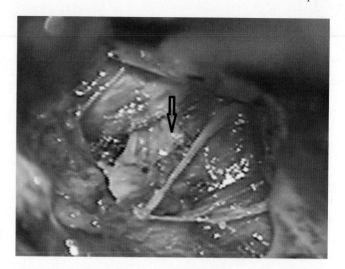

FIGURE 22-14
Annular defect (*arrow*) visualized after disc removal.

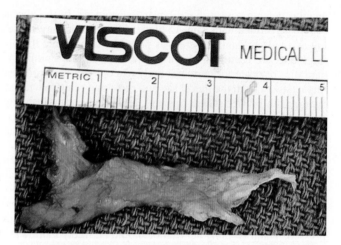

FIGURE 22-15
Large fragment.

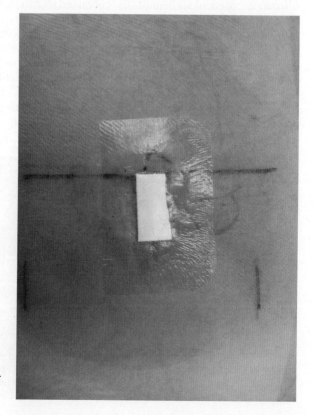

FIGURE 22-16
Dressing is applied after subcuticular absorbable stitch is placed.

POSTOPERATIVE MANAGEMENT

Lumbar microdiscectomy is routinely performed as an outpatient procedure barring complications. Oral analgesics are provided on an as-needed basis. The patient is encouraged to sit and walk as soon he or she is comfortable and the anesthetic has worn off. Normal activity may be resumed as tolerated except that patients are advised to avoid excessive trunk flexion, heavy lifting, and contact activities for 6 weeks. Physical therapy may be necessary depending on the patient's status before and after surgery.

RESULTS

Lumbar microdiscectomy is a very successful orthopedic procedure with greater than 90% of patients reporting good to excellent relief of leg pain and less than 10% recurrence of herniation (1,3,6,9). Patients can expect resolution of concordant radicular buttock and leg pain (7,10,11). Relief of lower back pain is less consistent. In general, patients with lower-level herniations do better than patients with upper lumbar herniations (4). Paracentral and foraminal herniations do better than central or extraforaminal herniations (2). Revision discectomy outcomes can be similar to the outcomes of primary discectomies, although there is a higher risk of spinal fluid leak. Relief of symptoms also closely correlates to the duration of time they were present preoperatively (5). Younger patients with recent onset of symptoms (3 to 6 months) experience rapid and more substantial improvement in pain and neurologic function (8). Older patients with long-standing symptoms experience more delayed relief, which is often incomplete. Patients with symptoms greater than 6 months typically have poorer outcomes whether treated operatively or nonoperatively though patients treated operatively still do better than those treated nonoperatively. Numbness often persists despite adequate decompression in patients with chronic symptoms.

COMPLICATIONS

Although many precautions are taken in preoperative planning, wrong-level surgery must always be a surgeon's main concern. Occasionally, the adjacent cephalad level is inadvertently exposed especially in obese patients with a lordotic lumbar spine. It can also occur in an older patient with significant degenerative disc disease resulting in loss of interspinous process distance. Difficulties in positioning and identifying landmarks may also contribute to increased risk of wrong-level surgery. Needle localization with indigo carmine dye is highly recommended in determining the correct level. Repeat radiographs with a Woodson elevator slipped under the cranial lamina but dorsal to the flavum or even a Penfield 4 dissector in place can also be obtained before the disc is incised. This is especially true if intraoperative findings do not correlate with those on the MRI. Additionally, the potential also exists for operating on the wrong side. The correct side of the patient's symptoms and precise location of disc herniation should be reconfirmed both when marking the patient in the preoperative area and prior to making incision as part of the WHO-sanctioned "time-out."

Anatomical variations may also lead to complications in localizing the correct operative level. Up to 10% of people have abnormal lumbar segmentation, with either four or more often six lumbar vertebrae as opposed to the usual five. Sagittal MRI findings must be matched up with plain lateral radiographs preoperatively to count up from the last formed disc space and determine which level requires the discectomy. Numbering individual segments on separate studies may lead to discrepancies and wrong-level exposure. In addition, we recommend labeling the levels on printed radiographs and correlating this with MRI findings both with the patient and at the time of dictation to decrease any discrepancies.

Other possible complications include inadequate decompression, spinal fluid leak, recurrent herniation, and postoperative wound infection. Spinal fluid leaks occur in up to 4% of primary surgery and up to 20% on revision discectomy. Recurrent herniation occurs 5% to 10% of the time, and postoperative wound infection is typically 1% to 2% with discitis 0% to 2% of the time. Rarer complications include great vessel injury with penetration of the anterior/lateral annulus or nerve root laceration.

CONCLUSION

The natural history of sciatica and radiculopathy secondary to lumbar disc herniations is generally quite favorable, with 6 to 12 weeks of conservative management typically allowing for resorption and subsequent pain relief in most cases. Patients that do not improve are candidates for operative intervention. Although many techniques are available for decompression, open lumbar microdiscectomy with the use of the operating microscope or loupe magnification remains the most common technique for addressing this pathology. Meticulous technique as described above can aid the surgeon in achieving successful outcomes in the vast majority of patients.

RECOMMENDED READING

1. Barrios C, Ahmed M, Arrotegui J, et al.: Microsurgery versus standard removal of the herniated lumbar disc. A 3-year comparison in 150 cases. *Acta Orthop Scand* 61: 399–403, 1990.
2. Carragee EJ, Han MY, Suen PW, et al.: Clinical outcomes after lumbar discectomy for sciatica: the effects of fragment type and annular competence. *J Bone Joint Surg Am* 85-A(1): 102–108, 2003.
3. Kahanovitz N, Viola K, McCulloch J: Limited surgical discectomy and microdiscectomy. A clinical comparison. *Spine* 14: 79–81, 1989.
4. Lurie JD, Faucett SC, Hanscom B, et al.: Lumbar discectomy outcomes vary by herniation level in the Spine Patient Outcomes Research Trial. *J Bone Joint Surg Am* 90: 1811–1819, 2008.
5. McCulloch JA, Young PH: *Essentials of spinal microsurgery*. Philadelphia, PA: Lippincott-Raven, 1998.
6. Nystrom B: Experience of microsurgical compared with conventional technique in lumbar disc operations. *Acta Neurol Scand* 76: 129–141, 1987.
7. Rhee JM, Schaufele M, Abdu WA: Radiculopathy and the herniated lumbar disc. Controversies regarding pathophysiology and management. *J Bone Joint Surg Am* 88: 2070–2080, 2006.
8. Rihn JA, Hilibrand AS, Radcliff K, et al.: Duration of symptoms resulting from lumbar disc herniation: effect on treatment outcomes. An analysis of the Spine Patient Outcomes Research Trial (SPORT). *J Bone Joint Surg Am* 93(20): 1906–1914, 2011.
9. Tullberg T, Isacson J, Weidenhielm L: Does microscopic removal of lumbar disc herniations lead to better results than the standard procedure? Results of a one-year randomized study. *Spine* 18: 24–27, 1993.
10. Weber H: The natural history of disc herniation and the influence of intervention. *Spine (Phila Pa 1976)* 19: 2233–2238, 1994.
11. Weinstein JN, Lurie JD, Tosteson TD, et al.: Surgical versus nonoperative treatment for lumbar disc herniation: four-year results for the Spine Patient Outcomes Research Trial (SPORT). *Spine (Phila Pa 1976)* 33: 2789–2800, 2008.

23 Lumbar Discectomy Using a Tubular Retractor System

Naderafshar Fereydonyan, Shyam A. Patel, and D. Greg Anderson

Lumbar microdiscectomy is the most commonly performed spinal operation (4). In 1909, Oppenheim and Krause described the removal of a herniated lumbar intervertebral disc using a midline posterior lumbar transdural approach, though they misunderstood the pathology and believed the disc herniation was a type of tumor (chondroma) (25). In 1934, Mixter and Barr (23) described the cause/effect relationship between lumbar disc herniation and sciatica. As surgical techniques evolved, extradural hemilaminectomy became the standard approach for retrieving herniated lumbar disc fragments. In an effort to improve surgical outcomes, there has been a general interest in reducing the iatrogenic surgical trauma to the muscles, ligaments, and joints surrounding the surgical site.

Over the years, there has been a trend toward less invasive surgical techniques for the treatment of lumbar disc herniations. Caspar and Yasargil separately described the concept of microdiscectomy in the 1970s (7,37). Kambin (17) used a modified arthroscope to perform lumbar discectomy. Foley and Smith (12) designed the microendoscopic (MED) system for lumbar discectomy in 1997. The second generation of the MED system was developed in 1999, allowing surgeons to address migrated herniated disc fragments and lateral recess stenosis (40). Various tubular retractor systems have been introduced in recent years, allowing microdiscectomy to be performed through progressively smaller surgical incisions. At least as equal in importance to the development of tubular retractor systems has been the improvement in viewing options including surgical endoscopes and operative microscopes. Using modern tubular retractor systems and surgical microscopes, the removal of herniated disc fragments has become a routine minor operation, commonly performed on an outpatient basis.

CLINICAL PRESENTATION

Symptoms

The most common symptoms of a lumbar disc herniation include radiating pain from the lumbar area to one or both extremities (following a dermatomal distribution), numbness or paresthesias, and muscle weakness. The symptoms generally begin abruptly; however, some patients may describe an evolution of pain in the lumbar spine, which progresses into the leg over a period of time. The symptoms may begin following some inciting event or during the course of normal daily life. In rare cases, patients may develop symptoms of saddle anesthesia and sphincter disturbance (cauda equina syndrome), which is considered to be a surgical emergency.

Physical Examination

The physical examination begins with a general inspection of the patient, which includes the gait and posture. Patients with severe radicular pain may avoid significant walking or present with a slightly flexed or side bent posture. Muscle spasm may be present in the acute phase of sciatica. The straight leg raise test (hip flexion with knee extension) may increase or reproduce the sharp, lancinating leg pain (10). A detailed neurologic examination is of paramount importance and should include motor, sensory, and reflex testing. Patients with symptoms of possible cauda equina syndrome should undergo rectal examination.

DIFFERENTIAL DIAGNOSIS

Many conditions may mimic the presentation of a lumbar disc herniation. The differential diagnosis includes tumors of the spinal column or neural elements, various forms of peripheral nerve pathologies (diabetic, entrapment, etc.), osteoarthritis of the lower extremity, instability of the lumbar spine, and spinal infections or fractures.

DIAGNOSIS AND IMAGING

The MRI is the imaging modality of choice for the evaluation of the lumbar spine in the setting of a patient suspected to have a lumbar disc herniation. It is important to know, however, that a considerable percentage of asymptomatic individuals will have abnormalities on lumbar MRI; hence, the symptoms and MRI findings must be carefully correlated (6).

For patients with contraindications to an MRI, CT myelography is an acceptable alternative (19). Plain radiographs, including dynamic flexion/extension films, are helpful in the diagnosis of lumbar instability or abnormalities of the lumbosacral segmentation.

In questionable cases or those with other related disease processes (e.g., diabetic patients), electromyography may also be helpful.

INDICATIONS

Most patients with symptomatic lumbar disc herniations will respond to nonsurgical treatment. In patients with acute, severe symptoms, a short course of bed rest (24 to 48 hours) may be helpful. Short-term oral analgesic medications may be used to control severe pain. Nonsteroidal anti-inflammatory drugs are often helpful in reducing symptoms. Less frequently, patients may require a short course of oral corticosteroids. In patients who fail to respond to initial treatments, lumbar epidural steroid injections may be considered. These procedures have been shown to reduce radicular symptoms in many patients (5). Some studies have suggested that patients who respond temporarily to a lumbar epidural steroid injection are more likely to have a favorable outcome with surgical treatment (31). Physical therapy, chiropractic treatment, and acupuncture have been promoted as treatment options for acute sciatica, although the quality of the data supporting these interventions is suboptimal.

The indications for a microendoscopic discectomy using a tubular retractor system are identical to those for a traditional open microdiscectomy. Patients with cauda equina syndrome or profound and severe and progressive motor weakness should be treated surgically in an urgent fashion (1,18,28).

The most frequent indication for surgery in the setting of a lumbar disc herniation is leg pain symptoms, which fail to respond adequately to nonsurgical care. Most experts agree that severe leg pain that has not responded adequately to a 6-week course of nonsurgical care constitutes a reasonable indication for surgical intervention. Other indications such as isolated sensory loss and isolated lower back pain in the setting of a lumbar disc herniation do not have substantial evidence-based support for a surgical approach at the current time.

Contraindications and Special Situations

Although there are no absolute contraindications to lumbar discectomy with a tubular retractor system, certain situations are best approached by experienced hands.

For example, compared to nonobese patients, morbidly obese patients present a greater technical challenge, although the theoretical advantages of a smaller surgical dissection in this patient population are substantial. Morbidly obese patients require the surgeon to consider the distance from skin to spine relative to the length of the available retractor system. Open field MRI may allow the surgeon to measure this distance during the preoperative planning session. Most tubular retractor systems have maximal lengths of 90 to 100 mm. Distances from skin to spine that are longer than this will require a "cut down" in order for the tube to be docked on the spine. Although the difficulty of such a case is increased, in experienced hands, the efficacy of a minimally invasive approach is supported in the literature (36).

Revision discectomy presents another technical challenge. Due to adhesions, the rate of dural tear is increased regardless of the surgical approach. Again, with experience, revision surgery is feasible; however, such cases are not recommended for surgeons early in the learning curve of tubular retractor-based surgery (22).

ADVANTAGES AND DISADVANTAGES OF USING A TUBULAR RETRACTOR SYSTEM

The primary goals of microdiscectomy using a tubular retractor system are not different from those of a traditional open microdiscectomy. It is critical that the surgeon achieve adequate decompression of the neural elements and remove all free disc material regardless of the approach. Using a tubular retractor system, surgery can theoretically be done with less dissection of the paraspinal soft tissues, reduced retractor pressure, more sparing of multifidus muscle, and a reduced devascularization of the area (16). Multiple studies regarding tubular-based microdiscectomy have suggested advantages of this approach including decreased postoperative pain, more rapid postoperative mobilization, decreased hospital stay, decreased narcotic usage, decreased surgical blood loss, and a quicker return to work or normal activities (9,14,40). Schick et al. (32) reported less root irritation during tubular retractor-based microdiscectomy compared to open microdiscectomy using intraoperative EMG monitoring. Arts et al. in a randomized clinical trial compared muscle injury between tubular-based microdiscectomy and conventional microdiscectomy. In this study, they measured the cross-sectional area of the multifidus muscle following surgery and failed to find a significant difference between the groups (2).

The steep learning curve of microdiscectomy using a tubular retractor system has been proposed as a potential disadvantage of the procedure. During the learning curve phase, a surgeon should anticipate longer operative times and potentially higher complication rates. Nowitzke et al. and Rong et al. have suggested that the length of the learning curve is approximately 30 cases, although it is logical to assume that various surgeon-related factors may affect this length (24,29).

TECHNIQUE

Minimally invasive lumbar discectomy, using a tubular retractor system, may be performed with either general or epidural anesthesia depending the surgeon's preference. The patient is positioned prone on a radiolucent spinal frame, and a standard sterile preparation and draping of the surgical field are performed. The site of incision is determined by first palpating and marking anatomic landmarks including the spinous processes, the intercrestal line, and the posterior superior iliac spines. An 18-gauge spinal needle is introduced at the site of the proposed surgical incision, and lateral C-arm fluoroscopy imaged is obtained to ensure that the site of the proposed incision is optimally placed to reach the lumbar disc herniation (Fig. 23-1). Next, an incision, equal in length to the diameter of the tubular retractor, is placed approximately 2.5 cm lateral to the midline. In an obese patient, a more

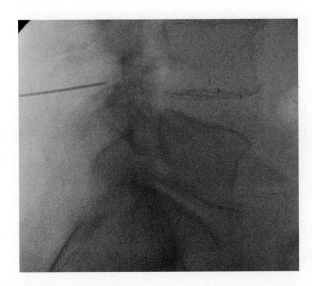

FIGURE 23-1

Fluoroscopic confirmation of the level of surgery.

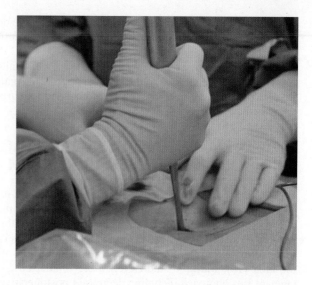

FIGURE 23-2
Subperiosteal dissection with a Cobb elevator.

lateral incision should be used. The skin and thoracolumbar fascia are sharply incised to reach the muscular compartment. Next, a small Cobb elevator is introduced through the incision and docked against the medial lamina. Gentle subperiosteal dissection with the Cobb is used to separate the soft tissue from the bone, preparing the bony docking site for the tubular retractor (Fig. 23-2). Sequential dilators are then introduced through the incision and docked against the medial lamina (Fig. 23-3). The initial dilator is used to palpate the caudal edge of the lamina, which is the preferred docking site. After serial dilation, a tubular retractor of appropriate length is selected and docked against the lamina and then secured to the table-mounted retractor holder (Fig. 23-4). Fluoroscopy is used to confirm proper positioning of tubular retractor prior to proceeding (Fig. 23-5).

Viewing can be achieved with an endoscope or microscope, although the authors find the operative microscope to provide superior three-dimensional visualization. After sterile draping, the operative microscope is brought into the field and focused on the operative field at the floor of the tubular retractor. Any remaining soft tissue overlying the lamina is cleared away using electrocautery to provide good visualization of the bony lamina. Next, a plane is developed between the inferior margin of lamina and underlying ligamentum flavum using an angled curette. The caudal aspect of the lamina is then resected using a Kerrison rongeur or high-speed drill to allow access to the site of the disc herniation (Fig. 23-6). The amount of bone removed will depend on the site of the herniation and the lumbar level. The ligamentum flavum is then released and resected as needed to gain access to the spinal canal (Fig. 23-7). A Woodson elevator is used to palpate the medial boarder of the pedicle, which is a useful landmark for localization within the spinal canal. The traversing nerve root is identified, and a plane beneath the nerve root is established.

At times, due to chronic inflammation or prior surgery, the plane along the nerve root may be difficult to establish due to adhesions. In these cases, careful dissection of the plane, starting cephalad or caudal to the site of the adhesions, may be required to free up the nerve root and allow

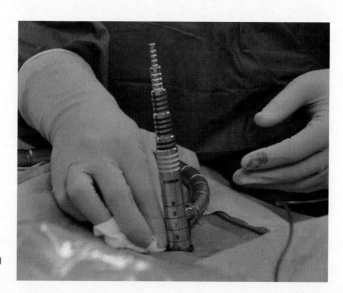

FIGURE 23-3
Sequential dilators used to establish the corridor for the tubular retractor.

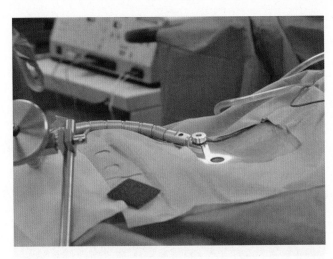

FIGURE 23-4

Tubular retractor secured to the table.

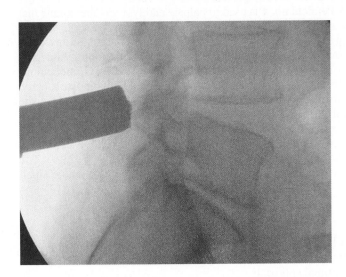

FIGURE 23-5

Tubular retractor position confirmed by fluoroscopy.

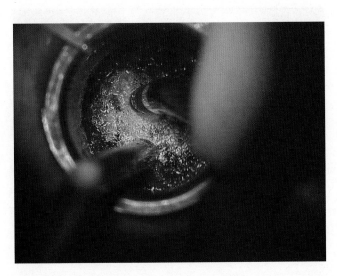

FIGURE 23-6

Laminotomy using a high-speed drill.

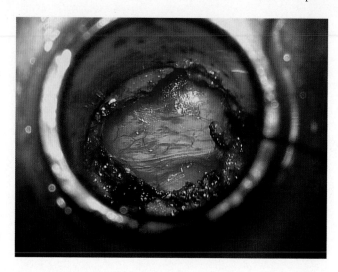

FIGURE 23-7

Exposure of the nerve root and dural
sac following laminoforaminotomy.

access to the ventral aspect of the epidural space. Once the nerve root is adequately mobilized, it is retracted, and the ventral epidural space is explored to identify the disc herniation. With contained herniations, it is preferred to work through the already-present annular disruption, if possible, rather than create a new annular incision. A Penfield no. 4 is used to palpate and lyse any membrane that overlies the site of the herniated disc, and all loose herniated material is evacuated (Fig. 23-8). The disc space is explored through the preexisting annular defect to ensure the absence of any additional loose fragments within the space. Also, the spinal canal is "swept" with a long 90-degree ball-tipped probe to be sure that no migrated disc material has been missed. Next, meticulous hemostasis is achieved. Any active bleeding from epidural veins is controlled with bipolar cautery. Any bleeding from bony edges is controlled with a light coating of bone wax. Irrigation of the site is performed, followed by withdrawal of the tubular retractor. The tubular retractor is withdrawn slowly with careful evaluation of the soft tissue along the site of the operative tract to ensure that no significant bleeders are missed. Any bleeding encountered during tube withdrawal is controlled by bipolar cautery. The fascia and skin are then closed with absorbable sutures (Fig. 23-9). The subcutaneous tissues are injected with local anesthetic to reduce postoperative pain, and a small bandage is applied.

Far Lateral Herniations

Far lateral herniations make up 7% to 12% of all lumbar herniations (11). In the past, there has been controversy regarding the optimal approach to access a far-lateral lumbar herniation. Fortunately, a tubular retractor system provides an optimal approach.

The surgical setup is identical to that described above. The site of the incision, however, is significantly more lateral and should be positioned about 2 cm lateral to the lateral margin of the facet joint or 5 cm lateral to the midline. The exact site may vary depending on the size of the patient,

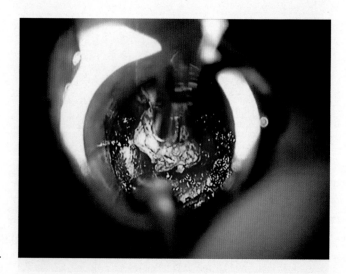

FIGURE 23-8

Disc material evacuation.

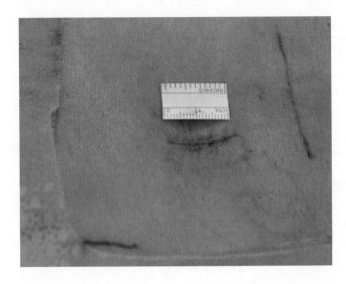

FIGURE 23-9

Final surgical incision for a two-level surgical procedure.

and a more exact estimate of the location of the incision can be measured from the preoperative MRI study. A spinal needle is introduced along the proposed site of the surgical incision. Anteroposterior and lateral fluoroscopy are used to confirm the location prior to making the surgical incision. Following incision and serial dilation, the tubular retractor is docked at the base of the caudal transverse process and secured to the operating table.

Under microscopic visualization, residual soft tissues are removed so that the transverse process and intertransverse membrane are identified. The intertransverse membrane is then released from its bony attachments, and the undersurface of the pars interarticularis is palpated to identify the location of the exiting nerve root. The lateral margin of the disc space is also identified medially in the so-called triangular working zone. It is typical to encounter multiple venous bleeders during this approach, and meticulous use of bipolar electrocautery should be used to maintain a dry surgical field. Not uncommonly, a small portion of lateral aspect of superior articular process will need to be drilled away to gain access to the caudal portion of the foramen. The location of the disc fragment can vary, but is most often found just ventral to the exiting nerve root. By sweeping beneath the nerve root with a small ball-tipped probe, the free disc material can often be identified and evacuated. Disc material lodged within the foramen may also be removed by sweeping along the foramen from cranial to caudal using the small ball-tipped prove. If a defect in the annulus is seen, this area can be explored for additional free disc material. If significant foraminal stenosis is present, additional bone from the superior articular process can be removed to enlarge the neural foramen. Care should be taken to minimize manipulation of the dorsal root ganglion and exiting nerve root as overmanipulation of this structure may lead to postoperative symptoms of radiculitis. After decompression of the exiting nerve root, the surgical steps are identical to that described above.

CONVERSION TO AN OPEN TECHNIQUE

If adequate decompression cannot be achieved via the tubular retractor, the surgeon may convert to an open technique although this is very rarely needed in experienced hands.

Even in the setting of a dural tear, it is preferable to perform an adequate repair, working through the tubular retractor, as the lack of significant wound dead space is helpful in reducing the risk of a persistent cerebrospinal fluid leak or durocutaneous fistula. Dural repair techniques are demanding when working through a tubular retractor system but are achievable using a micropituitary instrument as a needle driver and an arthroscopic knot pusher (8,35). Other techniques have been also described, such as the use of surgical clips, working through a minimally invasive approach (34).

POSTOPERATIVE MANAGEMENT

Following lumbar microdiscectomy with a tubular retractor system, patients are generally mobilized and discharged on the same day as surgery. Patients are encouraged to begin a walking program immediately and to resume normal daily activities as tolerated. A rehabilitation program incorporating core muscle strengthening and aerobic conditioning is initiated within weeks following surgery.

COMPLICATIONS

Dural Tears

Dural tears are a relatively common occurrence during spinal surgery with an incidence of up to 13.7% for lumbar spinal procedures (27,38–40). Although Tel et al. reported a higher rate of dural tears with minimally invasive lumbar surgery, inferior outcomes were not found (21). Due to the lack of substantial wound dead space, there appears to be a reduced incidence of major cerebral spinal fluid (CSF) leakage or wound breakdown. Several studies have shown no long-term impact on patient outcome when successful management of dural tears is achieved (38).

Inadequate Decompression

Persistent symptoms due to inadequate decompression or residual herniated disc material can occur with any form of lumbar decompression. In the event of this type of complication, it is best to proceed with reexploration of the site to achieve an adequate decompression before substantial scarring has had time to unify.

Surgical Site Infection

Infection rates following tubular access surgery are low. O'Toole et al. (26) found only 0.22% postoperative surgical site infections in 1,274 patients following minimally invasive surgical (MIS) procedures. In the rare event of a wound infection, treatment with debridement and antibiotic therapy should be instituted.

Neural Injury

Nerve root injury can generally be prevented with careful surgical technique. Prevention is paramount, because treatment options are limited for this problem.

RESULTS

Various studies have reported the clinical outcomes of MIS decompression in comparison to the traditional open lumbar discectomy. Smith et al. retrospectively reviewed 16 consecutive cases of recurrent lumbar disc herniations treated with a tubular retractor system. In his series, there were two cases with dural tears treated with dural sealant without any long-term consequence. Approximately 80% (13 cases) had excellent or good outcome (modified McNab criteria), and the remaining three cases had fair outcomes. There were no cases of delayed instability (33). Salame and Lidar reported a retrospective analysis of 31 patients treated for far-lateral disc herniations using a tubular retractor system and operative microscope. They found a low rate of complications with this approach and achieved significant improvement in SF-36 and VAS scores for back and leg pain (30). Harington and French reported the results of two groups of patients treated by either midline microdiscectomy or a minimally invasive approach for a one-level disc herniations. They found no difference in terms of surgical time, blood loss, or complications (14). German et al. (13) also found no significant differences in the operative time, rate of cerebrospinal fluid leak, or the need for a physical therapy consultation when comparing surgery with and without a minimally invasive approach. Lee et al. reported similar rates of dural tear, nerve root injury, reherniations, and wound complications for MIS discectomy using tubular retractor system in comparison to traditional lumbar microdiscectomy. There was, however, a statistically significant reduction in the length of hospital stay and reduced narcotics usage with the MIS approach (20). Arts et al. compared tubular microdiscectomy and conventional microdiscectomy in a prospective, randomized controlled trial. Outcomes were measured with the Roland Morris disability questionnaire, VAS for back and leg pain, and a self-reported recovery (measured on a 7-point Likert scale). The surgical technique for both groups of patients used a midline incision of 25 to 30 mm in length, with lateral retraction of the incision for the tubular retractor cohort. They found no statistically significant differences in outcome between the groups although there were more favorable mean scores reported on several scales for the conventional microdiscectomy group (20). A criticism of the Arts et al. study is the altered surgical technique in the tubular retractor group: Using a midline rather than paramedian incision would logically increase the soft tissue stretch necessary to place the tubular retractor and produce an abnormal trajectory of visualization. Hormuzdiyar et al. performed a meta-analysis, which included six trials and 837 patients (388 cases randomized to an MIS approach and 449 cases with an open approach). Although incidental durotomies were significantly more frequent in the MIS group, total complication rates were not significantly different. No difference in leg pain relief was found between the two techniques (3,15).

CONCLUSION

Advances in surgical instrumentation, retractor systems, and operative microscopes have allowed surgeons to perform lumbar discectomy routinely using a tubular retractor system and operative microscope. Although the tubular retractor approach does have a learning curve, there are a number of theoretical advantages with this approach, which make the procedure worth considering. In experienced hands, long-term outcomes are comparable to conventional microdiscectomy. However, a reduction in postoperative pain, hospitalization, recovery time, and blood loss is achievable with this technique.

RECOMMENDED READING

1. Ahn UM, Ahn NU, et al.: Cauda equina syndrome secondary to lumbar disc herniation: a meta-analysis of surgical outcomes. *Spine* 25: 1515–1522, 2000.
2. Arts M, Brand R, et al.: Does minimally invasive lumbar disc surgery result in less muscle injury than conventional surgery? A randomized controlled trial. *Eur spine J* 20(1): 51–57, 2011.
3. Arts MP, Brand R, van den Akker ME, et al.: Tubular diskectomy versus conventional microdiskectomy for sciatica. *JAMA* 302(2): 149–158, 2009.
4. Atlas SJ, Keller RB, Robson D, et al.: Surgical and nonsurgical management of lumbar spinal stenosis: four-year outcomes from the maine lumbar spine study. *Spine* 25: 556–562, 2000.
5. Baldwin NG: Lumbar disc disease: the natural history. *Neurosurg Focus* 13(2): E2, 2002.
6. Boden SD, Davis TS, et al.: Abnormal resonance scans of the lumbar spine in asymptomatic subjects: a prospective investigation. *J Bone Joint Surg Am* 72: 403–408, 1990.
7. Caspar W: A new surgical procedure for lumbar disc herniation causing less tissue damage through a microsurgical approach. *Adv Neurosurg* 4: 74–80, 1977.
8. Chou D, Wang VY, et al.: Primary dural repair during minimally invasive microdiscectomy using standard operating room instruments. *Neurosurg* 64(5): 356–359, 2009.
9. Cole JS, Jackson TR: Minimally invasive lumbar discectomy in obese patients. *Neurosurg* 61(3): 539–544, 2007.
10. Deville WL, van der Windt DA, et al.: The test of Lasegue: systematic review of the accuracy in diagnosing herniated discs. *Spine* 25: 1140–1147, 2000.
11. Epstein NE: Evaluation of varied surgical approach used in the management of 170 far-lateral lumbar disc herniations: indications and results. *J Neurosurg* 83(4): 648–656, 1995.
12. Foley KT, Smith MM: Microendoscopic discectomy. *Tech Neurosurg* 3: 301–307, 1997.
13. German JW, Adamo MA, Hoppenot RG, et al.: Perioperative results following lumbar discectomy: comparison of minimally invasive discectomy and standard microdiscectomy. *Neurosurg Focus* 25: E20, 2008.
14. Harington JF, French P: Open versus minimally invasive lumbar discectomy: comparison of operative times, length of hospital stay, narcotic use, and complications. *Minim Invasive Neurosurg* 51: 30–35, 2008.
15. Hormuzdiyar HD, Stephen PJ, et al.: The efficacy of minimally invasive discectomy compared with open discectomy: a meta-analysis of prospective randomized controlled trials. *J Neurosurg Spine* 16(5): 452–462, 2012.
16. Huang TJ, Ven-Wei-Hsu R, et al.: Less systemic cytokine response in patients following microendoscopic versus open lumbar discectomy. *J Orthop Res* 23(2): 406–411, 2005.
17. Kambin P: Arthroscopic microdiscectomy. *J Arthroplasty* 8: 287–295, 1992.
18. Kohles SS, et al.: Time dependent surgical outcomes following cauda equina diagnosis: comment on a meta-analysis. *Spine* 29(11): 1281–1287, 2004.
19. Kretzscmar K: Degenerative diseases of the spine. The role of myelography and myelo-CT. *Eur J Radiol* 27(3): 229–234, 1998.
20. Lee P, Liu JC, Fessler RG: Perioperative results following open and minimally invasive single-level lumbar discectomy. *J Clin Neurosci* 18(12): 1667–1670, 2011.
21. Macio T, Allessio L, et al.: Higher risk of dural tears and recurrent herniation with lumbar microendoscopic discectomy. *Eur Spine J* 19: 443–450, 2010.
22. Matsumoto M, Ishii K, et al.: Microendoscopic discectomy for recurrent lumbar disc herniation. *Asian J Endosc Surg* 3(2): 77–82, 2010.
23. Mixter WJ, Barr JS: Rupture of the intervertebral disc with involvement of spinal canal. *N Engl J Med* 211: 210–215, 1934.
24. Nowitzke AM, et al.: Assessment of the learning curve for lumbar microendoscopic discectomy. *Neurosurgery* 56(4): 755–762, 2005.
25. Oppenheim H, Krause F: Uber einklemmung bzw: strangulation der cauda equina. *Dtsch Med Wochenschr* 35: 697–700, 1909. Serial solutions.
26. O'Toole JE, Eichholz KM, Fessler RG: Surgical site infection rates after invasive spinal surgery. *J Neurosurg Spine* 11: 471–476, 2009.
27. Podichetty VK, Spears J, Isaacs RE, et al.: Complications associated with minimally invasive decompression for lumbar spinal stenosis. *J Spinal Disord Tech* 19: 161–166, 2006.
28. Qureshi A, Sell P: Cauda equina syndrome treated by surgical decompression, the influence of timing on surgical outcome. *Eur Spine J* 16(12): 2143–2151, 2007.
29. Rong LM, et al.: Spinal surgeons' learning curve for lumbar microendoscopic discectomy: a prospective study of our first 50 and latest 10 cases. *Chin Med J (Engl)* 121(21): 2148–2151, 2008.
30. Salame K, Lidar Z. Minimally invasive approach to far lateral lumbar disc herniation: technique and clinical results. *Acta Neurochir (Wien)* 152(4): 663–668, 2010.
31. Schaufele MK, Hatch L, Jones W: Interlaminar versus transforaminal epidural injections for the treatment of symptomatic lumbar intervertebral disc herniations. *Pain Physician* 9: 361–366, 2006.
32. Schick U, Dohnert J, Richter A, et al.: Microendoscopic lumbar discectomy versus open surgery: an intraoperative EMG study. *Eur Spine J* 11: 20–26, 2002.
33. Smith SJ, Ogden TA, Shafizadeh S, et al.: Clinical outcome after microendoscopic discectomy for recurrent lumbar disc herniation. *J Spinal Disord Tech* 23(1): 30–34, 2010.

34. Song D, Part P: Primary closure of inadvertent durotomies utilizing the U-clip in minimally invasive spinal surgery. *Spine* 36(26): E1753–E1757.
35. Than KD, Wang AC, Etame AB, et al.: Postoperative management of incidental durotomy in minimally invasive lumbar spine surgery. *Minim Invasive Neurosurg* 51(5): 263–266, 2008.
36. Tomazino A, et al.: Tubular microsurgery for lumbar discectomies and laminectomies in obese patients: operative results and outcomes. *Spine* 34(18): E664–E672, 2009.
37. Yasargil MG: Microsurgical operation of herniated lumbar disc. *Adv Neurosurg* 4: 81, 1977.
38. Wang JC, Bohlman HH, Riew KD: Dural tears secondary to operations on the lumbar spine: management and results after a two-year-minimum follow-up of eighty-eight patients. *J Bone Joint Surg Am* 80(12): 1728–1732, 1998.
39. Wood GW: Lower back pain and disorders of intervertebral disc. In: Canale ST, ed. *Campbell's operative orthopaedics*. 9th ed. St. Louis, MO: Mosby, 1998: 3014–3092.
40. Wu X, Zhuang S, Mao Z, et al.: Microendoscopic discectomy for lumbar disc herniation: surgical technique and outcome in 873 consecutive cases. *Spine* 31: 2689–2694, 2006.

24 Transpedicular Fixation: Open

Mark S. Eskander, Jesse L. Even, and James D. Kang

Roy-Camille et al. (7) introduced the idea of transpedicular screw fixation to the forefront of spinal surgery in 1963. Since then, open transpedicular fixation techniques are one of the most utilized in the treatment of a variety of spinal disorders. Pedicle screw fixation can rigidly control the three columns of the spine but needs an intact pedicle to do so. Some of the indications for transpedicular fixation include resisting translational instability, resisting axial instability, and controlling complex deforming forces (5,6).

INDICATIONS

There are many instances where transpedicular fixation is utilized by the surgeon to treat a particular problem. A clear understanding of the clinical problem and a patient's particular anatomy will determine when to use transpedicular fixation techniques (4). The following are some disease processes that are amenable to transpedicular fixation.

1. Degenerative disease
   a. Spondylolisthesis
   b. Disk degeneration (after multiple herniations)
   c. Degenerative scoliosis
2. Trauma
3. Deformity
   a. Scoliosis
   b. Kyphosis
4. Tumor
   a. Metastatic
   b. Primary
5. Malunion (flatback syndrome, angular deformities after prior surgery)
6. Osteomyelitis (if infection is under control and spine is unstable)
7. Cervical 7 pedicle screw (when the C7 lateral mass is disrupted after foraminotomy)

While transpedicular fixation of the spine has many uses and indications, there are several circumstances where it is contraindicated and may be a detriment to the patient and the spinal reconstruction construct.

CONTRAINDICATIONS

1. Osteopenia/osteoporosis
2. Atrophic/dystrophic pedicles
3. Congenital absence of pedicles
4. Fractures that disrupt the pedicle
5. Active infection

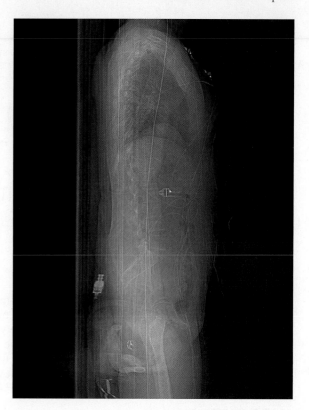

FIGURE 24-1

Lateral scout view from her CT scan. This scan illustrates her kyphotic deformity from her burst fractures at L3 and L4.

PREOPERATIVE PREPARATION

As with all areas of spinal surgery, preoperative planning is essential. After a thorough history and physical examination, complete radiographic evaluation of the spine is next. This is a case of a 20-year-old female who fell off a roof and sustained L3 and L4 burst fractures. The plan for this patient was a posterior spinal fusion (PSF) L2 to Ilium with iliac crest bone graft (ICBG), repair of traumatic durotomy, and reduction of retropulsed fragments from the canal. The patient's preoperative studies are shown; Figure 24-1 is a lateral scout view from her computerized tomography (CT) scan. This scan illustrates her kyphotic deformity from her burst fractures at L3 and L4. Figure 24-2 is a midsagittal CT showing the severity of the burst fractures with special attention to the canal compromise at L4 and the loss of lordosis. There are also some minor compression fractures at

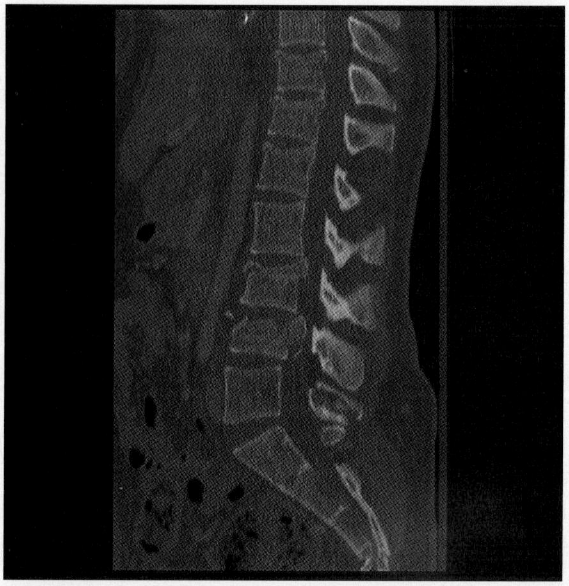

FIGURE 24-2

Midsagittal CT showing the severity of the burst fractures with special attention to the canal compromise at L4 and the loss of lordosis. There are also some minor compression fractures at T11–L1.

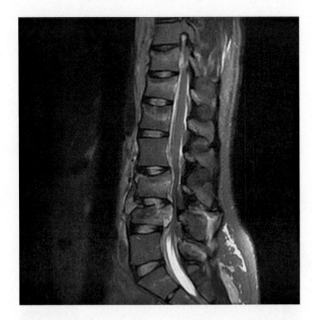

FIGURE 24-3

Midsagittal T2-weighted MRI showing burst fractures with significant canal compromise at L4.

T11–L1. Figure 24-3 is a midsagittal T2-weighted magnetic resonance imaging (MRI) showing burst fractures with significant canal compromise at L4.

Typically, our patients will have anteroposterior (AP) and lateral (flexion and extension) plain radiographs. Often more advanced imaging will ensue. This can include MRI and CT with and without myelography. If the cervical spine is being evaluated, a CT angiogram is preferred to help understand the vasculature in the neck. It is also important to note the alignment of the patient's spine when positioned on the operating room table with a cross-table lateral radiograph. This image is very useful to gauge the trajectory of the screw placement intraoperatively. This is particularly helpful in the setting of instability, secondary to trauma; infection; or tumor, where restoring spinal alignment is of the upmost importance. It is also helpful after performing osteotomies to visualize the correction that was obtained.

TECHNIQUE

Patient Positioning

The patient is gently flipped onto the Jackson table in the prone position. The pads of the Jackson frame support the chest and the iliac wings, allowing for gravity-assisted reduction of the fractured spine. The knees are slightly flexed with pads under each knee. The face is held in a prone view headrest with foam cushions. The eyes are free from any contact and pressure points. The arms are positioned on arm holders with padding. The palms are placed in the pronated position, and the elbows are flexed at 90 degrees. The shoulders are abducted and externally rotated to 90 degrees but forward flexed to 20 degrees to keep tension off of the brachial plexus.

Approach

After being prepped and draped, a midline incision with a no. 10 blade is then made from the bottom of L1 down to the sacral junction. This incision is then taken down to the fascia level using a Bovie electrocautery device. The fascia is then divided to expose the posterior aspect of the spinous process and lamina of L2, L3, L4, L5, and S1 as well as the sacral alar area. A Richardson retractor is then utilized to pull tension on the muscular attachments on the facet capsules, while the Bovie is used to carefully dissect the tissues of off the capsule and to further the exposure out to the transverse process. The transverse processes of L2 through L5 are exposed along with the sacral ala of S1. The posterior aspect of the posterior superior iliac spine (PSIS) is then also exposed through the same midline incision. After the exposure is completed, a Kocher is placed at the L3 spinous process and a lateral x-ray was then taken to confirm levels. Figure 24-4 is a lateral plain radiograph showing the restoration of lordosis after positioning on Jackson table in the prone position. At this time, a dural repair and fracture reduction are performed. Figure 24-5 is a postoperative midsagittal CT scan showing reduction of retropulsed bone from the canal.

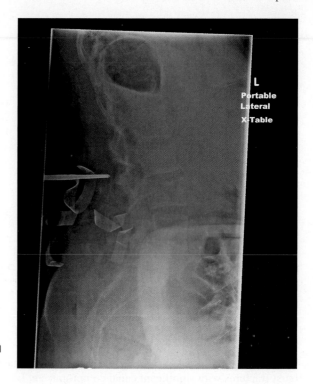

FIGURE 24-4

Lateral plain radiograph showing the
restoration of lordosis after positioning on
Jackson table in the prone position.

Bone Graft

Autogenous ICBG has been the gold standard in spinal fusion surgery against which all other grafting materials must be measured. Other authors have investigated the use of allograft, ceramics, and biologics such as bone morphogenetic protein (8).

We utilize a separate oblique incision over the posterior iliac wing, but the original midline incision may be subcutaneously mobilized to expose the iliac crest thereby avoiding another incision. The posterior iliac spine is identified along with the iliac crest too anteriorly, because the cluneal vessels and nerve may be inadvertently encountered. In addition, as the dissection is carried toward the sciatic notch, caution must be exercised to avoid injury to the superior gluteal artery. When cut, this artery may retract into the pelvis, making hemostasis difficult.

Corticocancellous strips of iliac crest are obtained with osteotomes, and much of the cancellous is obtained with gouges. The largest of cancellous bone is usually found directly under the PSIS.

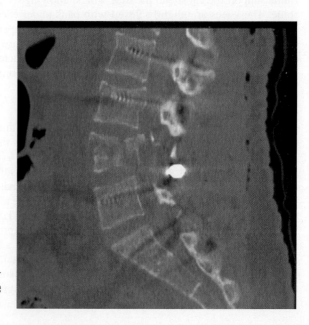

FIGURE 24-5

Postoperative midsagittal CT scan showing reduction of retropulsed bone from the
canal.

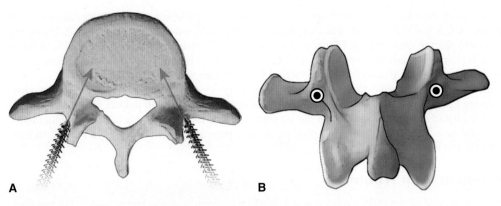

FIGURE 24-6

A: Axial view for the starting point and trajectory for pedicle screw placement.
B: AP view for the starting point and trajectory for pedicle screw placement.

During the bone harvest, care is taken to avoid entering the sacroiliac joint, because this may be a source of persistent pain postoperatively. Once the bone graft is obtained, bone wax and dry Gelfoam are used to achieve hemostasis from the bleeding bony surfaces, and the wound is closed in layers over a Hemovac drain.

Instrumentation (L2–S1)

With the laminae thoroughly exposed out to the facets, one must be careful to not damage the facet joint immediately above the most cephalad screw, in our case the L1–L2 facet joint. In this case, which is a bit unusual, there are two burst fractures at L3 and L4. We elected to stabilize these fractures by instrumenting from L2 into the ilium. We again looked at our intraoperative lateral radiograph to determine the trajectory of our screw placement and to make sure the fractures had fallen back into a normal lumbar lordosis.

A 4-mm bur was used to identify the starting point (Figs. 24-6A and B, 24-7A) for the L2 pedicle screw on the right side first, which was then cannulated using a pedicle finder (Fig. 24-7B). Prior

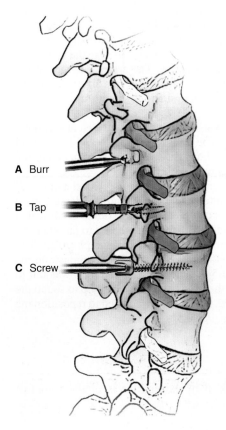

A Burr

B Tap

C Screw

FIGURE 24-7

A: Diagram illustrating the lateral starting point for the bur. **B:** Diagram illustrating the lateral starting point for the pedicle finder. **C:** Diagram illustrating the lateral starting point for the pedicle screw.

to screw insertion, a ball tip feeler is used to make sure that there are no pedicle violations of our channels. A 6.5 × 40 mm screw was then placed on the right side of L2 (Fig. 24-7C). Using the same technique, the contralateral L2 pedicle screw was also placed as well as bilateral L3, bilateral L5, and bilateral S1 pedicle screws. The pedicles at L4 are skipped due to fracture comminution. S1 pedicle screws were placed bicortically using 7.5 × 45 mm screws.

In the case of degenerative spines where a laminectomy is performed as well, we recommend first performing the laminectomy. Subsequently, with an open canal, one can palpate the pedicles using the Woodson and be sure the screws are placed anatomically. Extra caution is used when placing the screws, and avoidance of the inferior medial position is paramount in avoiding injury to the traversing and exiting roots (10).

Instrumentation (Ilium)

With the underside of the PSIS exposed in our midline incision, a 4-mm bur is used to bur the starting point of the pelvic fixation in the medial aspect of the posterior iliac crest. This is then carefully guided in between the inner and outer tables of the pelvis using a pedicle finder. A window into the PSIS from ICBG harvest allows for guidance of the pedicle finder between the inner and outer tables easily on the right side. The left side however is done with a blind technique, using the right as a template for the trajectory of the corresponding iliac screw. A tap is used to carefully sound this trajectory. A 7.5 × 80 mm screw is placed in the right side of her ilium for pelvic fixation. The contralateral iliac screw is also placed. An appropriate size rod is bent to lordotic posture, cut into appropriate length, and placed dorsally to span from L2 through ilium, and caps were then placed to secure the screw rod interface and finally tightened with a torque limiting driver. We then placed a cross-link between the L3 and L5 pedicle screws.

Posterior Arthrodesis

Careful exposure of all bony landmarks is of importance. We want good visualization of the lamina, pars, facet joints with undisrupted capsule, and the transverse processes. The exposure of the pars will prevent an inadvertent resection during decompression. This is most important in the setting of noninstrumented fusions. A pars resection may lead to iatrogenic instability. Just lateral to the pars is the artery of the pars, which can be controlled with a Bovie or bipolar cautery device. One must carefully preserve the facet capsule to minimize instability (1). When using instrumentation, it is not problematic to resect the hypertrophic joints and capsule.

A Richardson retractor can be used to help expose the transverse processes or the ala as dissection is carried laterally over the facet joints. It is important at this point to remember the anatomic relationships. The transverse process of L4, for example, is located slightly cephalad to the pars and lateral to the L3–L4 facet joint. It is also within this region that the most significant arterial bleeding can occur via the transverse process artery. The artery emerges at the upper aspect of the junction of the transverse process with the pedicle (4). This artery should be cauterized at this point as inadvertent injury may lead to retraction and difficulty in controlling after the fact.

The intervening muscle and soft tissue between the transverse processes are cleared at this point to allow for a clean trough for the placement of bone graft. The transverse process and lateral wall of the facets are decorticated using the high-speed 4-mm bur. For fusions into the sacrum and ilium, we decorticate the posterior aspect of posterior iliac crest as well as the sacrum.

The autograft bone that was obtained from the right iliac crest is carefully morselized and mixed with the allograft cancellous bone. The bone graft is then scattered and packed into the dorsal lateral gutters to span from L2 through pelvis to ensure that there is complete coverage of the decorticated areas. It is important to meticulously pack the bone graft underneath the screw heads to facilitate the posterior arthrodesis from L2 through pelvis. We then obtain PA and lateral radiographs to confirm good position of the hardware and fracture alignment (9). Figures 24-8 and 24-9 demonstrate the final construct with PA and lateral plain radiographs. The L5 pedicle screw on the right was felt to be too inferior based on this plain radiograph. We removed the screw and used a ball tip to sound the path, and no defects in the cortical pedicular wall were noted. However, we decided to reposition the screw in a more cephalad orientation.

PEARLS AND PITFALLS

1. Optimal positioning and padding of the patient and their extremities is of the foremost importance.

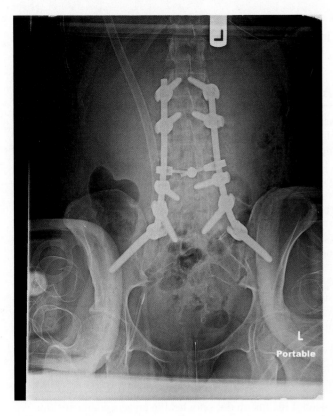

FIGURE 24-8

Final PA plain film showing hardware position. The L5 pedicle screw on the right was felt to be too inferior based on this plain radiograph.

2. Careful inspection of how the patient lays on the table is critical for proper fusion position.
3. Careful exposure of all relevant anatomy will avoid an errant hardware placement.
4. Careful preoperative planning so that all imaging studies have been reviewed and all of the materials/instrumentation for the case are available.

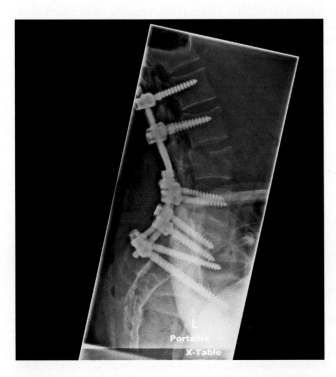

FIGURE 24-9

Final lateral plain film showing hardware position. The L5 pedicle screw on the right was felt to be too inferior based on this plain radiograph.

5. Having a backup plan in place in case the instrumentation is inadequate. Being able to adjust from one plan to another in a seamless fashion is a key to avoiding surgical complications.

POSTOPERATIVE MANAGEMENT

1. We routinely use Hemovac drains for instrumented lumbar fusions. The drain can be pulled after 24 to 48 hours or less than 50 mL/shift of output. If there is a dural tear, the drain can be left in longer to continue to decompress the subfascial space.
2. After a sterile dressing is applied, the patient is logrolled onto the hospital bed.
3. The head of the bed can be elevated to 30 to 60 degrees. (Keep patient flat for 24 hours if dural repair was performed.)
4. Patients are ambulatory day 1 after surgery. They work with therapists for the next few days in the hospital.
5. In an uncomplicated hospital course, patients typically leave for home after 3 to 5 days.
6. Patients will have either a corset for comfort or a thoracic lumbar sacral orthosis (TLSO) if they had larger reconstructive surgery.
7. Patients will have a narcotic supply for 6 weeks after surgery.
8. Patients may drive 1 month after surgery.
9. Patients should avoid lifting greater than 10 pounds in the 1st month.
10. Patients can return to a desk job at 1 month, light duty labor jobs at 3 to 6 months, and heavy duty labor jobs at 6 to 12 months.

COMPLICATIONS

1. Hardware failure—May require revision if the fusion does not heal in an acceptable position
2. Dural tear—Adequate repair and bed rest typically resolve this issue. However, if there is a persistent symptomatic leak, a dural patch and shunt may be needed to seal the defect.
3. Infection—Usually serial washouts and treatment with IV antibiotics will resolve the infection. In cases where the infection is refractory to these methods, removal of instrumentation may be necessary to fully eradicate the infection.
4. Wound dehiscence—Often application of wet to dry dressing changes or a vacuum-assisted closure devise can be helpful in achieving closure by secondary intention. A careful evaluation of the patient's nutrition status is needed in these situations to optimize wound healing along with a possible plastic surgery consultation.
5. Deep vein thrombosis/pulmonary embolism (DVT/PE)—These issues may be treated with Coumadin in cases that show substantial clotting. Generally, it is safe to anticoagulate at 72 hours after surgery, but one must be vigilant for formation of a compressive hematoma in the epidural space.
6. Nerve root injury—Identification on CT scan of the aberrant screw and repositioning of the offending agent (typically malpositioned screw)
7. Adjacent segment disease—Careful handling of the facet above the fusion level may help to avoid this problem. This is a known issue that needs to be monitored over the next few years with serial radiographs. It can occur at a rate of 10% in 10 years but can occur sooner in some situations.

RESULTS

As with all cases in spine surgery, the expectation of a positive outcome is dependent on a number of factors including patient selection, presenting diagnosis, expectation of patient/surgeon, and optimal surgical techniques. With modern techniques for posterior spinal fusions using ICBG, one can expect 85% to 90% fusion rates (2,3).

RECOMMENDED READING

1. Boden SD, Wiesel SW: Lumbosacral segmental motion in normal individuals. Have we been measuring instability properly? *Spine* 15: 571–576, 1990.
2. France JC, Yasemski MJ, Lauerman WC, et al.: A randomized prospective study of posterolateral lumbar fusion: outcomes with and without pedicle screw instrumentation. *Spine* 24: 553–560, 1999.
3. Kang J, An H, Hilibrand A, et al.: Grafton and local bone have comparable outcomes to iliac crest bone in instrumented single level lumbar fusions. *Spine* 37(12): 1083–1091, 2012.

4. MacNab I, Dall D: The blood supply to the lumbar spine and its application to the technique of intertransverse lumbar fusion. *J Bone Joint Surg Br* 53: 628–638, 1971.
5. McAfee PC, Weiland DJ, Carlow JJ: Survivorship analysis of pedicle spinal instrumentation. *Spine* 16(8 Suppl): S422–S427, 1991.
6. Puno RM, Bechtold JE, Byrd JA III, et al.: Biomechanical analysis of transpedicular rod systems. A preliminary report. *Spine* 16: 973–980, 1991.
7. Roy-Camille R, Sallant G, Mazel C: Internal fixation of the lumbar spine with pedicle screw plating. *Clin Orthop* 203: 7–17, 1986.
8. Urist MR, Dawson E: Intertransverse process fusion with the aid of chemosterilized autolyzed antigen-extracted allogeneic (AAA) bone. *Clin Orthop* 154: 97–113, 1981.
9. Weinstein JN, Spratt KF, Spengler DM, et al.: Spinal pedicle fixation: reliability and validity of roentgenogram-based assessment and surgical factors on successful screw placement. *Spine* 13: 1012–1018, 1988.
10. Zindrick MR, Wiltse LL, Doornik A, et al.: Analysis of the morphometric characteristics of the thoracic and lumbar pedicles. *Spine* 12: 160–166, 1987.

25 Transpedicular Fixation: Minimally Invasive

Siddharth B. Joglekar and James D. Schwender

P edicle screw instrumentation has a history that spans less than 50 years since the first description of pedicle screw plating by Raymond Roy-Camille in 1970 (28). Owing to their biomechanical and clinical superiority, pedicle screws have become the spinal anchors of choice for fusion over the last two decades. More recently, less invasive paramedian and percutaneous pedicle screw placement has become widely used to reduce the surgical trauma of the erector spinae musculature. Percutaneous pedicle screw insertion may be traced back to Magerl (17) who first described the "fixateur externe" for the lumbar spine in 1980 and 1984. This technique included percutaneous insertion of posted Schanz screws into the pedicles followed by external bridging of the construct with rods. While the first description of percutaneous pedicle screw instrumentation followed just 10 years after introduction of pedicle screws, it has taken the next three decades for surgeons to develop it into a safe and universally acceptable technique.

Mini-open placement of screws through the transsacrospinalis posterolateral portal with the help of specialized retractor systems has also become a popular minimally invasive spine (MIS) technique. The development of MIS screw placement techniques has been paralleled by the development of radiologic and computer-aided guidance systems to improve accuracy of screw placement.

INDICATIONS

Minimally invasive pedicle screw placement can be used to stabilize the spine in almost every situation where open placement of screws is indicated including degenerative, traumatic, infectious, and neoplastic etiologies. In obese patients in whom open placement would be challenging, MIS screw placement may be preferable.

CONTRAINDICATIONS

There are no absolute contraindications to minimally invasive placement of pedicle screws. MIS pedicle screws would be relatively contraindicated in the following situations:

1. Lack of technical expertise or adequate experience
2. Lack of imaging or navigation equipment when percutaneous placement is being considered
3. Severe deformities of the spine, sclerotic pedicles, very narrow pedicles, and very long multisegment fixations when MIS techniques have been assessed to be technically unsafe or challenging on the preoperative planning
4. When MIS techniques may be noncompatible with the pathology being treated, for example, neoplastic disorders or infections

313

PREOPERATIVE PREPARATION

Careful preoperative planning is essential with a complete history and physical examination along with the aid of radiographs and three-dimensional (3D) imaging. The following factors need to be considered carefully in the preoperative plan:

1. Medical clearance for surgery
2. The indication for surgery to treat the appropriate pathology
3. Type of fusion considered: posterolateral and/or interbody
4. Type of screws (tulip heads versus posted)
5. Type of approach (mini-open versus percutaneous)
6. Type of bone graft (allograft versus iliac crest graft versus biologics)
7. Type of retractor systems (expandable versus tubular)
8. Instrumentation system to be utilized and availability of all specialized equipment and instruments
9. Type of rods and rod introduction system
10. Type of navigation/imaging guidance
11. Need for neuromonitoring
12. Pedicle morphology: size and angulation of the pedicles

   Anatomy of the pedicle in terms of angulation, size, and pedicle length is variable throughout the spine (20,36,39). Pedicles in the thoracic region are significantly smaller and more variable in size and shape than those found in the lumbar region. The transverse diameter is generally much smaller than the vertical diameter for each pedicle, which demands much greater screw placement accuracy in the transverse plane at each level. Transverse pedicle diameters in the thoracic spine are reported to range from 4.5 to 7.8 mm with an increasing trend from T1 to T12, whereas the pedicle angulations in the transverse plane vary from 0 to 30 degrees with a decreasing trend from T1 to T12 (6,36,39). In the lumbar spine, the transverse pedicle diameter gradually increases from L1 to L5 (7.4 to 18.3 mm), and the transverse plane lumbar pedicle angle increases from L1 to L5 (25 to 40 degrees) (5).

TECHNIQUE

There are two main techniques in use for MIS screw placement:

1. Mini-open placement
2. Percutaneous screw placement

   There are further variations in each technique based on the imaging/navigation technique utilized. The following variations may be possible:

I. Mini-open placement through a tubular retractor system:
   a. Free-hand screw insertion with direct anatomic visualization
   b. Image-guided screw placement (C-arm) without navigation for assistance
   c. Image-guided screw placement (C-arm or CT scan) with computer-aided navigation for assistance
II. Percutaneous screw placement relies on image-guided techniques, and free-hand insertion is not possible. Navigated and nonnavigated insertion is possible.

Mini-Open Pedicle Screw Placement

Mini-open MIS fusions utilize the surgical corridor as described by Wiltse et al. (37) between the multifidus and longissimus paraspinal muscles (Fig. 25-1). This trajectory is ideal for both pedicle screw placement and decompression and fusion techniques.

   Fluoroscopy is used to make the appropriate skin incisions. The skin incisions are made 2.5 cm in vertical length and 4 to 5 cm off midline. Sequential dilators are then passed through the fascia and docked onto the facet joint. A tubular retractor (typically 22 or 26 mm) is then docked and secured over the dilators. The use of an expandable retractor allows the blades to expand cephalad or caudad creating a corridor for pedicle screw placement (Fig. 25-2). Soft tissue is cleared to expose the standard pedicle screw entry points. Screws can be placed using a variety of methods including free hand, under C-arm guidance, or utilizing navigation depending upon surgeon preference. In addition, both posted and tulip-style pedicle screws can be used if working through the tubular retractor systems that are available.

   Surgeon preference dictates the sequence of steps during a minimally invasive fusion. Early on in a surgeon's experience, it may be easiest to place the pedicle screw tracts first prior to the decompression or facetectomy. This will preserve "normal" anatomy to help orient the surgeon to

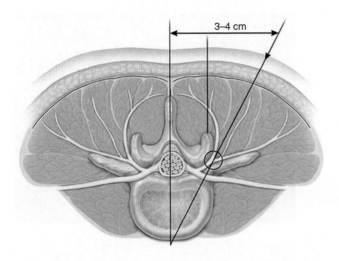

FIGURE 25-1

Schematic diagram of the lumbar spine in the axial plane.

the anatomic starting points. However, it is the author's experience that it is more efficient to perform the transforaminal lumbar interbody fusion (TLIF) followed by appropriate decompression prior to screw tract preparation and screw placement. This minimizes the surgical exposure during the portion of the procedure that requires the most expansion of the modular retractor and thereby helps to limit muscle creep (Fig. 25-3).

The major advantage of this technique versus the percutaneous screw technique is the ability to directly visualize the bony anatomy, thus reducing the requirement of fluoroscopy. In addition, facet joint and posterolateral fusion can be accomplished through the same tubular retractor that the pedicle screws are placed.

Percutaneous Pedicle Screw Placement

Pedicle screws can be safely and effectively placed percutaneously, thus avoiding the additional dissection required for the placement of traditional and mini-open pedicle screws. Percutaneous pedicle screw placement has the advantage of less muscle damage and less potential damage to the medial branch nerve (innervation of the multifidus) and can be used effectively over long-segment fusions. The placement of percutaneous pedicle screws can require more operative time and more x-ray exposure for accurate placement. When using the fluoroscopic technique, the orientation of the C-arm beam is of critical importance. The anteroposterior (AP) images must be true AP images of each pedicle for screw placement (Fig. 25-4). The spinous process should be in the midline of the vertebral body, equally spaced between both pedicles. The superior and inferior endplates should be parallel, and the pedicles should be appropriately located at the caudal end of the ascending articular process. On the lateral view, the superior endplate should appear as one line, and the pedicles should overlap and thus appear as one (Fig. 25-5). True AP and lateral radiographs are of critical importance because small variance can produce erroneous placement of the pedicle screw.

The pedicle of interest is localized utilizing the AP fluoroscopic image. The skin is incised just lateral to the pedicle. The thoracolumbar dorsal fascia and muscle fascia are incised. A Jamshidi

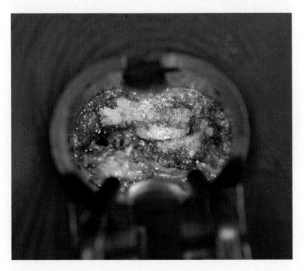

FIGURE 25-2

Exposed anatomy of the lumbar spine through a modular tubular retractor system.

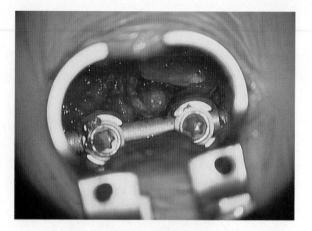

FIGURE 25-3

Completed decompression and TLIF with pedicle screws placed under direct visualization.

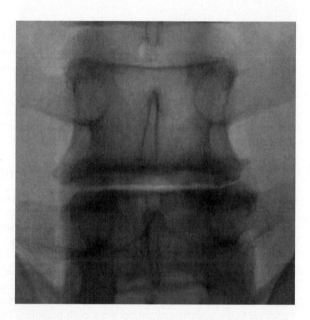

FIGURE 25-4

True AP of the lumbar spine.

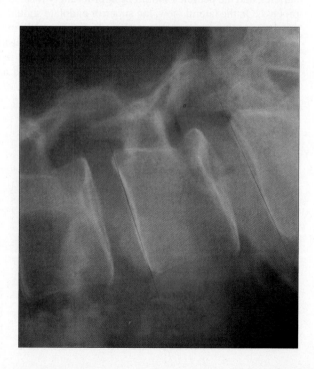

FIGURE 25-5

True lateral of the lumbar spine. Note the endplates are parallel and overlap.

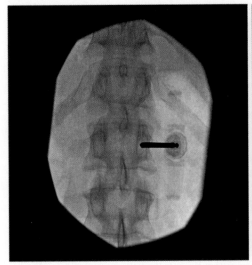
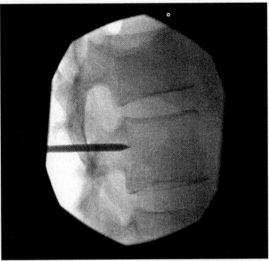

FIGURE 25-6

AP and lateral images with a Jamshidi trocar inserted. Note that the trocar tip remains within the confines of the pedicle on the AP when at the neurocentral junction on the lateral.

trocar is used to cannulate the pedicle. The ideal starting point is at the 10 o'clock and 2 o'clock positions on the left and right pedicles, respectively. The Jamshidi is slowly advanced a few millimeters into the pedicle. A lateral fluoroscopic image is obtained and should confirm that the Jamshidi is placed within the center of the pedicle. Under AP fluoroscopic imaging, the Jamshidi is advanced about 20 mm. The tip should stay lateral to the medial border of the pedicle. A lateral image is obtained and should show the tip of the Jamshidi at or past the neurocentral junction (Fig. 25-6). If so, the Jamshidi can be safely advanced to its desired depth. If the tip of the Jamshidi is at or medial to the medial border of the pedicle on the AP view and not yet passed the neurocentral junction on the lateral view, then it has likely breached the medial border of the pedicle.

After the Jamshidi is placed appropriately, a guidewire is passed. This is repeated at each pedicle. The pedicle screw is then placed over each guidewire, and then the appropriately sized rod is passed. It is critical to continue periodic lateral fluoroscopic visualization to avoid advancing the guidewire anteriorly. Avoid kinking of the guidewire, and remove any dried blood to minimize the risk of guidewire advancement while inserting the screw. In addition, remove the guidewire when the pedicle screw reaches the neurocentral junction.

When first performing these procedures, the authors encourage the liberal use of fluoroscopy or computer-aided navigation. With experience, radiographic exposure and operative time will diminish (Fig. 25-7).

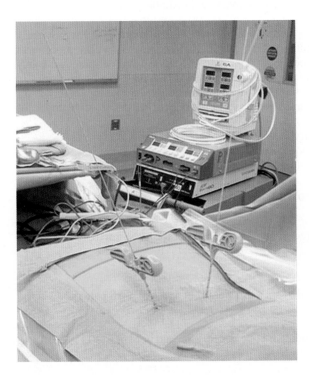

FIGURE 25-7

K-wires placed through the Jamshidi trocar prior to pedicle screw insertion.

PEARLS AND PITFALLS

1. When placing pedicle screws through the MIS tubular retractor technique, remember to move the retractor for accurate visualization of the required bony anatomy. Do not let the retractor dictate what you see and do.
2. When first placing screws through a tubular retractor, expose the pars and the medial portion of the transverse process clearly.
3. Pedicle screw tracks may be easier to prepare prior to performing the decompression and facetectomy when more bony landmarks are present.
4. When placing percutaneous screws, fluoroscopic images must be "perfect" AP and lateral views. Otherwise, percutaneous screw placement may be aberrant.
5. Start simple in terms of complexity of case selection.

POSTOPERATIVE MANAGEMENT

The postoperative rehabilitation plan for these patients is similar to an open pedicle screw placement technique with the exception that mobilization and discharge of the patients may be accelerated as a result of the reduced pain and need for narcotics due to the minimally invasive approach. Wound care strategies may be followed as per the surgeon preference. Bracing needs should be individualized based on the pathology treated and the strength of the fixation construct. We usually do not recommend the use of brace immobilization for instrumented spinal fusions.

COMPLICATIONS

1. Early technical complications are more common with initial learning curve.
2. Radiation exposure to patient, operative team, and surgeon.

    It is variable depending on the body site examined, experience, type of shielding, distance, time of exposure, type of intraoperative imaging and guidance system used, and the surgical technique. In general, with the use of biplanar fluoroscopy for intraoperative imaging, it takes 417 single-level cases for the torso and 1,471 single-level cases for the extremity in order to exceed the annual allowed radiation dose limits (2,25,26). Average exposure to a patient in a single-level procedure ranges from 4.5 to 7.8 cGy compared to the threshold limit of 200 cGy for radiation-related side effects (2,25,33). Exposure to radiation doses of 50 to 100 mSv (protracted exposure) or 10 to 50 mSv (acute exposure) has been postulated to increase the risk of certain types of cancers, and every effort should be made to keep radiation doses to a minimum (3).
3. Increased operative time to do the same type of procedure early in the learning curve.

    Both operative time and radiation exposure shorten with experience (25).
4. Increased costs and dependence on specialized equipment and technology.
5. Superior facet violation.

    A recent study showed a significantly higher overall facet violation grade and significantly greater incidence of high-grade facet joint violations ($P = 0.0059$) compared to open procedures when using a CT-based facet joint violation grading system (1). Up to 13.5% of percutaneously placed screws have been found to violate the superior facet (21). This may have implications in terms of future development of adjacent segment degeneration. However, the reduction of soft tissue trauma without exposure of the supraadjacent facet joint may offset the negative impact of percutaneous screw placement.
6. Incidental durotomy and neurologic injury.

    Should be no different after the technique is mastered.
7. Inadequate decompression or treatment of targeted pathology.

Results of MIS and Percutaneous Pedicle Screw Placement

1. Decreased blood loss

    Significant differences when compared to open procedures in terms of intraoperative blood loss (16)
2. Faster rehabilitation (15)
3. Less pain (15)

    Significant differences when compared to open procedures in terms of VAS pain scores at the 1st week postoperative (16).
4. Reduction in rate of infection
5. Minimize collateral soft tissue injury including muscle denervation and ischemia (10,11,18,31,34)

6. Can be safely done even in obese patients (22). The distance of skin entry point from the midline needs to be increased to account for increased thickness of soft tissues.

Comparison of Mini-Open and Percutaneous Pedicle Screws

The choice of which minimally invasive instrumentation technique to utilize is largely surgeon dependent. Regev et al. (27) compared mini-open pedicle screw insertion with percutaneous pedicle screw insertion on cadavers. After screw placement, the authors dissected out the medial branch nerve. The medial branch nerve originates from the dorsal rami of each spinal nerve and innervates the multifidus muscle. The medial branch nerve was transected in 84% of cases using the mini-open technique as compared to 20% of the percutaneous insertion technique. The clinical importance of this difference is unknown. However, in this cadaveric study, percutaneous pedicle screw insertion better preserved the segmental innervation of the multifidus compared to mini-open pedicle screw insertion.

There are no clinical studies that directly compare the use of pedicle screws placed through a tubular retractor (mini-open) to percutaneous pedicle screws. However, multiple studies have reported perioperative data regarding percutaneous and open screw insertion. Schizas et al. (29) reported their experience with 18 minimally invasive TLIFs using percutaneous pedicle screw fixation and compared this to 18 open TLIFs. The percutaneous pedicle screw patients used 2.7 cGy/cm^2 of radiation as compared to 1.8 cGy/cm^2 in the open TLIF group. The minimally invasive TLIF operative time averaged 4.3 hours in the last third of their experience compared to 5.1 hours in the open TLIF group. Their estimated blood loss was 456 mL compared to 961 mL in the open group ($P < 0.01$). Peng et al. (24) also reviewed their results of minimally invasive TLIFs. They used an average of 105 seconds of fluoroscopy. They had an average EBL of 150 mL and average operative time of 216 minutes. Neither of these studies reported any technical complications with minimally invasive TLIFs performed by percutaneous screws. Foley's (7) initial experience was similar with an average operative time of 290 minutes and estimated blood loss of 25 mL. He reported one technical complication of a loose locking plug, which required revision. Dhall et al. (4) compared minimally invasive TLIFs with traditional pedicle screws to open TLIFs. Their average EBL was 194 mL, and their average OR time was 199 minutes compared to an average EBL of 505 mL and average OR time of 237 minutes in the open group. There were two technical complications in the minimally invasive group with one misplaced pedicle screw and one case of interbody cage migration. The open group also had one misplaced screw. Schwender et al. (30) reported on their initial experience with minimally invasive TLIFs and percutaneous screw insertion. Their average operative time was 240 minutes, and the average EBL was 140 mL. In this series, there were two misplaced screws and interbody cage dislodgement. Park and Ha (23) compared 32 minimally invasive PLIFs with 29 open PLIFs. All minimally invasive cases were stabilized with percutaneous screws. The average OR time was longer for the minimally invasive cases compared to open, 191 and 150 minutes, respectively. The average EBL in the minimally invasive cases was 432 mL compared to 737 mL. There were two technical complications; one screw malposition and one interbody cage migration were reported in the minimally invasive group and none in the open group. These differences were not statistically significant.

In 2005, Kim et al. (13) compared longitudinal changes in multifidus cross-sectional area and trunk extension strength in both open and percutaneous pedicle screw constructs. The T2-weighted cross-sectional area of the multifidus muscle was recorded on preoperative and postoperative MRIs. Trunk extension strength was measured using a Medx. Multifidus cross-sectional area decreased from 1,140 to 800 mm^2 in open pedicle screw constructs as compared to percutaneous pedicle screw construction where multifidus area decreased from 1,320 to 1,270 mm^2. Trunk extension strength increased in both open and percutaneous pedicle screw constructs, but the improvements in strength were only statistically significant in the percutaneous pedicle screw group.

Overall, there are not enough comparative data to make any evidence-based decisions between the use of the mini-open technique of placing pedicle screws through tubular retractors and percutaneous pedicle screws. More clinical data are needed. The complication profile between minimally invasive pedicle screw instrumentation and open pedicle screw instrumentation appears similar. Minimally invasive pedicle instrumentation results in decreased blood loss, less pain in the early postoperative period, and less long-term injury to the multifidus muscle.

Comparison of Screw Insertion Technique: Fluoroscopic Versus Advanced Navigation

Multiple insertion techniques exist for the placement of percutaneous pedicle screws. Pedicle screws can be placed safely with conventional fluoroscopy or by computer navigation and 3D imaging. No technique is foolproof, and a recent meta-analysis of the literature demonstrated that, overall, the median placement accuracy using in vivo CT-based navigation techniques was 90.76% compared to

TABLE 25-1   Reports Regarding the Accuracy of the Various Image-Guided Techniques as well as Navigational Modalities

Study	Patient/Cadavers (N)	Pedicles Screws (n)	Levels	Intraop Imaging	Placement	Computer Navigation	Evaluation	Breach Percentage for Pedicles	Breach Percentage for Patients
Youkilis et al. (38)	65	224	T1–T12	None	Open	Yes	Postop CT	8.5 (3.6)	29 (12)
Nottmeier et al. (19)	184	951	T1–S1	O-arm/3D C-arm	Open	Yes	Postop CT	5.2 (0.7)	27.7 (3.8)
Smith et al. (32)	151	601	L1–S1	C-arm	PC	No	Postop CT	6.2 (3.7)	24.5 (14.5)
Heintel et al. (8)	111	502	T4–L5	C-arm	PC	No	Postop CT	(1.5)	(7.2)
Park et al. (21)	26	172	T1–S1	C-arm	PC	No	Postop CT	18 (2.9)	119 (19)
Raley and Mobbs (25)	88	424	T4–S1	C-arm	PC	No	Postop CT	9.7 (4)	46.5 (19.3)
Houten et al. (9)	52	205	L1–S1	O-arm	PC	Yes	O-arm	2.9 (1.4)	11.5 (5.7)
	42	141	L1–S1	C-arm	PC	No	Postop CT	7.8 (4.9)	264 (166)
Kim et al. (14)	110	488	L2–S1	C-arm	PC	No	Postop CT	23.6 (1.6)	104 (7.2)

Figures in brackets indicate critical or grade 3 pedicle breach percentages.

85.48% for two-dimensional fluoroscopy-based navigation (35). There are several reports regarding the accuracy of the various image-guided techniques as well as navigational modalities (Table 25-1).

One of the concerns with the use of fluoroscopy is radiation exposure to both the surgeon and the patient. Bindal et al. (2) prospectively recorded radiation exposure in 24 consecutive minimally invasive TLIF procedures. The mean fluoroscopy time was 1.69 minutes (101 seconds). The mean exposure was 76 mRem at the surgeon's dominant hand, 27 mRem under a lead apron, and 32 mRem at an unprotected thyroid level. The mean exposure to the patient's skin was between 59 and 78 mRem depending upon the orientation to the x-ray beam. According to Bindal et al., the radiation exposure to both surgeon and patients was relatively low. They extrapolated that it would take 194 cases to exceed the acceptable torso radiation limits. The radiation levels they observed also compared favorably to other fluoroscopic procedures such as percutaneous coronary interventions.

Nonetheless, all surgeons should be judicious and minimize radiation exposure to the patient, to the OR personnel, and to themselves. Computer-assisted navigation has been proposed as one means to reduce fluoroscopic use. Kim et al. (12) performed a two-phased cadaveric and prospective clinical review comparing navigation-assisted fluoroscopy and standard fluoroscopy use in minimally invasive TLIFs. In the cadaver study, they noted a longer setup time for navigation (9.7 minutes) compared to fluoroscopy (4.8 minutes). The mean fluoroscopic time was 42 seconds in the fluoroscopy group and 29 seconds in the navigation group. The average radiation exposure was undetectable in the navigation group and was 12.4 mRem in the fluoroscopic group. Clinically minimally invasive TLIFs with navigation used 57 seconds of fluoroscopy, and minimally invasive TLIFs with fluoroscopy used 147 seconds. They reported no cases of screw malposition in either group, and blood loss, operating time, and hospital stay were similar in both groups.

Navigation-assisted placement of pedicle screws is gaining popularity around the United States. Early data suggest that navigation can be used safely for percutaneous pedicle screw placement. However, caution is warranted when known identifiable landmarks are not visualized. The data that navigation provides are only as good as the data it collects. Visual arrays can be dislodged causing the navigation to error. Surgeon vigilance is required.

KEY POINTS

1. Minimally invasive pedicle screw instrumentation is associated with less blood loss and shorter hospital stays, but longer initial operative times.
2. Minimally invasive instrumentation has a lower infection rate than open instrumentation.
3. Both mini-open and percutaneous pedicle screw insertion techniques have comparable complication rates.
4. Technical complications have been comparable in minimally invasive instrumentation and open instrumentation.

RECOMMENDED READING

1. Babu R, Park JG, Mehta AI, et al.: Comparison of superior level facet joint violations during open and percutaneous pedicle screw placement. *Neurosurgery* 71(5): 962–970, 2012.
2. Bindal RK, Glaze S, Ognoskie M, et al.: Surgeon and patient radiation exposure in minimally invasive transforaminal lumbar interbody fusion. *J Neurosurg Spine* 9(6): 570–573, 2008.
3. Brenner DJ, Doll R, Goodhead DT, et al.: Cancer risks attributable to low doses of ionizing radiation: assessing what we really know. *Proc Natl Acad Sci U S A* 100(24): 13761–13766, 2003.
4. Dhall SS, Wang MY, Mummaneni PV: Clinical and radiographic comparison of mini-open transforaminal lumbar interbody fusion with open transforaminal lumbar interbody fusion in 42 patients with long-term follow-up. *J Neurosurg Spine* 9(6): 560–565, 2008.
5. Ebraheim NA, Rollins JR Jr, Xu R, et al.: Projection of the lumbar pedicle and its morphometric analysis. *Spine (Phila Pa 1976)* 21(11): 1296–1300, 1996.
6. Ebraheim NA, Xu R, Ahmad M, et al.: Projection of the thoracic pedicle and its morphometric analysis. *Spine (Phila Pa 1976)* 22(3): 233–238, 1997.
7. Foley KT, Holly LT, Schwender JD: Minimally invasive lumbar fusion. *Spine (Phila Pa 1976)* 28(15 suppl): S26–S35, 2003.
8. Heintel TM, Berglehner A, Meffert R: Accuracy of percutaneous pedicle screws for thoracic and lumbar spine fractures: a prospective trial. *Eur Spine J* 22(3): 495–502, 2013.
9. Houten JK, Nasser R, Baxi N: Clinical assessment of percutaneous lumbar pedicle screw placement using the O-arm multidimensional surgical imaging system. *Neurosurgery* 70(4): 990–995, 2012.
10. Hyun SJ, Kim YB, Kim YS, et al.: Postoperative changes in paraspinal muscle volume: comparison between paramedian interfascial and midline approaches for lumbar fusion. *J Korean Med Sci* 22(4): 646–651, 2007.
11. Kawaguchi Y, Matsui H, Tsuji H: Back muscle injury after posterior lumbar spine surgery. A histologic and enzymatic analysis. *Spine (Phila Pa 1976)* 21(8): 941–944, 1996.
12. Kim CW, Lee YP, Taylor W, et al.: Use of navigation-assisted fluoroscopy to decrease radiation exposure during minimally invasive spine surgery. *Spine J* 8(4): 584–590, 2008.
13. Kim DY, Lee SH, Chung SK, et al.: Comparison of multifidus muscle atrophy and trunk extension muscle strength: percutaneous versus open pedicle screw fixation. *Spine (Phila Pa 1976)* 30(1): 123–129, 2005.
14. Kim MC, Chung HT, Cho JL, et al.: Factors affecting the accurate placement of percutaneous pedicle screws during minimally invasive transforaminal lumbar interbody fusion. *Eur Spine J* 20(10): 1635–1643, 2011.
15. Kotani Y, Abumi K, Ito M, et al.: Mid-term clinical results of minimally invasive decompression and posterolateral fusion with percutaneous pedicle screws versus conventional approach for degenerative spondylolisthesis with spinal stenosis. *Eur Spine J* 21(6): 1171–1177, 2012.
16. Ma YQ, Li XL, Dong J, et al.: Comparison of percutaneous versus open monosegment instrumentation in the treatment of incomplete thoracolumbar burst fracture. *Zhonghua Yi Xue Za Zhi* 92(13): 904–908, 2012.
17. Magerl FP: Stabilization of the lower thoracic and lumbar spine with external skeletal fixation. *Clin Orthop Relat Res* 189: 125–141, 1984.
18. Mayer TG, Vanharanta H, Gatchel RJ, et al.: Comparison of CT scan muscle measurements and isokinetic trunk strength in postoperative patients. *Spine (Phila Pa 1976)* 14(1): 33–36, 1989.
19. Nottmeier EW, Seemer W, Young PM: Placement of thoracolumbar pedicle screws using three-dimensional image guidance: experience in a large patient cohort. *J Neurosurg Spine* 10(1): 33–39, 2009.
20. Panjabi MM, O'Holleran JD, Crisco JJ III, et al.: Complexity of the thoracic spine pedicle anatomy. *Eur Spine J* 6(1): 19–24, 1997.
21. Park DK, Thomas AO, St Clair S, et al.: Percutaneous lumbar and thoracic pedicle screws: a trauma experience. *J Spinal Disord Tech* 2012 Mar 27. [Epub ahead of print].
22. Park Y, Ha JW, Lee YT, et al.: Percutaneous placement of pedicle screws in overweight and obese patients. *Spine J* 11(10): 919–924, 2011.
23. Park Y, Ha JW: Comparison of one-level posterior lumbar interbody fusion performed with a minimally invasive approach or a traditional open approach. *Spine (Phila Pa 1976)* 32(5): 537–543, 2007.
24. Peng CW, Yue WM, Poh SY, et al.: Clinical and radiological outcomes of minimally invasive versus open transforaminal lumbar interbody fusion. *Spine (Phila Pa 1976)* 34(13): 1385–1389, 2009.
25. Raley DA, Mobbs RJ: Retrospective computed tomography scan analysis of percutaneously inserted pedicle screws for posterior transpedicular stabilisation of the thoracic and lumbar spine: accuracy and complication rates. *Spine (Phila Pa 1976)* 37(12): 1092–1100, 2012.
26. Rampersaud YR, Foley KT, Shen AC, et al.: Radiation exposure to the spine surgeon during fluoroscopically assisted pedicle screw insertion. *Spine (Phila Pa 1976)* 25(20): 2637–2645, 2000.
27. Regev GJ, Lee YP, Taylor WR, et al.: Nerve injury to the posterior rami medial branch during the insertion of pedicle screws: comparison of mini-open versus percutaneous pedicle screw insertion techniques. *Spine (Phila Pa 1976)* 34(11): 1239–1242, 2009.
28. Roy-Camille R, Roy-Camille M, Demeulenaere C: Osteosynthesis of dorsal, lumbar, and lumbosacral spine with metallic plates screwed into vertebral pedicles and articular apophyses. *Presse Med* 78(32): 1447–1448, 1970.
29. Schizas C, Tzinieris N, Tsiridis E, et al.: Minimally invasive versus open transforaminal lumbar interbody fusion: evaluating initial experience. *Int Orthop* 33(6): 1683–1688, 2009.
30. Schwender JD, Holly LT, Rouben DP, et al.: Minimally invasive transforaminal lumbar interbody fusion (TLIF): technical feasibility and initial results. *J Spinal Disord Tech* 18: S1–S6, 2005.
31. Sihvonen T, Herno A, Paljarvi L, et al.: Local denervation atrophy of paraspinal muscles in postoperative failed back syndrome. *Spine (Phila Pa 1976)* 18(5): 575–581, 1993.
32. Smith ZA, Sugimoto K, Lawton CD, et al.: Incidence of lumbar spine pedicle breach following percutaneous screw fixation: a radiographic evaluation of 601 screws in 151 patients. *J Spinal Disord Tech* 2012 Jun 7. [Epub ahead of print].
33. Synowitz M, Kiwit J: Surgeon's radiation exposure during percutaneous vertebroplasty. *J Neurosurg Spine* 4(2): 106–109, 2006.
34. Taylor H, McGregor AH, Medhi-Zadeh S, et al.: The impact of self-retaining retractors on the paraspinal muscles during posterior spinal surgery. *Spine (Phila Pa 1976)* 27(24): 2758–2762, 2002.
35. Tian NF, Xu HZ: Image-guided pedicle screw insertion accuracy: a meta-analysis. *Int Orthop* 33(4): 895–903, 2009.
36. Vaccaro AR, Rizzolo SJ, Allardyce TJ, et al.: Placement of pedicle screws in the thoracic spine. Part I: morphometric analysis of the thoracic vertebrae. *J Bone Joint Surg Am* 77(8): 1193–1199, 1995.

37. Wiltse LL, Bateman JG, Hutchinson RH, et al.: The paraspinal sacrospinalis-splitting approach to the lumbar spine. *J Bone Joint Surg Am* 50(5): 919–926, 1968.
38. Youkilis AS, Quint DJ, McGillicuddy JE, et al.: Stereotactic navigation for placement of pedicle screws in the thoracic spine. *Neurosurgery* 48(4): 771–778, 2001; discussion 778–779.
39. Zindrick MR, Wiltse LL, Doornik A, et al.: Analysis of the morphometric characteristics of the thoracic and lumbar pedicles. *Spine (Phila Pa 1976)* 12(2): 160–166, 1987.

26 Transforaminal Posterior Lumbar Interbody Fusion

Jeffrey A. Rihn, Sapan D. Gandhi, and Todd J. Albert

Lumbar fusion is used to successfully treat many pathologies of the lumbar spine that cause instability and neurologic compromise, including tumor, trauma, infection, and most commonly, degenerative conditions. Lumbar fusion can be performed postero-laterally, anteriorly, or both. Posterolateral fusion is achieved between the transverse processes and across the facet joints. Anterior fusion is achieved within the interbody space. A number of approaches to lumbar interbody fusion have been described including poste-rior, transforaminal, direct lateral, and anterior. The posterior lumbar interbody fusion (PLIF) was thought to be first introduced by Cloward (5). While this technique increased in popularity because of its ability to achieve 360-degree arthrodesis from a posterior approach, it requires significant neural retraction for disc space preparation and cage/bone graft insertion. The transforaminal lumbar interbody fusion (TLIF) technique, a slight modification of the PLIF, was introduced by Harms in 1993 and has become the most common approach for obtaining a combined anterior and posterolateral fusion through a single posterior incision (8). The benefit of the TLIF over the PLIF is that it involves a unilateral approach to disc space preparation and cage/bone graft inser-tion that can be achieved with minimal retraction of the traversing nerve root. Numerous publi-cations have reported the safety and efficacy of the TLIF approach to achieving a lumbar fusion (2,7,12,19,22,27,29). This chapter describes the surgical technique of the TLIF and the associated perioperative considerations.

INDICATIONS/CONTRAINDICATIONS

Previously reported indications for the TLIF include lumbar spondylolisthesis (both degenera-tive and isthmic), degenerative scoliosis, recurrent disc herniation, and degenerative disc disease (DDD). To maximize potential benefit from surgery, confirmatory imaging should correspond to the patient's symptoms and signs. In patients with considerable disc collapse or spondylolisthesis, ante-rior column support in the form of an interbody cage may be needed to adequately address the spinal pathology and may improve the chances of obtaining a successful fusion (i.e., greater surface area for fusion compared to a posterolateral fusion alone). Distraction of the interbody space through placement of an interbody cage can indirectly decompress the foramen in cases of severe neurofo-raminal stenosis. In cases of degenerative scoliosis, insertion of the interbody cage on the side of the concavity of the curve can help neutralize the disc space and restore a more normal alignment.

The transforaminal approach to interbody fusion is not possible to perform in patients with conjoined nerve roots, as the low take off of the exiting nerve root does not allow for the trans-foraminal approach to the disc space. Conjoint nerve roots can typically be identified on preop-erative MRI. If it is unilateral, then the TLIF can be performed from the contralateral side. If the conjoint nerve roots are bilateral, then an anterior approach should be performed for the inter-body fusion. Similarly, TLIF in patients with recurrent disc herniation and scar tissue formation can be challenging, as the traversing nerve root of the affected level is often bound by scar tissue and difficult to mobilize enough to safely perform the interbody fusion. Patients with considerable osteoporosis or bony destruction from tumor or infection are typically not considered candidates for a TLIF, although reports of treating discitis/osteomyelitis using this approach have appeared in the literature (30). Intact endplates are important when performing a TLIF. Endplate destruction by the pathologic process or endplate violation at the time of the procedure will lead to subsidence of the interbody cage and potentially a less desirable result.

PREOPERATIVE PREPARATION

Prior to surgery, imaging studies (i.e., plain radiographs, MRI, and/or CT scan) should be carefully reviewed and used to generate a surgical plan. Patient pathology (e.g., recurrent disc herniation, pars defects, degree of spondylolisthesis and collapse, sacral doming, pedicle anomalies) and variations in patient anatomy (e.g., lumbosacral variations that affect numbering of lumbar vertebrae, conjoint nerve root) should be clearly identified. Patients with isthmic spondylolisthesis, particularly in higher grade slips, may have dysmorphic pedicles or doming of the sacrum that makes the TLIF approach challenging (Fig. 26-1A–F). The pedicles can be dysmorphic, with a very small diameter,

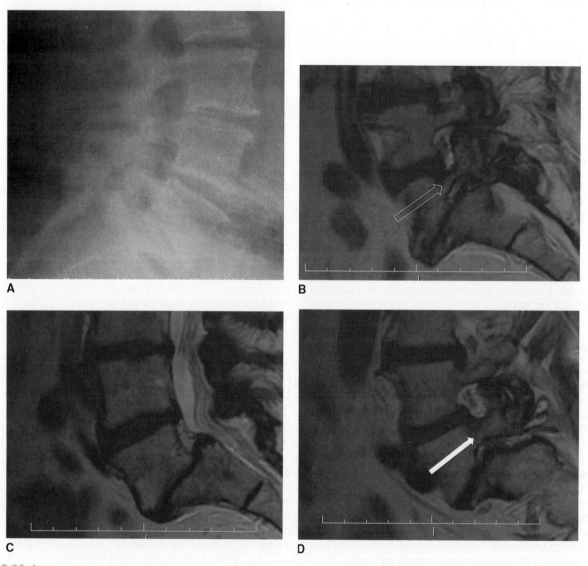

FIGURE 26-1

A: Later plain lumbar radiograph of a 59-year-old female patient with a grade II isthmic spondylolisthesis at L5–S1 with significant disc collapse. The L5 pedicles appear very narrow on the lateral radiograph. Right parasagittal **(B)**, midsagittal **(C)**, and left parasagittal **(D)** T2-weighted lumbar MRI demonstrate a dysmorphic, very small pedicle on the right side (*open arrow*, **B**). The left pedicle (*closed arrow*, **D**) appears to be of sufficient size for instrumentation. Severe L5–S1 neuroforaminal stenosis is noted in the parasagittal images **(B,D)**. The patient underwent an L5–S1 TLIF and posterolateral decompression and fusion L4–S1. The right L5 pedicle intraoperatively could not be instrumented due to the small size of the pedicle.

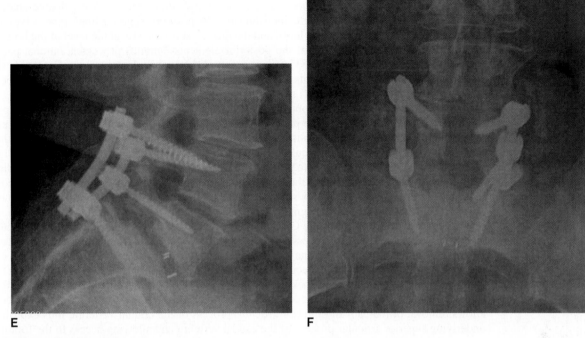

E   F

FIGURE 26-1 (*Continued*)

Lateral **(E)** and anteroposterior **(F)** postoperative plain radiographs demonstrate the interbody cage in the anterior one-third of the L5–S1 interspace, with some restoration of disc height and a 30% reduction of the spondylolisthesis.

that can preclude screw placement. This is not an uncommon finding at the L5 level in cases of a high-grade L5/S1 isthmic spondylolisthesis. In these cases, it may be necessary to instrument and fuse up to the L4 level to allow adequate stabilization. Furthermore, significant sacral doming can make cage placement difficult. The shape of the endplates of the involved level(s) should be clearly defined on preoperative imaging, and a plan for cage placement and positioning should be made in the preoperative planning stages. In very high-grade spondylolisthesis (grade IV), the degree of slippage and endplate deformity may preclude interbody fusion. In these cases, an alternative procedure is often preferable, in which case a fibular strut allograft is inserted, from either a posterior or anterior approach, through the L5 and S1 bodies and across the L5/S1 disc space. The details of this procedure are beyond the scope of this chapter.

Bone graft options should be considered in the preoperative planning stages, and a discussion of such should be had with the patient. The options for bone grafting include local autograft bone, iliac crest autograft bone, allograft bone, demineralized bone matrix, synthetic bone graft material (e.g., beta tricalcium phosphate), and/or recombinant bone morphogenetic protein-2 (rhBMP-2). There is no perfect bone graft option, and each of the above options has both benefits and downsides. Iliac crest bone graft has traditionally been considered the gold standard for lumbar spine fusion. However, high rates of donor-site complications and increased operative time have led to a shift toward alternatives to iliac crest autograft (22). Graft extenders used in combination with autologous bone graft or recombinant bone morphogenetic protein-2 (rhBMP-2)–soaked collagen sponges may help increase fusion rates and decrease rates of pseudarthrosis. The use of rhBMP-2 for TLIF is considered "off-label" in regard to its FDA status. While rhBMP-2 seems to improve fusion rates and decrease donor-site complications, it has been associated with complications such as vertebral osteolysis and postoperative radiculitis (22,23).

TECHNIQUE

Patients are typically positioned on a radiolucent Jackson table with the abdomen hanging free and with all bony and soft tissue protuberances well padded. Allowing the abdomen to hang free reduces venous pressure and minimizes blood loss. An additional benefit of the Jackson table is that it is radiolucent, thus allowing intraoperative fluoroscopy and/or plain radiographic images in both the anteroposterior and lateral views to confirm instrumentation and interbody cage placement. The Jackson table also allows for a lordotic lumbar alignment that helps to prevent fusing the involved levels in a kyphotic position.

After prepping and draping, a longitudinal incision is made in the midline over the spinous processes of the involved levels. Intraoperative fluoroscopy/radiographic and/or palpable anatomical landmarks can be used to localize the incision site. The posterior superior iliac spine is typically at the level of the L5–S1 interspinous level, and the iliac crest is typically at the level of the L4 spinous process. Subperiosteal dissection of the posterior elements (spinous processes, lamina, pars, and transverse processes) of the involved levels is accomplished using electrocautery. Great care should be taken to not violate the facet joints adjacent to involved levels during the exposure. Intraoperative fluoroscopy/radiography should be used to confirm the surgical level.

Once an adequate exposure is obtained, attention is turned toward the decompression portion of the procedure. The nature of the pathology dictates the nature and extent of the decompression. When treating an isthmic spondylolisthesis, a Gill laminectomy is performed by removing the spinous process, lamina, inferior articular processes, and pars of the involved level as one fragment of bone, that is, the Gill fragment (e.g., L5 in the case of an L5–S1 isthmic spondylolisthesis) (6). This is accomplished by dividing the interspinous ligaments above and below the involved level (e.g., L4–L5 and L5–S1 interspinous ligaments), the bilateral facet capsules, and any ligamentum flavum attachments to the Gill fragment. The Gill fragment can typically be removed as a single bony fragment. The removal of the Gill fragment exposes the underlying epidural fat and dura, as well as the superior articular processes of the caudal level involved in the spondylolisthesis (e.g., S1 superior articular processes in an L5–S1 isthmic spondylolisthesis). When performing a TLIF for a unilateral pathology (e.g., recurrent disc herniation, foraminal disc herniation, facet cyst) or a degenerative scoliosis that does not require a full laminectomy, an osteotomy is performed through the pars and lamina of the cranial vertebra of the involved disc level. Such an osteotomy allows removal of the pars and inferior articular process of the cranial vertebra, thus exposing the underlying superior articular process of the caudal vertebra and allowing access to the foramen on the side from which the TLIF is to be performed. Once the superior articular process is exposed, the ligamentum flavum is removed, and the underlying pedicle of that superior articular process is skeletonized using a Kerrison rongeur. This allows identification of the exiting and traversing nerve roots of the involved level.

The triangle through which the TLIF is performed is defined by the inferior border of the exiting nerve root, the lateral border of the traversing nerve root, and the pedicle and posterior aspect of the superior endplate of the caudal vertebra (Fig. 26-2). There are usually epidural veins overlying the disc space in this triangle that should be divided using bipolar electrocautery. If excessive bleeding is encountered that cannot be controlled with the bipolar, thrombin-soaked Gelfoam or Floseal (Baxter, Deerfield, IL) can be used to obtain hemostasis. The traversing nerve root is gently retracted medially using a nerve root retractor. If present, the disc herniation is removed, and the annulus is incised using a no. 15 blade scalpel. Great attention should be given to the exiting nerve root to avoid injury. Excessive manipulation of the dorsal root ganglia of the exiting nerve root can lead to postoperative neurogenic pain. In cases of spondylolisthesis and significant disc collapse, there

FIGURE 26-2

Drawing that demonstrates the triangle (*dotted black triangle*) through which the TLIF is performed. The borders of the triangle are composed of the exiting nerve root of the cranial level (*solid black arrow*), the superior endplate and the skeletonized pedicle of the caudal vertebral body and the skeletonized pedicle of the (*open arrow*), and the thecal sac and traversing nerve root (*dotted arrow*).

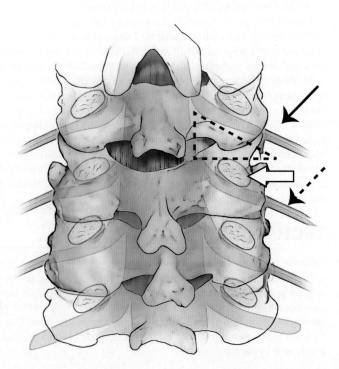

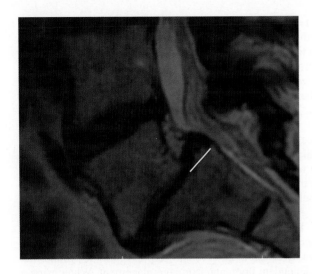

FIGURE 26-3

T2-weighted sagittal MRI of a patient with a grade II isthmic spondylolisthesis. The *white line* demonstrates the "lip" of bone that should be removed using a Kerrison rongeur. Removal of this bone will allow for a more direct approach to the intervertebral space and will simplify disc removal and cage placement.

is often a bony lip arising from the superior endplate of the inferior vertebral body of the involved level (Fig. 26-3). After entering the disc space with a scalpel, this bony lip should be removed using a Kerrison rongeur. Removal of this lip will facilitate disc removal and cage placement. Through the annulotomy, the intervertebral space is debrided free of all accessible disc and cartilaginous material back to bleeding endplate bone. This is accomplished using a series of curved and straight curettes and/or chondrotomes, endplate scrapers, double-angled curettes, and straight and angled pituitary rongeurs. The double-angled curette is effective in removing the contralateral disc and cartilaginous material (Fig. 26-4). There are numerous designs of instruments used to remove disc and cartilaginous material from the disc space. The manufacturer providing the implants typically makes these instruments available to the surgeon. The surgeon should be familiar with the options when it comes to disc space preparation instruments and should choose those with which he/she is most comfortable. Cadaver studies have reported that approximately 70% of the disc can be removed through a unilateral TLIF approach (11,13). When preparing the disc space, great care should be made to avoid violation of the anterior and the anterolateral annulus in order to avoid injury to the large blood vessels that travel across this area (i.e., aorta, inferior vena cava, common iliac artery, and veins). A recent MRI study by Vaccaro et al. (25) documented the close proximity of these vessels in relation to the lower lumbar disc spaces when the patient is in the prone position.

During disc space preparation, a lamina spreader is placed between the remaining lamina/spinous processes of the involved level for distraction of the interspace. In the case of isthmic spondylolisthesis, when a Gill laminectomy is performed, the lamina spreader is placed on the lamina of the next cranial vertebra. Alternatively, pedicle screws can be placed contralateral to the side on which

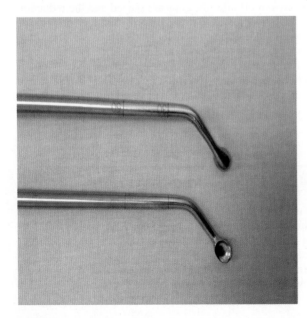

FIGURE 26-4

The double-angled curette allows for removal of disc and cartilaginous material contralateral to the side from which the TLIF is performed. There are two separate curettes that allow preparation of both vertebral endplates of the involved level.

the TLIF is being performed and distraction can be obtained across the pedicle screws. Each instrumentation system should include such a pedicle screw–based distraction device. Distraction allows for adequate disc space preparation. Distraction and disc space preparation is also facilitated by the use of serial dilators. Such dilators are inserted serially (from small to large) until the disc space is adequately distracted and a "good fit" is noted with the dilator. The size of the largest dilator should correspond to the size of the cage. After the disc space has been adequately prepared and dilated, however, a trial is placed to confirm the size. The size of a cage can range from 7 to 14 mm, depending on the degree of disc collapse.

Prior to inserting the cage, the interspace should be inspected to ensure that bleeding endplate bone is exposed on both involved vertebral body endplates. The bone graft material can then be impacted into the disc space and packed within the opening of the selected cage. The cage is secured to an inserting device and then is impacted using a mallet into the interbody space. The traversing nerve root should be gently retracted medially, and the location of the exiting nerve root should be monitored during cage insertion. After the cage is in a relatively acceptable position, the insertion device is detached and removed. The final position of the cage can be adjusted using a mallet and straight and/or curved impactors. The curved cage should rest horizontally across the anterior one-third of the disc space. Studies by Kwon et al. (17) and Kepler et al. (15) found that restoration of lordosis and disc height are dependent upon anterior cage placement. When using a bullet-shaped cage, the cage should be inserted diagonally across the disc space from ipsilateral to contralateral. An impactor can then be used to tamp the posterior aspect of the bullet-shaped cage so that the cage rests in a more horizontal position in the anterior one-third of the intervertebral space. When there is asymmetric disc collapse (e.g., degenerative scoliosis), the bullet-shaped cage can be inserted in a more vertical fashion on the collapsed side in order to neutralize the disc space.

After placing the cage, pedicle screws can be placed according to the preferred technique of the surgeon. Prior to the final tightening of the caps onto the rod, a compression device can be used to apply gentle compression across the pedicle screws ipsilateral to the side from which the TLIF was performed. This gentle compression will decrease the risk that the cage will dislodge into the spinal canal. Cage and screw position should be confirmed using intraoperative fluoroscopy or plain radiography.

When a significant spondylolisthesis exists, reduction can be accomplished using the pedicle screws. The reduction either can be performed after the cage is inserted or can be performed over a dilator, with the cage inserted after the reduction is performed and the rods are tightened into place. In order to obtain a reduction, bilateral pedicle screws are inserted into the involved vertebral bodies. It is essential that a secure purchase be obtained in order to perform a reduction. Performing a reduction with poor screw purchase (e.g., osteoporotic bone, redirected screw with subpar purchase) can lead to screw pullout. Due to the nature of the underlying pathology, the screws in the cranial vertebra will sit anterior to the screws of the caudal vertebra. Rods are then contoured such that the rods are fully seated in the caudal vertebral screws and are not fully seated in the cranial vertebral screws due to their anterior position. The caudal caps are placed and tightened, and then, using a reduction device over the cranial vertebral screws, the cranial vertebral screws are reduced to the rod, and the cranial caps are placed and tightened (Fig. 26-5). A variety of such reduction devices and techniques exist. Some manufactures have screws with extended threaded tabs that assist in this reduction technique and that then can be broken off after the caps are placed and the reduction is complete (Fig. 26-6). Some surgeons prefer to use plates that are placed over the screw posts for reduction (Fig. 26-7). In patients with a high grade II or grade III spondylolisthesis, it is often necessary to place screws in the vertebra above the listhesed vertebral body (e.g., L4 in an L5–S1 spondylolisthesis) in order to obtain a reduction. In this case, the rods are placed into the S1 and L4 screws, and then the L5 screws are reduced to the rod using a reduction device. The L4 screws can be left in and the fusion extended, or the L4 screws can subsequently be removed (one side at a time) after the reduction is complete (Fig. 26-8A–E).

PEARLS AND PITFALLS

- Preoperative imaging should be evaluated for abnormal pedicle morphology and the presence of a conjoint nerve root.
- Excessive retraction of the traversing nerve root or manipulation of the dorsal root ganglion of the exiting nerve root should be avoided as this can result in neuropathic pain.
- Violation of the anterior and anterolateral annulus fibrosus can place the anterior vascular structures at risk for injury and should be avoided.
- In cases of spondylolisthesis, there is often a "lip" of bone on the superior endplate of the caudal vertebra that needs to be removed to allow adequate access to the intervertebral body space for disc removal and cage placement.

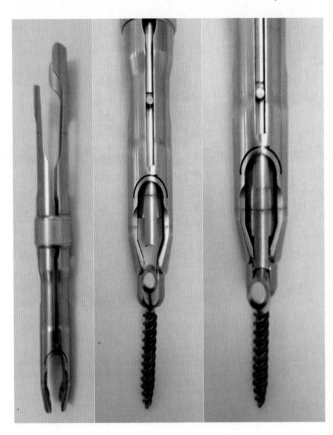

FIGURE 26-5

Photographs of a reduction clip (Flex clip, Depuy Spine, Inc. Raynham, MA) that can be placed over the rod and clipped to the screw. A device then threads down the clip and reduces the rod to the screw. A cap can then be inserted down the center of the device and treaded into the screw over the rod.

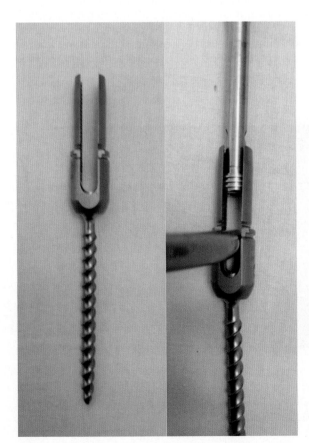

FIGURE 26-6

Photographs of the extended tab screw (Depuy Spine Inc., Raynham, MA) that can be used to assist reduction of the spondylolisthesis. The rod is placed into the screw, and the cap can be placed down the extended threaded tabs, over the rod, thus reducing the rod to the screw. The extended tabs can then be broken off.

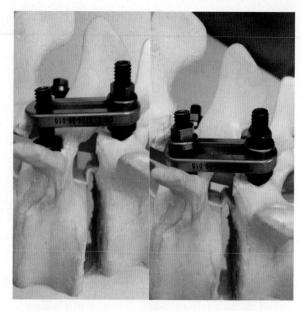

FIGURE 26-7

Photographs depicting the use of posted screws and plates (Expedium offset, Depuy Spine Inc., Raynham, MA) to obtain reduction in a spondylolisthesis. The plate is placed over the posted pedicle screws of both vertebral bodies of the involved level. A nut is threaded onto the post of the caudal screw and tightened.
A nut is then threaded onto the post of the cranial screw and tightened, thus reducing the plate to the screw and reducing the spondylolisthesis.

- Several techniques exist for performing a reduction of a spondylolisthesis when performing a TLIF. The surgeon should be familiar with available options and have the appropriate instrumentation available.
- A laminar spreader and/or pedicle-based distraction devices are essential for providing distraction of the involved level to allow for adequate disc space preparation and cage insertion.
- The cage should be positioned in the anterior one-third of the intervertebral space to maintain/restore lordosis and disc height.

POSTOPERATIVE MANAGEMENT

Postoperatively, the patient is maintained on intravenous antibiotics for 6 to 24 hours (including the preoperative dose). If a subfascial drain was used, it is maintained until the output is less than 30 mL per 8-hour shift. Unless a durotomy occurred, early ambulation is encouraged after surgery. Sequential compression devices can be used to minimize the risk of deep venous thrombosis. Barring postoperative complication, patients can typically be discharged on the second or third postoperative

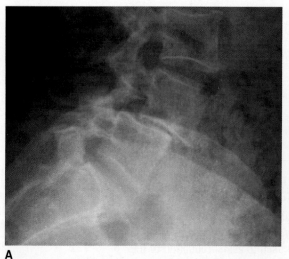

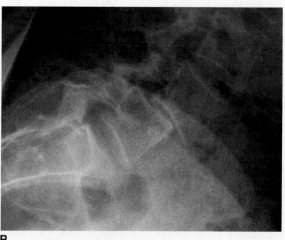

A   **B**

FIGURE 26-8

A–D: Neutral **(A)** and flexion **(B)** lateral plain radiograph of a 55-year-old female with a significant degenerative spondylolisthesis of L4–L5. There is considerable collapse of the L4–L5 interspace and increased segmental kyphosis on the flexion radiograph **(B)**.

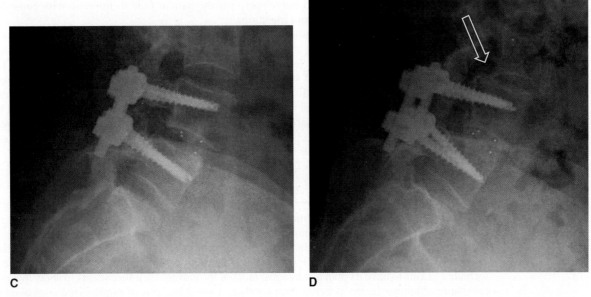

C   D

FIGURE 26-8 (*Continued*)

This patient underwent an L4–L5 laminectomy and TLIF. Prior to performing the laminectomy, a lamina spreader was used for distraction. After interbody cage insertion and screw placement, the rods were placed into the screws, caps were tightened onto the L5 screws, and then reduction clips were placed over the L4 screws and the reduction clips were used to reduce the spondylolisthesis over the cage. The postoperative lateral radiograph **(C)** shows significant reduction and restoration of disc height. Unfortunately, the patient presented with increased back and anterior thigh pain 2 years after surgery, and the 2-year postoperative lateral radiograph **(D)** demonstrates adjacent-level degenerative spondylolisthesis (*open arrow*).

day. The use of a postoperative brace is somewhat controversial. The authors prefer to use an off-the-shelf lumbosacral orthosis for 6 weeks when the patient is out of bed for support of the core muscles.

The authors prefer to see patients at 2 weeks, 6 weeks, 3 months, and 1 year after surgery and then annually. Plain radiographs may be obtained at follow-up to ensure the location and integrity of the instrumentation and to assess for fusion. A solid bony fusion is indicated by the presence of bridging trabecular bone in the interbody space and/or posterolateral space, the absence of any loosening around the instrumentation (i.e., "haloing"), and the absence of motion when comparing lateral flexion and extension radiographs. When patients present with symptoms (i.e., back pain and/or radiculopathy) in the postoperative period, CT scan can be used to further assess fusion and/or instrumentation placement. It can be somewhat difficult to assess interbody fusion using plain radiography, particularly at the L5–S1 level, due to overlap of the ilium. CT scan provides a more accurate assessment.

COMPLICATIONS

Several studies have previously reported complications associated with the TLIF procedure (4,19,21,22,26,27). Reported complications include death, pulmonary embolus, pneumonia, myocardial infarction, excessive bleeding, infection, malpositioned instrumentation, nerve root injury, dural tear, postoperative radiculitis, ectopic bone formation, vertebral osteolysis, bone graft donor site–related problems (e.g., pain, infection, wound complications), nonunion, and adjacent-level disease. Postoperative radiculitis, ectopic bone formation, and vertebral osteolysis following the use of rhBMP-2 in the TLIF procedure have received attention in the literature. The incidence of postoperative radiculitis is reported to be as high as 16% and is thought to be related to a hyperinflammatory response to the rhBMP-2 (21,22). Placement of the rhBMP-2 in the anterior one-third of the interbody space and creating a barrier (e.g., a hydrogel sealant, Duraseal, Covidien, Mansfield, MA) between the rhBMP-2 sponge and the exposed neural elements can minimize the risk of postoperative radiculitis (19,22). Vertebral osteolysis has been reported to occur in up to 18% of patients who undergo TLIF with rhBMP-2 (18,22). The osteolysis that forms around the interbody cage can be associated with increased back and/or leg pain. Fortunately, the symptoms and radiographic findings associated with osteolysis seem to be self-limiting, with no affect on outcome or fusion rate. Ectopic bone has been reported to occur 2% to 21% of patients who undergo TLIF with rhBMP-2 (14,22). This can cause severe radiculopathy. It is diagnosed on CT scan and may necessitate revision decompression of the affected nerve root(s) if the patient fails to improve with conservative treatment, such as selective nerve root injections.

The reported rate of nonunion following the use of autograft or rhBMP-2 is relatively low (i.e., less than 5%). Although it may be asymptomatic, nonunion can present as increased back and/or leg pain. Lucency around the pedicle screws and absence of bridging trabecular bone on CT scan are evidence of nonunion. Revision surgery for nonunion should be reserved for those who remain symptomatic greater than 1 year after surgery. Adjacent-level disease has been well documented after arthrodesis of both the cervical and lumbar spine (9,24). Theoretically, fusion of a level in the spine causes increased loads on adjacent levels, therefore accelerating their degeneration. However, there is some debate whether adjacent-level degeneration occurs as a direct result of arthrodesis or whether it is just a natural progression of DDD (10).

RESULTS

The TLIF procedure has been reported to be safe and effective for the treatment of a wide range of lumbar pathology, including isthmic spondylolisthesis, recurrent disc herniation, foraminal disc herniation, degenerative scoliosis, and degenerative spondylolisthesis (2,7,12,19,22,27,29). The literature does not seem to favor TLIF over other techniques of lumbar fusion (1,16,29). While each technique seems to have its own advantages, most of the current literature seems to show that no one technique of lumbar fusion is better than another. A meta-analysis of randomized controlled trials and comparative observational studies comparing instrumented posterolateral fusion with instrumented PLIF by Zhou et al. (31) suggests that while there is no difference in clinical outcome, complication rate, operating time, and blood loss between the two methods, there is some evidence the instrumented PLIF achieves higher fusion rates and better spinal alignment. Subgroup analysis of the Spine Patient Outcomes Research Trial (SPORT) data did not find any consistent difference in outcomes between the different techniques of lumbar fusion for the treatment of degenerative spondylolisthesis (1). In addition, other smaller studies have not found any significant differences in clinical outcome between different methods of lumbar interbody fusion and traditional posterolateral fusion (3,28). Comparisons of TLIF and anterior lumbar interbody fusion seem to show little difference in outcomes for isthmic spondylolisthesis (16), while comparisons of PLIF to posterolateral fusion seem to show that PLIF is superior for isthmic spondylolisthesis (20). However, small study populations and inferior study designs limit the impact of these studies.

CONCLUSIONS

The TLIF allows for a combined interbody and posterolateral fusion through a single posterior approach. The approach to the disc space is made more laterally than the traditional PLIF approach. This theoretically minimizes retraction of the traversing nerve and the dura during discectomy and insertion of the interbody device. While the TLIF is a safe approach that is effective in relieving back and leg pain in certain settings, clinical data do not support the superiority of this technique over other established methods of lumbar fusion. The surgeon should be aware of the reported complications associated with the TLIF procedure when counseling the patient preoperatively, particularly if the "off-label" use of rhBMP-2 is considered as a bone graft option.

RECOMMENDED READING

1. Abdu WA, Lurie JD, Spratt KF, et al.: Degenerative spondylolisthesis: does fusion method influence outcome? Four-year results of the spine patient outcomes research trial. *Spine (Phila Pa 1976)* 34(21): 2351–2360, 2009.
2. Adogwa O, Parker SL, Davis BJ, et al.: Cost-effectiveness of transforaminal lumbar interbody fusion for Grade I degenerative spondylolisthesis. *J Neurosurg Spine* 15(2): 138–143, 2011.
3. Audat Z, Moutasem O, Yousef K, et al.: Comparison of clinical and radiological results of posterolateral fusion, posterior lumbar interbody fusion and transforaminal lumbar interbody fusion techniques in the treatment of degenerative lumbar spine. *Singapore Med J* 53(3): 183–187, 2012.
4. Burneikiene S, Nelson EL, Mason A, et al.: Complications in patients undergoing combined transforaminal lumbar interbody fusion and posterior instrumentation with deformity correction for degenerative scoliosis and spinal stenosis. *Surg Neurol Int* 3: 25, 2012.
5. Cloward RB: The treatment of ruptured lumbar intervertebral discs by vertebral body fusion. I. Indications, operative technique, after care. *J Neurosurg* 10(2): 154–168, 1953.
6. Gill GG, Manning JG, White HL: Surgical treatment of spondylolisthesis without spine fusion; excision of the loose lamina with decompression of the nerve roots. *J Bone Joint Surg Am* 1955;37-A(3): 493–520.
7. Hackenberg L, Halm H, Bullmann V, et al.: Transforaminal lumbar interbody fusion: a safe technique with satisfactory three to five year results. *Eur Spine J* 14(6): 551–558, 2005.
8. Harms J, Jeszenszky D: The unilateral transforaminal approach for posterior lumbar interbody fusion. *Orthop Traumatol* 2: 88–89, 1998.

9. Hilibrand AS, Carlson GD, Palumbo MA, et al.: Radiculopathy and myelopathy at segments adjacent to the site of a previous anterior cervical arthrodesis. *J Bone Joint Surg Am* 81(4): 519–528, 1999.

10. Hilibrand AS, Robbins M: Adjacent segment degeneration and adjacent segment disease: the consequences of spinal fusion? *Spine J* 4(6 Suppl): 190S–194S, 2004.

11. Huh HY, Ji C, Ryu KS, et al.: Comparison of SpineJet XL and Conventional Instrumentation for Disk Space Preparation in Unilateral Transforaminal Lumbar Interbody Fusion. *J Korean Neurosurg Soc* 47(5): 370–376, 2010.

12. Humphreys SC, Hodges SD, Patwardhan AG, et al.: Comparison of posterior and transforaminal approaches to lumbar interbody fusion. *Spine (Phila Pa 1976)* 26(5): 567–571, 2001.

13. Javernick MA, Kuklo TR, Polly DW Jr. Transforaminal lumbar interbody fusion: unilateral versus bilateral disk removal—an in vivo study. *Am J Orthop* 32(7): 344–348, 2003; discussion 348.

14. Joseph V, Rampersaud YR: Heterotopic bone formation with the use of rhBMP2 in posterior minimal access interbody fusion: a CT analysis. *Spine (Phila Pa 1976)* 32(25): 2885–2890, 2007.

15. Kepler CK, Rihn JA, Radcliff KE, et al.: Restoration of lordosis and disk height after single-level transforaminal lumbar interbody fusion. *Orthop Surg* 4(1): 15–20, 2012.

16. Kim JS, Lee KY, Lee SH, et al.: Which lumbar interbody fusion technique is better in terms of level for the treatment of unstable isthmic spondylolisthesis? *J Neurosurg Spine* 12(2): 171–177, 2010.

17. Kwon BK, Berta S, Daffner SD, et al.: Radiographic analysis of transforaminal lumbar interbody fusion for the treatment of adult isthmic spondylolisthesis. *J Spinal Disord Tech* 16(5): 469–476, 2003.

18. Lewandrowski KU, Nanson C, Calderon R: Vertebral osteolysis after posterior interbody lumbar fusion with recombinant human bone morphogenetic protein 2: a report of five cases. *Spine J* 7(5): 609–614, 2007.

19. Mummaneni PV, Pan J, Haid RW, et al.: Contribution of recombinant human bone morphogenetic protein-2 to the rapid creation of interbody fusion when used in transforaminal lumbar interbody fusion: a preliminary report. Invited submission from the Joint Section Meeting on Disorders of the Spine and Peripheral Nerves, March 2004. *J Neurosurg Spine* 1(1): 19–23, 2004.

20. Musluman AM, Yilmaz A, Cansever T, et al.: Posterior lumbar interbody fusion versus posterolateral fusion with instrumentation in the treatment of low-grade isthmic spondylolisthesis: midterm clinical outcomes. *J Neurosurg Spine* 14(4): 488–496, 2011.

21. Rihn JA, Makda J, Hong J, et al.: The use of RhBMP-2 in single-level transforaminal lumbar interbody fusion: a clinical and radiographic analysis. *Eur Spine J* 18(11): 1629–1636, 2009.

22. Rihn JA, Patel R, Makda J, et al.: Complications associated with single-level transforaminal lumbar interbody fusion. *Spine J* 9(8): 623–629, 2009.

23. Rowan FE, O'Malley N, Poynton A: RhBMP-2 use in lumbar fusion surgery is associated with transient immediate postoperative leg pain. *Eur Spine J* 21(7): 1331–1337, 2012.

24. Sears WR, Sergides IG, Kazemi N, et al.: Incidence and prevalence of surgery at segments adjacent to a previous posterior lumbar arthrodesis. *Spine J* 11(1): 11–20, 2011.

25. Vaccaro AR, Kepler CK, Rihn JA, et al.: Anatomical relationships of the anterior blood vessels to the lower lumbar intervertebral discs: analysis based on magnetic resonance imaging of patients in the prone position. *J Bone Joint Surg Am* 94(12): 1088–1094, 2012.

26. Villavicencio AT, Burneikiene S, Bulsara KR, et al.: Perioperative complications in transforaminal lumbar interbody fusion versus anterior-posterior reconstruction for lumbar disc degeneration and instability. *J Spinal Disord Tech* 19(2): 92–97, 2006.

27. Villavicencio AT, Burneikiene S, Nelson EL, et al.: Safety of transforaminal lumbar interbody fusion and intervertebral recombinant human bone morphogenetic protein-2. *J Neurosurg Spine* 3(6): 436–443, 2005.

28. Wu Y, Tang H, Li Z, et al.: Outcome of posterior lumbar interbody fusion versus posterolateral fusion in lumbar degenerative disease. *J Clin Neurosci* 18(6): 780–783, 2011.

29. Yan DL, Pei FX, Li J, et al.: Comparative study of PILF and TLIF treatment in adult degenerative spondylolisthesis. *Eur Spine J* 17(10): 1311–1316, 2008.

30. Zaveri GR, Mehta SS: Surgical treatment of lumbar tuberculous spondylodiscitis by transforaminal lumbar interbody fusion (TLIF) and posterior instrumentation. *J Spinal Disord Tech* 22(4): 257–262, 2009.

31. Zhou ZJ, Zhao FD, Fang XQ, et al.: Meta-analysis of instrumented posterior interbody fusion versus instrumented posterolateral fusion in the lumbar spine. *J Neurosurg Spine* 15(3): 295–310, 2011.

27 Mini-ALIF

Thomas A. Zdeblick

INDICATIONS/CONTRAINDICATIONS

Indications

In selected patients, anterior lumbar interbody fusion (ALIF) is indicated for the treatment of symptomatic degenerative discs. Additional indications include pseudoarthrosis, spondylolisthesis (either isthmic or degenerative), lateral listhesis, and scoliosis. These deformity indications are typically coupled with posterior instrumentation as well. Although every case must be individualized, certain generalizations regarding indications can be made. Appropriate symptoms of degenerative disc disease include an aching low back pain that is typically present in the midline and over the sacroiliac joints after activity. On occasion, radiation into the buttocks may occur. Plain radiographs typically show loss of disc space height, endplate sclerosis, endplate osteophytes, and loss of lordosis. Magnetic resonance imaging (MRI) scans typically show loss of disc hydration and peri–endplate edema. Annular tears or a high-intensity zone is not sufficient in most cases to warrant fusion. Discography, although controversial, may be utilized to confirm a concordant pain response.

ALIF procedures are typically indicated for one- or, rarely, two-level disc degeneration. Clinical results, at least for fusion, of three-level or more procedures have been less than ideal. In my practice, I limit the indications for ALIF for disc degeneration to patients younger than 65. There are several reasons for this. As patients become older, osteoporosis and thinning of the endplates occur. This makes interbody devices less stable. Also, the retraction of the great vessels required for anterior lumbar spine exposure poses a greater risk to the older patient. Complications such as embolism, thrombosis, leg ischemia, and swelling are more common in older patients.

Postdiscectomy collapse is an excellent indication for ALIF. In these cases, however, the surgeon should expect to find a greater amount of adhesion surrounding the anterior annulus. Prior disc space infection is not necessarily a contraindication, as long as the infection has been adequately treated and systemic markers have returned to normal.

Isthmic spondylolisthesis is best reduced via ALIF. Following complete discectomy, sequential distracters placed within the disc space provide excellent mechanical force to reduce the translational deformity. Indirectly, foraminal stenosis is decompressed as well via distraction. Posterior instrumentation is typically placed following reduction. In cases with disc collapse and spondylolisthesis, stand-alone ALIF may be indicated.

In long deformity constructs ending at the sacrum, many surgeons prefer ALIF at the L5–S1 junction to improve fusion rate and prevent distal hardware failure. ALIF also works quite well to treat pseudoarthrosis of poster lumbar fusions. The large surface area and excellent vascular supply of the vertebral endplates readily enable fusion healing.

Contraindications

The placement of anterior cages is contraindicated with active infection. Although anterior approach and débridement with bone grafting can be performed in cases of active infection, metallic implants are not recommended. Stand-alone ALIF procedures are not recommended in cases of osteoporosis or osteopenia with thinning of the endplates. Previous anterior spinal surgery is a relative contraindication due to the presence of adhesions along the great vessels, which makes their dissection much more difficult. These cases must be individualized. Other previous abdominal surgery is not a contraindication to this approach. Midline incisions for laparotomy or Pfannenstiel incisions for gynecologic procedures have not proved to be a contraindication to the mini-open approach. Prior retroperitoneal radiation treatment is a contraindication. Extensile abdominal wall reconstruction, however—for instance, mesh repair of hernia—does make the approach much more difficult. Morbid obesity is a contraindication.

TECHNIQUE

The patient is positioned supine on the operative table. I do not place a lumbar bolster to hyperextend the spine. I find this can lead to foraminal compression or, rarely, femoral nerve palsy. A radiolucent operating table is utilized, the patient is placed in slight Trendelenburg position, and I often roll the table toward the right during the approach. This helps facilitate the retraction of the peritoneal contents from left to right. All patients undergoing ALIF receive a mild bowel preparation the night before surgery. This consists of a single enema and one bottle of GoLYTELY. This not only helps during the retraction but also helps prevent postoperative ileus. I have found that a bowel preparation given preoperatively greatly facilitates early patient discharge.

The appropriate level for skin incision is marked under guidance of both anteroposterior and lateral fluoroscopy (Fig. 27-1A). Using the lateral view, the surgeon marks on the anterior abdomen the direct line of extension from the disc space to be operated upon. If a two-level procedure is performed, the incision is centered between the two levels but closer to the more inferior of the two disc spaces. For single-level procedures, a 6- to 7-cm transverse skin incision is utilized. For two-level procedures, a 9- or 10-cm oblique incision is made. Alternatively, a paramedian vertical skin incision can be used as well. I prefer the horizontal skin incision purely for cosmetic reasons. I typically stand on the patient's right side, working toward myself for the left-to-right exposure. The fluoroscopy equipment is brought in and left in place superior to the surgeon (Fig. 27-1B).

L5–S1 Exposure

A 7-cm transverse skin incision is made beginning 1 cm to the right of midline and extending 6 cm to the left of the midline. Fluoroscopy is used to locate this incision. Typically, for L5–S1, this incision is located two to three fingerbreadths above the pubic symphysis. Sharp dissection is carried out through skin and subcutaneous tissue, and the anterior rectus sheath is exposed. The anterior rectus sheath is incised transversely with a no. 10 blade (Fig. 27-2). Alternatively, this can be incised vertically paramedian. Care is taken not to disturb the muscle fibers lying beneath.

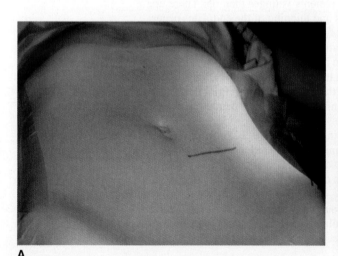

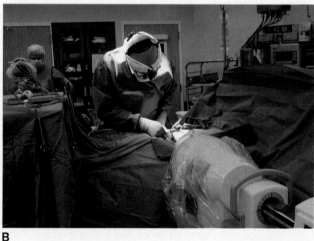

A   **B**

FIGURE 27-1

A: The skin incision is marked with the use of fluoroscopy. This photograph shows an incision for L4–L5 beginning in the midline and extending 7 cm to the left. L4–L5 is typically one to two fingerbreadths below the umbilicus. The incision for L5–S1 is typically two to three fingerbreadths above the pubic symphysis. **B:** The typical operating room setup. The patient lies supine with the arms out to the side. A radiolucent operating table is utilized. During the exposure, the surgeon stands on the patient's right side. This enables the surgeon to dissect free the left common iliac vein with greater ease. If the surgeon desires, he or she can switch to the left side for the instrumentation portion of the procedure. Fluoroscopy equipment generally stays superior and is brought down in place for lateral views as needed.

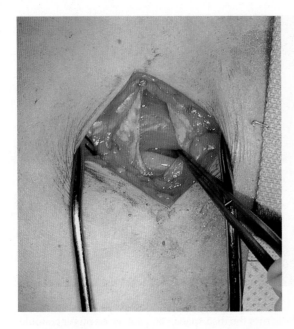

FIGURE 27-2

After the skin incision, the anterior rectus sheath is incised horizontally. Care is taken not to disturb the underlying fibers of the rectus abdominis muscle. Blunt dissection is then carried out in the midline between the heads of the right and left rectus muscles.

The midline between the heads of the rectus muscle is then located using blunt dissection. Using Kitner dissectors and a finger and working from the midline, the surgeon develops the preperitoneal space underlying the left rectus muscle (Figs. 27-3 and 27-4). A small finger retractor is slipped under the rectus muscle, and it is elevated. The surgeon can now bluntly dissect underneath the rectus muscle, along the posterior rectus sheath, until the arcuate line is palpated inferiorly and laterally.

Blunt dissection inferior to the arcuate line allows entry into the retroperitoneal space. For more extensile exposure, the posterior rectus sheath can be divided superiorly from the arcuate line. This must be done carefully, with scissors, as the peritoneum is tightly bound to the posterior sheath. A thin Deaver retractor is then slipped into this space, and the peritoneum is retracted from left to right. The peritoneal reflection along the lateral abdominal wall must be mobilized bluntly using Kitner in a "paddling" fashion. The left ureter is then identified, which ensures that the surgeon is indeed operating within the retroperitoneal space. Typically, I retract the ureter along with the peritoneum in a left-to-right direction. Blunt dissection alone is continued until the promontory of the sacrum is palpable. The Deaver retractor is then placed into a mechanical holder to ensure that the peritoneum is maintained in its position.

Complete exposure of the L5–S1 disc space requires mobilization of the left common iliac vein and the middle sacral artery and vein (Fig. 27-5A and B). This must be done without disturbing the presacral plexus of nerves. Often these nerves are visible. They run vertically across the disc space in a plane that is superficial to that of the middle sacral artery and vein. I begin by bluntly dissecting

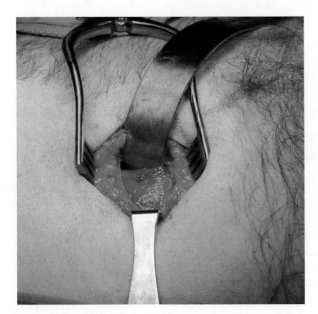

FIGURE 27-3

The preperitoneal space is developed in the space underlying the left rectus abdominis muscle. This is done with Kitner dissectors and finger dissection.

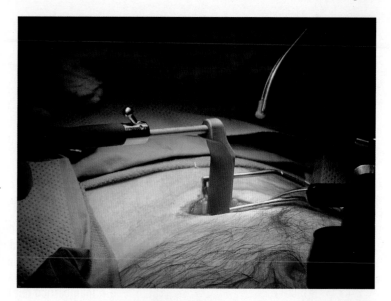

FIGURE 27-4

The arcuate line is usually palpable, and blunt dissection can continue inferior to the arcuate line. In this manner, the retroperitoneal space is identified, and the ureter and psoas muscle are visualized.

this presacral plexus of nerves from left to right across the disc space. No cautery or bipolar should be used while this nervous plexus is mobilized. The middle sacral artery and vein lie in a plane directly adherent to the anterior annulus.

Typically, there are two veins and a single artery. Care should be taken while these are mobilized, to make sure that they are not mistaken for the presacral nervous plexus (Fig. 27-5C). These vessels are mobilized with a fine right-angled dissector and clips applied and then divided. Cautery must be avoided. Blunt dissection with Kitner elevators can then be performed across the disc space.

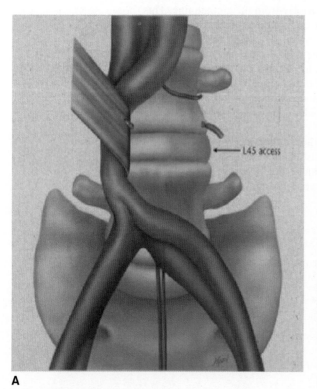

A

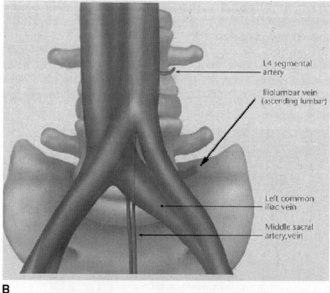

B

FIGURE 27-5

A: This drawing shows a typical vascular pattern overlying the L4–L5 and L5–S1 disc spaces. Exposure of the L4–L5 disc space requires retraction of the aorta and the inferior vena cava from left to right. In order to mobilize these vessels, the iliolumbar (ascending lumbar) vein must be located along the lateral aspect of the left common iliac vein. This is typically a short, thick vein that drains from under the psoas muscle into the left common iliac vein. Once this vein is ligated, adequate mobilization is possible. **B:** Diagram showing the retraction possible at L4–L5 once the iliolumbar vein is ligated. On occasion, the segmental vessels at L4 require ligation as well.

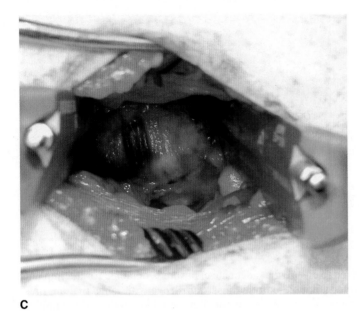

FIGURE 27-5 (*Continued*)

C: At L5–S1, the middle sacral artery and vein are ligated, and the left common iliac vein is elevated superiorly and laterally. This position is then maintained by retractors.

C

I typically expose the left side of the disc space first. This requires elevation of the left common iliac vein. This vein must be carefully mobilized with Kitner elevators.

The inferior edge of the vein, once it exsanguinates, can be difficult to visualize. Retraction needs to be applied and then let off periodically so that the vein fills with blood and becomes visible. There are typically small perforating veins that go directly from the disc space into the left common iliac vein. These need to be taken down with bipolar cautery and divided sharply. Occasionally, adhesions between the annulus and iliac vein are present. Sharply dividing the superficial layer of the annulus and retracting this with the vein are safer than attempting to peel the vein from the annulus. A retractor blade can then be placed underneath the left common iliac vein as it is elevated and retracted laterally. Once it is above the endplate of L5, it is held in place with a K-wire or staked screw (Fig. 27-6). If a K-wire alone is used, I place a red rubber catheter over the K-wire to protect the vessel and impact this into the vertebral body of L5. I now use a retractor, which has a lipped blade that is secured in place with a threaded screw. The table should now be rolled back to the neutral position. Similarly, the right side of the disc space is now exposed bluntly and a retractor placed into the right side of the L5 vertebral body (Fig. 27-7). Alternatively, these retractors can be placed in mechanical holding arms. A thin malleable retractor can then be placed anterior to the sacrum, which now allows full exposure of the L5–S1 disc space.

Anteroposterior and lateral fluoroscopic views are taken to confirm the level and to locate the midline of the disc space. The midline is then marked on the inferior edge of the L5 endplate.

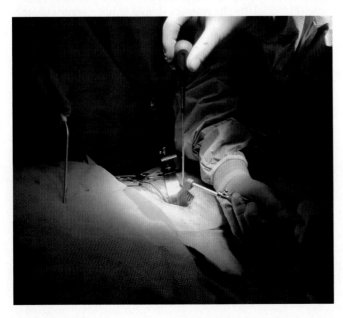

FIGURE 27-6

After mobilization of the appropriate great vessels, retraction is held in place by fixed and staked retractor blades.

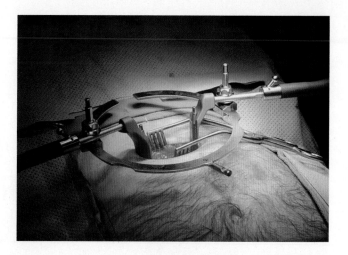

FIGURE 27-7

Once both retractor blades are in place, a thin malleable retractor can be placed inferiorly. The retractor blades are then hooked to a self-retaining ring, which is fastened to the operating table. This allows for a stable retraction system for minimally invasive exposure.

Appropriate templates are then utilized to ensure that adequate exposure is obtained for the implants to be used. For cage insertion, I prefer a double-barreled insertion sleeve with tangs that are present within the disc space. Each manufacturer's specific instructions should be followed for implant insertion. Appropriate-sized templates are used to determine whether adequate annular exposure has been accomplished. This annular exposure is then marked, and an anterior annulotomy is performed with a no. 10 blade.

Once the anterior annulus is resected, a complete discectomy is performed (Fig. 27-8). Long sharp elevators are used to remove disc material from the endplates. Long curettes are then used to remove the remainder of the endplate cartilage and disc material. It is important that dissection be carried out posteriorly back to the posterior longitudinal ligament. Particularly in cases of disc space collapse, release of the posterior annulus is required so that distraction occurs throughout the disc space and not just anteriorly. This prevents postoperative foraminal stenosis. Recurrent disc herniations may also be retrieved at this stage through posterior annular defects. This is done with fine-angled curettes. Disc space distracters can be impacted unilaterally to allow greater access within the disc space (Fig. 27-9). Lateral fluoroscopy is utilized to monitor disc space distraction. I plan to restore disc height to match the normal disc height of the adjacent level.

After completed discectomy, resection of endplate cartilage, and posterior release, the disc space is now ready for cage, bone graft, or arthroplasty insertion. The details of the implant insertion are specific to the implant being utilized. However, there are general principles to follow. Fluoroscopic guidance needs to be utilized throughout the procedure to ensure accurate placement. For threaded cages, the double-barreled sleeve is inserted along with the double distraction plugs. The lateral fluoroscopic view should ensure the distraction occurs in a parallel manner, that is, that the endplates remain parallel to each other. If the disc space is distracting only anteriorly, additional posterior release of annulus or posterior longitudinal ligament needs to be performed. In addition, the double-barreled sleeve needs to be aligned directly with the endplates at L5 and S1. The reamers are then sequentially passed on either side (Fig. 27-10). The reamers should remove approximately 1 to 1.5 mm of bone from either endplate. Fluoroscopy is utilized to ensure that this reaming is

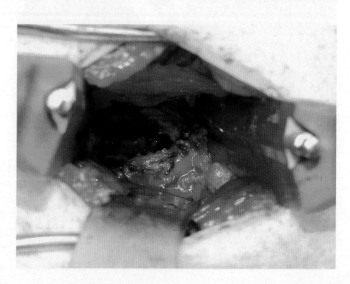

FIGURE 27-8

A complete (en bloc) discectomy is performed. The anterior annulus is incised, and all endplate cartilage and disc material are removed by using a combination of elevators, curettes, and rongeurs. The posterior annulus is removed as well.

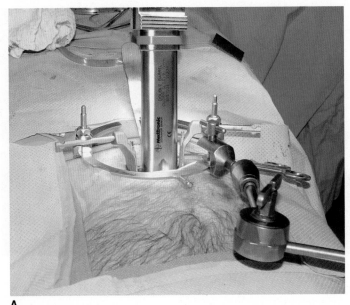
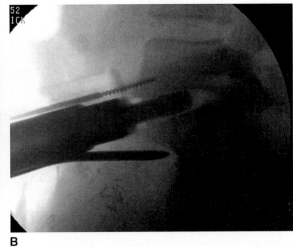

A   B

FIGURE 27-9

A: The disc space is now sequentially distracted up to its final height. This final height is determined by templates and cage dimensions. **B:** Lateral fluoroscopic view of the distractor in place. Note the parallel distraction of the endplates.

symmetric. I typically ream 6 mm deeper (more posterior) than the length of the cage chosen. After removal of the reamers, the endplate can be directly inspected. Ideally, the weight-bearing shoulder of the cage should contact intact endplate. Centrally, the endplate should be resected to expose bleeding cancellous bone. If this has not been accomplished, a fine-angled curette can be utilized at this point to deepen the central channel in the endplate. I prefer to use a tapered threaded titanium cage, which is self-tapping. The cage is prefilled with either autologous cancellous bone or an appropriate bone graft substitute (Fig. 27-11). These cages are now threaded in place sequentially. They should not be countersunk. On the lateral fluoroscopic image (Fig. 27-12), the anterior weight-bearing headwall of the cages should be in alignment with the anterior cortex of the L5

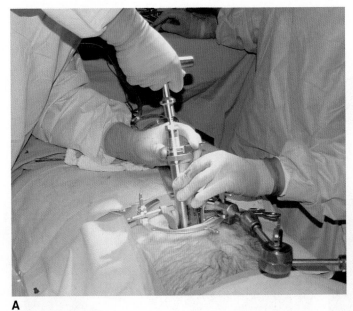
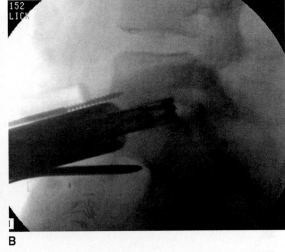

A   B

FIGURE 27-10

A: Each endplate is then prepared. This can be done with curettes or reamers (as shown). Approximately 1 to 1.5 mm of bone should be removed from either endplate. **B:** This fluoroscopic image shows a reamer symmetrically removing bone from the L5 and S1 endplates.

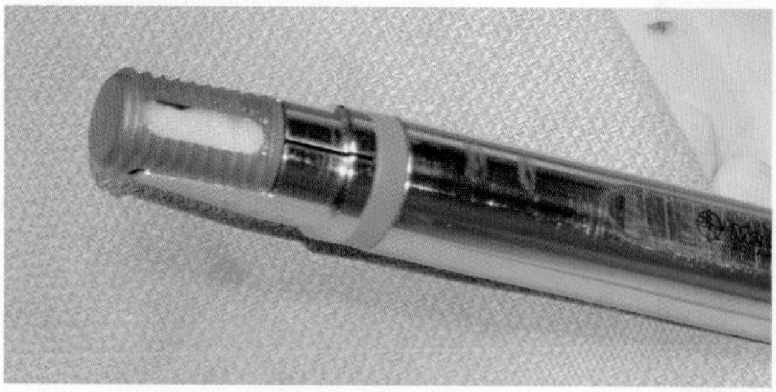

A

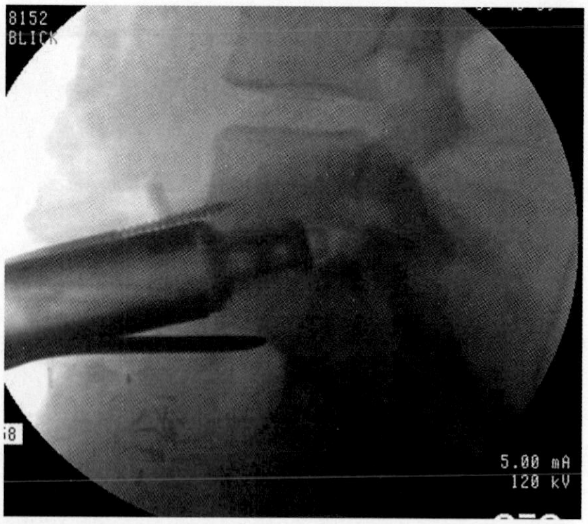

B

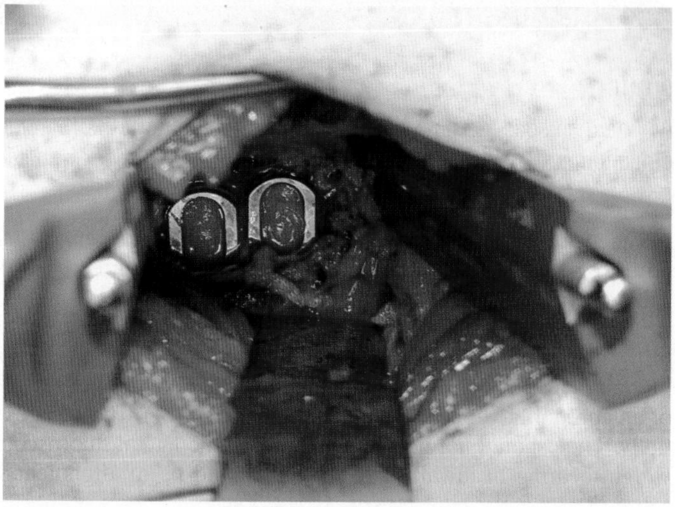

C

FIGURE 27-11

A: The cage can be prefilled with either iliac crest bone graft or a bone graft substitute. **B:** Lateral fluoroscopic image of the first cage in place. The distraction plug is then removed and the second cage threaded to the identical depth. **C:** Cages in vivo.

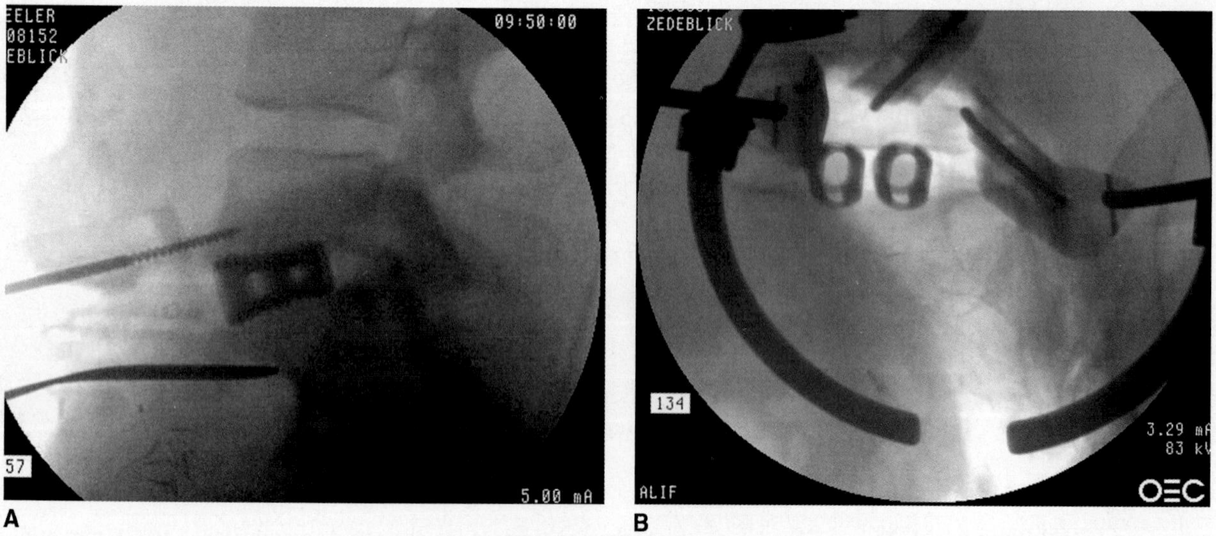

A B

FIGURE 27-12

A: Final lateral fluoroscopic images showing excellent cage placement at L5–S1. **B:** Final anteroposterior view.

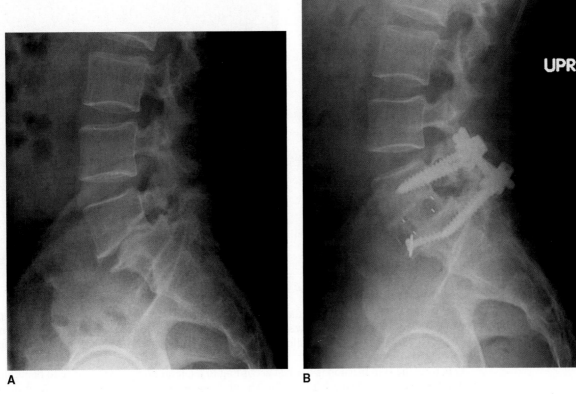

FIGURE 27-13

A: Lateral radiograph demonstrating L5–S1 isthmic spondylolisthesis. **B:** Lateral radiograph postoperatively. The spondylolisthesis has been reduced via ALIF with a PEEK spacer, followed by minimally invasive posterior fixation.

vertebral body. Once cage position is verified on the anteroposterior and lateral fluoroscopic images, additional material, either bone graft or bone substitute, can be packed within, between, and lateral to the cages (Fig. 27-13).

With impacted ring-style implants (PEEK, allograft bone, or metal), the procedure is similar except that distraction needs to be maintained to initiate insertion. There are commercially available instruments to assist in this. These typically maintain distraction through thin-bladed paddles and "slide" the graft in place along the paddles. I prefer to use a thin Cobb elevator placed laterally within the disc space, rotated on edge, to hold distraction while I transition from the final distraction plug to the impacted implant. The ring-style implant can be further secured with a screw/washer placed into the sacrum as a buttress.

In isthmic spondylolisthesis, ALIF is useful in reducing the translational slip. A complete anterior annular excision and discectomy are performed. The endplates need to be smoothed using a burr, particularly with a domed sacrum. Sequential distraction up to a predetermined height is then accomplished. Typically, I strive to achieve the height of the adjacent disc space (Fig. 27-13A and B). An impacted ring-style implant is preferred. Percutaneous or minimally invasive posterior instrumentation can then be performed.

Before closure, the retractor blades need to be carefully removed. Iliac vessel retraction is required during retractor blade removal. Once the surgeon has verified that there is no significant bleeding, closure is accomplished in layers: the anterior rectus sheath, subcutaneous tissue, and skin (Fig. 27-14). Postoperatively, patients typically wear only a soft binder for comfort after anterior interbody cage fusion. Nonimpact aerobic exercises begin at 4 weeks, and activities are increased progressively as tolerated.

L4–L5 Anterior Exposure

For L4–L5, anterior exposure is always more difficult. Preoperative assessment of the patient's computed tomographic or MRI scan enables the surgeon to visualize the vascular pattern. Typically, at L4–L5, the aorta has bifurcated into right and left iliac arteries. The inferior vena cava either is a single vessel or has just bifurcated into the iliac veins. The level of each of these bifurcations can be assessed on the MRI scan. In most cases, exposure at L4–L5 is accomplished by going left of all four

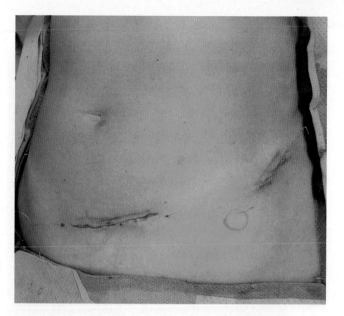

FIGURE 27-14

Skin closure is performed in a subcuticular manner. This leaves a pleasing cosmetic scar. For two-level cases, a slightly longer and more oblique incision is utilized.

vessels and retracting them across the disc space (Fig. 27-5). In the rare case of a high bifurcation, exposure can be accomplished between the bifurcations of the vessels, much as at L5–S1. In other rare cases, a very low bifurcation allows exposure by retraction of the aorta and inferior vena cava alone, as at L3–L4.

As before, the skin incision is marked according to a lateral fluoroscopic image to be in line with the L4–L5 disc space. The anterior rectus sheath is once again identified through blunt dissection and then sharply incised horizontally. For two-level procedures, this anterior rectus sheath incision can be Z-lengthened. This is done by extending a vertical incision superiorly in the midline and a lateral incision inferiorly at the lateral margin of the rectus sheath. Blunt dissection is then carried out in the midline between the heads of the rectus muscle, and the preperitoneal space is developed underneath the left rectus abdominis muscle. On occasion, the surgeon can still work bluntly inferior to the arcuate line to develop the retroperitoneal space. However, this does not generate adequate space to work at L4–L5 and certainly not at L3–L4. In these situations, the posterior rectus sheath needs to be incised in a vertical manner. This can be done either with fine scissors, working from the arcuate line superiorly, or by using a no. 15 blade to incise the posterior rectus sheath near its lateral border. These maneuvers can usually be performed via the midline approach. On occasion, the surgeon may need to work lateral to the left rectus muscle. The surgeon can then carefully dissect with fine scissors between the posterior rectus sheath and the underlying peritoneum to develop the potential space therein. Once this space is developed, a vertical incision in the posterior rectus sheath can be lengthened to provide adequate space. Once again, the retroperitoneal space is then entered lateral to the peritoneum, and a Deaver retractor is placed.

The mobilization of the great vessels is important at the L4–L5 disc space. With a self-retaining Deaver retractor placed at the edge of the L4–L5 disc, the surgeon can take time to examine the vasculature. Through blunt dissection, the left common iliac artery should be identified, as should the left common iliac vein. On occasion, the surgeon can mobilize these vessels across the disc space without any additional ligature. More commonly, however, the iliolumbar vein and possibly the L4 segmental vessels need to be divided. The iliolumbar vein is a very short, thick vein that comes into the left common iliac vein laterally, from underneath the psoas muscle. This vein tethers the left iliac vein and prevents it from being retracted across the spine. It needs to be identified and divided. I prefer to do this first with a fine right-angled clamp and by passing two silk ligatures around the vein. Next, I place a metal Ligaclip (Ethicon Inc., Somerville, NJ) distally and divide the vein. I then use a 5-0 monofilament suture in a baseball stitch across the stump of the divided iliolumbar vein proximally. This ensures that, during retraction, the surgeon does not lose control of this vein.

Blunt dissection can then begin lateral to the left common iliac artery and vein and worked across the L4–L5 disc space. Once again, if the vessels cannot be retracted beyond the midline, the L4 segmental artery and vein need to be located superiorly and divided. As before, when dissecting the inferior vena cava or left common iliac vein, the surgeon should be careful not to exsanguinate the vessel and injure its edge. Small perforating veins are often present between the L4 and L5 disc annulus and the inferior vena cava. These should be located, cauterized with bipolar cautery, and sharply divided. Once the vessels are adequately mobilized from left to right across the L4–L5 disc space, the self-retaining retractor blades, protected K-wires, or both can be placed in the vertebral body of

L4 to maintain retraction. Laterally, the retractor is placed medial to the psoas muscle. The sympathetic chain should be identified and protected. The surgeon must remember that once these great vessels are in the retracted position, the remainder of the procedure should be performed rapidly and efficiently to minimize the amount of retraction time. If the table was rolled toward the right for the approach, it should, at this point, be rolled into the flat position for the remainder of the procedure.

Disc Arthroplasty

As before, fluoroscopy is utilized to locate the midline of the disc space, which is appropriately marked. A complete discectomy is then be performed, again using curettes to remove endplate cartilage and disc material. For arthroplasty, care should be taken to remove all of the posterior annulus and, if necessary, a portion of the posterior longitudinal ligament in order to perform a posterior release. It is imperative, when the disc is distracted, that all portions of the endplate are mobilized. The surgeon can check this with handheld disc space distractors. The bony endplate should remain intact. The surgeon can then appropriately prepare the endplates for arthroplasty by using the device-specific cutting jig, which will mark the location of the endplate fin or keel. The actual insertion tool is then applied, the disc space is distracted, and the prosthesis is placed. In general, the disc prosthesis should be placed posteriorly within the disc space.

POSTOPERATIVE MANAGEMENT

After stand-alone cage arthroplasty, patients are ambulated the same afternoon. They wear only a soft abdominal binder. Clear liquids and a light meal are given in the evening after surgery, and most patients are discharged home the following morning. Nonimpact aerobic exercises begin 4 weeks after surgery, and light weight lifting can begin at 6 weeks.

COMPLICATIONS

The rectus abdominis muscle is innervated from its lateral nerves. If multilevel approaches are used, it is possible to denervate this muscle. Great care should be taken to stay medial (i.e., in the midline) to the rectus muscle whenever possible. If lateral dissection is required, the surgeon should take care to find the segmental innervation and preserve it. For three levels or more, it is better to approach the spine laterally through a flank approach and leave the rectus abdominis muscle alone.

The ureter should be identified in the retroperitoneal space and protected. The ureter is prone to injury, particularly at L4–L5. Inadequate visualization at L4–L5 most commonly results from the inability to ligate the iliolumbar vein. If this vein is not ligated, excessive stretch will be necessary to be placed upon the left iliac vein, and inadequate exposure will result. Vascular injuries are most commonly tears of the left common iliac vein. If these occur, an immediate tamponade should be provided with a sponge stick. Usually, these tears can be repaired with a 5-0 monofilament suture. In rare instances, a backing pledget is required in their repair. For complex repairs, the assistance of a vascular surgeon is necessary. When placing self-retaining retractors, it is very important to ensure that the vein is adequately protected beforehand. Similarly, before each step in the procedure, particularly before reaming and cage placement, the surgeon should recheck that the vein has not worked its way out from under the retractor.

Bladder injury is rare. In revision cases or following mesh herniorrhaphy, the bladder may become adherent to the abdominal wall and be prone to injury even with blunt dissection. Early recognition and immediate repair are essential should these occur.

Improper cage or arthroplasty placement usually is a result of poor exposure. Orientation to the midline and the use of fluoroscopy greatly enhance positioning. Ideally, the implants should be centered on the midline, and a minimal amount of reaming from either endplate should be performed. Appropriate implant sizing is based on preoperative templating and intraoperative measurements. Postoperative cage displacement is usually caused by inadequate bone stock (as in osteoporosis), excessive instability (e.g., as in spondylolisthesis), or inappropriate cage sizing.

Retrograde ejaculation may occur in men following ALIF. This incidence is low and appears to depend greatly on surgical technique. Certainly, retroperitoneal exposure lowers this risk when compared to transperitoneal exposure. All cautery near the presacral nervous plexus should be avoided. Minimal peridiscal exposure, always blunt, is also helpful.

It is controversial as to whether implant choice or bone graft substitute use affects the incidence of retrograde ejaculation. Over the past 10 years, using titanium cages and rhBMP-2, the author's incidence of RE is less than 1%.

Mini-open anterior approaches to the spine carry low rates of morbidity; in our series, vascular repair was necessary in fewer than 2% of cases, and bladder or ureter injury is even more rare.

Retrograde ejaculation may occur if damage to the presacral plexus occurs. With the open retro-peritoneal approach, this problem is much less frequent than with transperitoneal or laparoscopic approaches. In our series, it has occurred in just one case in more than 200.

RESULTS

The treatment of disc degeneration with cage ALIF has met with variable success. Patient selection is key. Single-level procedures are, in general, more successful than multilevel procedures. Collapsed disc spaces are more amenable to surgical treatment than are "dark discs" with positive discograms. For single-level collapsed discs, a 90% clinical success rate is possible (Figs. 27-15 to 27-17).

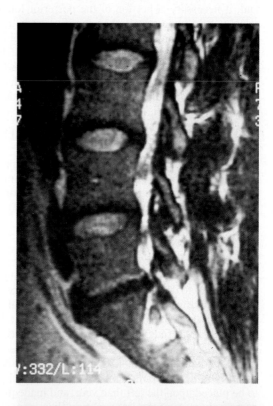

FIGURE 27-15

This sagittal MRI scan shows marked disc degeneration at L5–S1. Note the disc space collapse and modic changes on either side of the endplate.

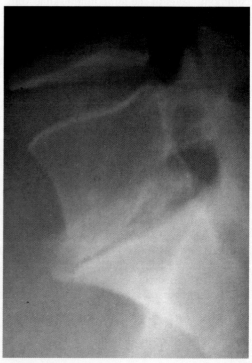

FIGURE 27-16

Preoperative lateral radiograph demonstrating marked collapse and degeneration of the L5–S1 disc space. This resulted in chronic, aching low back pain.

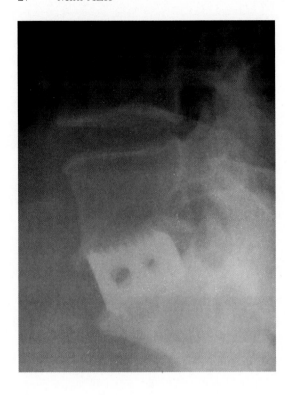

FIGURE 27-17

Postoperative lateral radiograph showing the distraction of the degenerative disc. This results in increased foraminal size. The interbody devices are shown in place, maintaining the distraction and allowing fusion.

RECOMMENDED READING

1. Blumenthal SL, Baker J, Dossett A, et al.: The role of anterior lumbar fusion for internal disc disruption. *Spine* 13: 566–569, 1988.
2. Boden SD, Zdeblick TA, Sandhu HS, et al.: The use of rhBMP-2 in interbody fusion cages. Definitive evidence of osteoinduction in humans: a preliminary report. *Spine* 25: 376–381, 2000.
3. Flynn JC, Price CT: Sexual complications of anterior fusion of the lumbar spine. *Spine* 9: 489–491, 1984.
4. Harmon PH: Anterior excision and vertebral fusion operation for intervertebral disc syndromes of the lower lumbar spine: three to five year results in 244 cases. *Clin Orthop* 26: 107–127, 1963.
5. Kuslich SD, Ulstrom CL, Griffith SL, et al.: The Bagby and Kuslich method of lumbar interbody fusion: history, techniques, and 2-year follow-up results of a United States prospective, multicenter trial. *Spine* 23: 1267–1279, 1998.
6. Mahvi DM, Zdeblick TA: A prospective study of laparoscopic spinal fusion: technique and operative complications. *Ann Surg* 224: 85–90, 1996.
7. Stauffer RN, Coventry MB: Anterior interbody lumbar spinal fusion. *J Bone Joint Surg Am* 54: 756–768, 1972.
8. Zdeblick TA: Laparoscopic spinal fusion. *Orthop Clin North Am* 29: 635–645, 1998.
9. Zucherman JF, Zdeblick TA, Bailey SA, et al.: Instrumented laparoscopic spinal fusion: preliminary results. *Spine* 20: 2029–2034, 1995.

28 Lumbar Disc Arthroplasty

Darren R. Lebl, Federico P. Girardi, Alexander P. Hughes, and Frank P. Cammisa Jr.

INDICATIONS

For many years, lumbar spinal fusion has been considered the "gold standard" treatment for degenerative disc disease (DDD) that fails conservative therapy. Reports of symptomatic adjacent segment disease (ASD) at the levels cephalad or caudal to a fusion have been estimated to occur in as many as 16% of patients at 5 years and 36% of patients at 10 years postoperatively (4). As such, lumbar total disc replacement (TDR) has become a widely performed operation in many parts of the world with encouraging early to midterm outcomes (10). FDA approval in 2004 of the Charité (11) (Depuy Spine, Raynham, MA) and in 2006 of the Prodisc-L (12) (Synthes Spine, West Chester, PA) has expanded TDR utilization in the United States for the treatment of one-level DDD from L3–S1 (Prodisc-L) to L4–S1 (Charité). At present, the indications and optimal selection of patients for TDR remain a topic of ongoing debate.

Generally, skeletally mature patients with chronic discogenic low back pain (LBP) due to DDD that is unresponsive to a minimum of 6 months of conservative measures such as physical therapy, weight loss, activity modification, pain management, and injections may be considered for lumbar TDR. Clinical history of symptomatic DDD that is consistent with physical examination and imaging studies is important for appropriate patient selection. A lack of clear consistency between these methods of evaluation may signal involvement of other disease processes considered in the differential diagnosis, psychiatric disorders, secondary gain issues, or narcotic pain medication dependency.

CONTRAINDICATIONS

Active infection, clinically significant facet joint arthropathy, metal (or polyethylene) allergy to the TDR device material, morbid obesity, rheumatologic disorders, clinically significant central or lateral recess stenosis, and greater than grade 1 spondylolisthesis are absolute contraindications to lumbar TDR. Current FDA approval recommends TDR be avoided in patients with objective osteopenia or osteoporosis (T-score less than −1) (12). Greater than 3 mm of anterolisthesis, 11 degrees of scoliosis, bilateral pars defects, and iatrogenic instability following posterior decompression are also contraindications to lumbar TDR (12).

PREOPERATIVE PREPARATION

Preoperative preparation of the candidate for lumbar TDR includes patient education, thorough history and physical examination to rule out any of the above potential contraindications, and study of preoperative radiography. Preoperative CT scan permits analysis of the morphology of the patient's bony endplates at the planned TDR level for preoperative consideration of device sizing. Variations in sacral morphology or endplate irregularities may preclude stable fixation of the metallic TDR endplate. MRI will help to evaluate any retrovertebral disc material or foraminal stenosis that requires surgical decompression. Concordant pain on provocative discography may provide

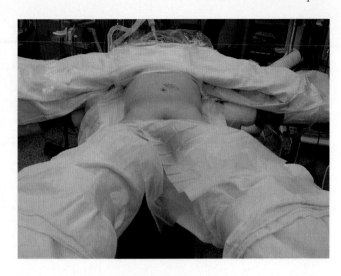

FIGURE 28-1

Proper supine patient positioning for lumbar TDR with arms abducted 90 degrees and legs abducted and all appropriate pressure points are padded. Surgical drapes are placed proximally at the xiphoid process and distally at the pubic symphysis for exposure of the entire abdomen.

additional information to the practitioner to aid in patient selection; however, it has not been shown to be highly predictive of identifying bona fide intradiscal lesions causing chronic LBP (2) and may accelerate disc degeneration at the control levels (1). As such, the authors do not recommend routine discography as part of the preoperative imaging studies. Preoperative lumbar spine MRI and CT may be reviewed to determine the level of aortic and iliac bifurcation and to screen for the presence of any vascular anomalies that may complicate the exposure.

TECHNIQUE

Patient Positioning and Setup

Following the induction of general endotracheal anesthesia, the patient is positioned in the "da Vinci position"—supine with the arms abducted 90 degrees and the legs abducted (Fig. 28-1). Patient positioning should allow for C-arm positioning circumferentially around the operative table. A lateral fluoroscopic image taken prior to prepping and draping with a radiographic marker at the site of the planned skin incision will ensure the exposure is at the appropriate level (Figs. 28-2 and 28-3). Anatomic variations in the patient's sacropelvic anatomy (pelvic incidence = pelvic tilt + sacral slope) may preclude safe surgical approach to the operative disc space. The abdominal region is prepped and draped from the xiphoid process to the symphysis pubis and laterally to the anterior axillary line.

Surgical Exposure

Routine anterior retroperitoneal approach to the lumbar spine is performed by 4 to 6 cm left-sided paramedian transverse skin incision for single-level cases. A right-sided approach may alternatively be performed in the setting of prior abdominal surgery. Many spine surgeons perform this approach assisted by a vascular access surgeon. The external oblique fascia is identified and is incised just to the left of midline to allow blunt finger elevation and mobilization of the rectus sheath laterally or

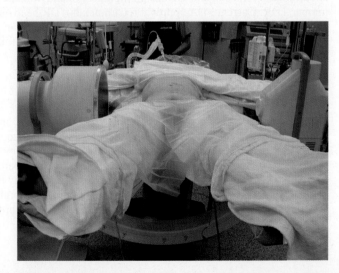

FIGURE 28-2

Lateral fluoroscopic measurement is essential for proper exposure of the operative segment TDR balancing intraoperatively.

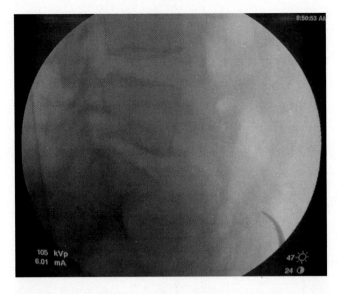

FIGURE 28-3

A radiopaque marker such as a curved hemostat placed over the region of the skin incision will ensure that the patient's lumbosacral anatomy permits safe and adequate exposure.

toward the midline (Fig. 28-4A and B). The posterior rectus sheath is incised longitudinally, and the peritoneal contents are gently swept medially by blunt manual dissection. The peritoneum is elevated away from the psoas muscle with care that the ureter remains medial along with the peritoneal contents. Iliac artery pulsations may be palpated, and the L5–S1 disc space can be exposed in the interval between the bifurcated iliac vessels. The middle sacral vessels may course through the midline on the anterior aspect of the L5–S1 disc space and require ligation. Gentle retraction of the iliac vessels laterally and superiorly is necessary for adequate exposure of L5–S1.

The approach to L4–L5 or L3–L4 may require ligation of the ascending iliolumbar vein as it drains from a cephalad direction into the common iliac vein on the left. The aorta and vena cava are gently mobilized medially from left to right to provide adequate midline exposure of the operative disc space. The disc is marked by a spinal needle or curved hemostat in the midline, and AP and lateral fluoroscopy are performed to determine the location of the midline and to ensure the correct operative level, respectively. AP fluoroscopy is used to mark the midline on the cephalad and caudal vertebral bodies with Bovie electrocautery for later TDR device positioning (Fig. 28-5).

Disc Space Preparation

A box-cut annulotomy is marked out through the anterior longitudinal ligament (ALL) and anterior annulus of the disc space using Bovie electrocautery and incised using a long-handle no. 10 scalpel (cutting the disc in a direction away from the iliac vessels). A sequence of pituitary rongeur,

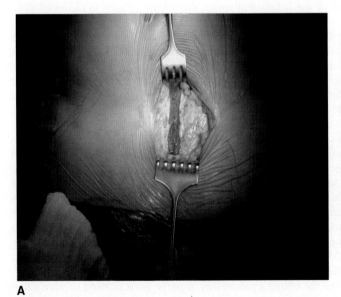

A

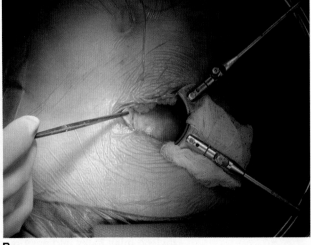

B

FIGURE 28-4

Approach through the rectus sheath **(A)** and mobilization **(B)** to expose the peritoneal contents.

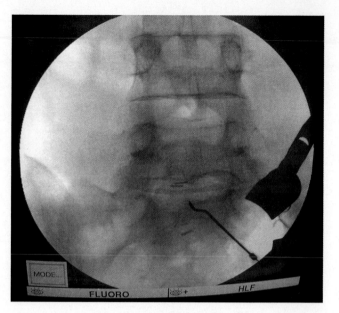

FIGURE 28-5

Spinal needle or curved hemostat is used to mark the midline on Ferguson AP imaging (shown), and lateral imaging will confirm the correct operative segment. Visualization of the pedicles at the operative segment will aid in correct determination of the AP plane.

Kerrison rongeurs, straight and curved curettes, and ring curettes is performed for completion of the discectomy. Removal of endplate cartilage is necessary (TDR devices rely on bony ingrowth/ongrowth to the device itself) and should be performed gently using a ring curette to expose bleeding, viable endplate bone. Resection of the posterior longitudinal ligament (PLL) is performed by placing a nerve hook underneath the longitudinal fibers in the midline to develop the interval between the PLL and the epidural space thereby allowing the footplate of a no. 2 or no. 3 Kerrison rongeur to be passed under the ligament for resection laterally toward the foramen. Thrombin-soaked Gelfoam and bipolar electrocautery are utilized to improve hemostasis of the endplate surfaces and in the epidural space during this portion of the procedure.

A small, curved curette may be gently placed into the neuroforamen posterolaterally to ensure that during flexion/extension and lateral bending of the motion-preserving device, impingement of the exiting nerve root does not occur. A meticulous discectomy is necessary for TDR procedures due to the possibility of any residual disc material to migrate or impinge on neural structures during the preserved motion of the functional spinal unit.

TDR Implantation

The implantation technique of the TDR is dependent on the design of the particular device. With any TDR device, optimal clinical results will be achieved when the axis of rotation of the TDR is approximated to the axis of rotation of the functional spinal unit. Arthroplasty in the axial skeleton does not permit intraoperative placement of the implanted TDR device through the patient's functional range of motion intraoperatively (as can be performed easily in arthroplasty in the appendicular skeleton). As such, TDR balancing in the lumbar spine relies on direct visualization of the disc space and prediction of the position of the TDR device during a physiologic range of motion. AP/Ferguson view and lateral fluoroscopy allow positioning of the TDR device in the mediolateral and anteroposterior planes, respectively. On the Ferguson view, the lumbar pedicles serve as landmarks for assessment of the rotation of the spine for optimal positioning of the device in the midline.

Under lateral fluoroscopic guidance, a vertebral body spreader may be utilized for distraction of the disc space (Fig. 28-6A). Trialing of the device is next performed, and the largest footprint size to maximize coverage of the host endplate is chosen to allow loading of the device on the strongest portion of the endplate bone (laterally in the apophyseal ring). Lordosis (Prodisc-L—6 or 11 degrees lordotic implants) should be chosen to match the patient's sagittal alignment as determined by preoperative imaging studies (Fig. 28-6B and C). Devices with a keel (Prodisc-L) utilize the trialing device as a cutting jig to guide the direction and depth of the chisel cuts. Chisel cuts are made in the midline as determined by the pedicles and marked previously on AP fluoroscopy. The Prodisc-L device is inserted with the endplates in a collapsed position and is later distracted for insertion of the polyethylene inlay (10-, 12-, or 14-mm height sizing options). Once the polyethylene inlay locks into position into the cobalt chrome tray, a nerve hook is used to verify that there is no gapping or step-off. Final implant position is confirmed on AP and lateral fluoroscopy (Fig. 28-7A–C).

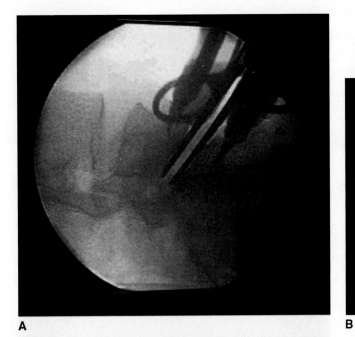

A

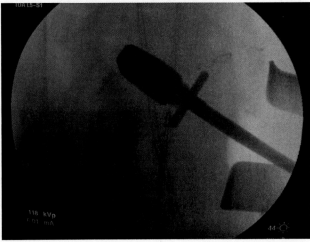

B

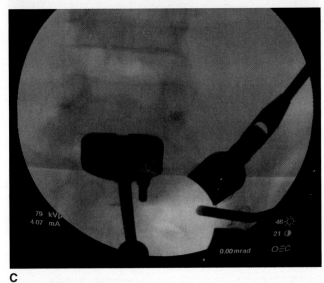

C

FIGURE 28-6

Disc space distraction may be necessary if the degenerative disc has lost its height preoperatively **(A)** and trialing in the lateral **(B)** and AP/Ferguson **(C)** views is utilized for proper implant balancing and positioning.

Wound Closure

Inspection of the anterior disc space and iliac vessels for meticulous hemostasis is recommended prior to wound closure. Deep retractors are removed, and the rectus sheath is closed with running no. 1 polydioxanone suture. Deep dermal closure is performed with interrupted 2-0 Vicryl sutures and skin closure completed with 3-0 Monocryl subcuticular stitch followed by Steri-Strips and sterile surgical dressing (Fig. 28-8A and B).

PEARLS AND PITFALLS

The initial and perhaps most common pitfall of lumbar TDR is improper patient selection. Degenerative changes such as sclerosis may falsely elevate dual-energy x-ray absorptiometry (DEXA) scores in the lumbar spine (8). Therefore, the authors' preferred method is to not rely solely on the lumbar DEXA T-score. In the scenario in which a T-score is within the normal range in the lumbar spine and the T-score values in the appendicular skeleton (hip, wrist) are suggestive of osteopenia or osteoporosis, TDR is not recommended.

The authors' preferred operative technique begins with the setup and positioning of the patient. Intraoperative lower extremity pulse oximetry recording is used to alert the surgeon of retractors that may be occluding, inducing thrombus formation, or damaging the adjacent iliac vessels. Intraoperative neuromonitoring is recommended in all patients to ensure that during device sizing and

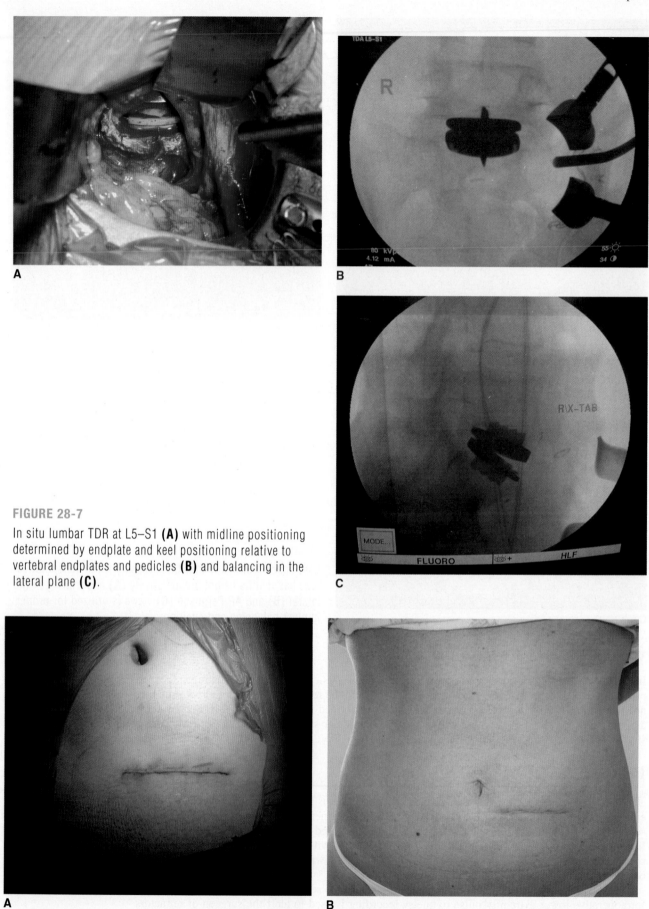

FIGURE 28-7

In situ lumbar TDR at L5–S1 **(A)** with midline positioning determined by endplate and keel positioning relative to vertebral endplates and pedicles **(B)** and balancing in the lateral plane **(C)**.

FIGURE 28-8

Transverse skin incision closed with 3-0 absorbable subcuticular suture **(A)** and 1-year follow-up of well-healed scar **(B)**.

implantation, distraction of the disc space does not result in a traction-related neurapraxia and to avoid direct impingement of the TDR device on the exiting nerve root.

During fluoroscopic confirmation of the operative level, the authors' preferred technique is to mark the ALL with a hemostat (as opposed to an intradiscal spinal needle) to avoid potential iatrogenic violation of a nonoperative spinal segment and potential acceleration of degeneration by the marking procedure itself. Wide surgical exposure with careful handling of the iliac vessels will allow complete and thorough discectomy with removal of the degenerated disc in its entirety. Following resection of the PLL, a small curved curette or ball-tipped probe may be placed behind the posterior margin of the vertebral body to remove any retrovertebral disc material and postero-laterally to ensure adequate foraminal decompression. Gentle endplate preparation (and avoidance of rasps or aggressive instruments to remove endplate cartilage) will help to avoid propagation of stress risers and later device subsidence. During device implantation, lateral fluoroscopy is utilized to avoid placement of the TDR endplates in relative extension or in an anterior position in the disc space to avoid the posterior component "fish-mouth" impingement seen commonly in clinically failed devices (5). Oversizing of the implant may also be avoided by lateral fluoroscopic visualization during trialing of the implant and comparison with preoperative templating.

POSTOPERATIVE MANAGEMENT

Neurovascular examination is the first step in the postoperative management of the TDR patient. Evaluation of lower extremity capillary refill, edema, temperature, and pulses allows assessment of the iliac vessels. Lower extremity sensorimotor examination will help rule out any distraction-related neurapraxia of the nerve roots at the operative segment. Patient is kept nil per os (NPO) until bowel function has returned, and then diet is advanced as tolerated. Early patient mobilization as tolerated (POD no. 0 to no. 1) will improve motility and speed the postoperative recovery. Upright AP, flexion, and extension x-rays allow early assessment of device positioning and performance under a physiologic load and during range of motion. Hospital length of stay is patient specific and may vary from 2 to 5 days.

COMPLICATIONS

Potential exposure-related complications related to major vascular injury during TDR are similar in incidence to those reported in the literature for anterior lumbar interbody fusion (ALIF) procedures in clinical reports and meta-analysis (less than 3% to 5%) (3,13). TDR requires improved visualization of the disc space for device balancing as compared to mini-ALIF techniques. As such, overaggressive retraction of the vessels should be avoided.

Postoperative ileus is a relatively common occurrence following anterior retroperitoneal or transperitoneal exposure of the lumbar spine and close monitoring of bowel function, and management of fluid/electrolyte status is imperative. The preoperative informed decision-making process should include the possibility of approach-related retrograde ejaculation (6), in particular, in younger male patients with future reproductive plans.

Undersizing of the TDR implant may result in hypermobility of the motion segment and endplate impingement of the TDR device. Smaller PE insert height (10 mm) and lower degrees of lordosis (6 degrees) have been associated with metallic endplate impingement in retrieved semiconstrained TDR devices.

International TDR retrieval study data have demonstrated clinical failure to occur in patients due to a variety of reasons including continued axial back pain, radicular symptoms, endplate collapse or implant subsidence, component migration, and polyethylene dislodgement (5). Device failure due to continued axial back pain may potentially be minimized by ensuring an adequately posterior position of the TDR device, which serves to unload the facet joints and permit a more physiologic load transfer to the vertebral bodies (9).

Wear particles of similar size to those generated by total hip and total knee replacements have been demonstrated following TDR (7). Nonetheless, polyethylene-induced osteolysis to date has been an infrequent problem following lumbar TDR, potentially due to the lack of a true joint synovium in the disc space (to contain the wear debris and induce an osteolytic cascade), and few reports of this phenomenon have been made at the present time.

RESULTS

Successful treatment of the patient afflicted by severe DDD with lumbar TDR may be evaluated by satisfactory fixation of the device to the host endplates; proper device balancing to avoid impingement of the TDR endplates or adjacent neurologic structures; improvement or maintenance of neurologic status; avoidance of subsidence, migration, or loosening; clinical improvement in symptoms;

a decrease in the incidence of ASD compared to fusion; and long-term follow-up. At present, it is the last of these criteria that remains to be reported.

Radiographic success in the FDA-IDE trial for the Prodisc-L device was defined as no radiographic evidence of device migration or subsidence greater than 3 mm, no loss of disc height greater than 3 mm, no extensive radiolucency along the implant/bone interface (less than 25% of the interface's length for each endplate defined as success), range of motion at the implanted level that is maintained or improved from the preoperative baseline, and no evidence of bony fusion (12).

Retrieval analysis of clinically failed Prodisc-L devices has demonstrated metallic endplate impingement, in particular, posteriorly, to be a common finding (5). Preservation of the ALL may avoid this extension imbalancing by transpsoas TDR from an extreme lateral approach, which has shown encouraging early results but remains to be studied in larger trials (5). Newer devices that are being implanted in parts of Europe (M6-L, Spinal Kinetics, Sunnyvale, CA) with a shock-absorbing capacity due to an artificial polymer nucleus and an artificial fiber annulus may more closely approximate the normal properties of the lumbar intervertebral disc than the semiconstrained ball-and-socket metal-on-polyethylene devices, and studies of these newer designs are under way.

RECOMMENDED READING

1. Carragee EJ, Don AS, Hurwitz EL, et al.: 2009 ISSLS Prize Winner: does discography cause accelerated progression of degeneration changes in the lumbar disc: a ten-year matched cohort study. *Spine (Phila Pa 1976)* 34(21): 2338–2345, 2009.
2. Carragee EJ, Lincoln T, Parmar VS, et al.: A gold standard evaluation of the "discogenic pain" diagnosis as determined by provocative discography. *Spine (Phila Pa 1976)* 31(18): 2115–2123, 2006.
3. Fantini GA, Pappou IP, Girardi FP, et al.: Major vascular injury during anterior lumbar spinal surgery: incidence, risk factors, and management. *Spine (Phila Pa 1976)* 32(24): 2751–2758, 2007.
4. Ghiselli G, Wang JC, Bhatia NN, et al.: Adjacent segment degeneration in the lumbar spine. *J Bone Joint Surg Am* 86-A(7): 1497–1503, 2004.
5. Lebl DR, Cammisa FP, Girardi FP, et al.: In vivo functional Performance of failed prodisc-L devices-retrieval analysis of lumbar total disc replacements. *Spine (Phila Pa 1976)* 37(19): E1209–E1217, 2012.
6. Lindley EM, McBeth ZL, Henry SE, et al.: Retrograde ejaculation following anterior lumbar spine surgery. *Spine (Phila Pa 1976)* 37(20):1785–1789, 2012.
7. Punt IM, Austen S, Cleutjens JP, et al.: Are periprosthetic tissue reactions observed after revision of total disc replacement comparable to the reactions observed after total hip or knee revision surgery? *Spine (Phila Pa 1976)* 37(2): 150–159, 2012.
8. Rand T, Seidl G, Kainberger F, et al.: Impact of spinal degenerative changes on the evaluation of bone mineral density with dual energy x-ray absorptiometry (DXA). *Calcif Tissue Int* 60(5): 430–433, 1997.
9. Rundell SA, Auerbach JD, Balderston RA, et al.: Total disc replacement positioning affects facet contact forces and vertebral body strains. *Spine (Phila Pa 1976)* 33(23): 2510–2517, 2008.
10. Tropiano P, Huang RC, Girardi FP, et al.: Lumbar total disc replacement. Seven to eleven-year follow-up. *J Bone Joint Surg Am* 87(3): 490–496, 2005.
11. US. Food and Drug Administration—Department of Health & Human Services: Charite Total Disc Replacement—P040006 Approval Letter. October 26, 2004; Available from: http://www.accessdata.fda.gov/cdrh_docs/pdf4/p040006a.pdf.
12. US. Food and Drug Administration—Department of Health & Human Services: Prodisc-L Total Disc Replacement—P050010 Approval Letter. August 4, 2006; Available from: http://www.accessdata.fda.gov/cdrh_docs/pdf5/p050010a.pdf.
13. Wood KB, Devine J, Fischer D, et al.: Vascular injury in elective anterior lumbosacral surgery. *Spine (Phila Pa 1976)* 35(9 Suppl): S66–S75, 2010.

29 Lateral Lumbar Interbody Fusion

Neil Badlani and Frank M. Phillips

INDICATIONS

Lateral lumbar interbody fusion (LLIF) is a relatively new technique that allows for interbody
fusion and anterior column support through a minimally invasive, transpsoas approach. Like any
interbody fusion, it allows for increased surface area for fusion, restoration of disc and foraminal
height, and potential correction of both sagittal and coronal plane deformities (4,8,13). It is there-
fore indicated when interbody fusion and anterior column support or reconstruction is desired in
the thoracic or lumbar spine, proximal to L5–S1. Examples of this include
Instability/low-grade spondylolisthesis
Sagittal or coronal deformity correction
Degenerative disc pathology, that is, discogenic low back pain or postdiscectomy axial back pain
Foraminal stenosis treated though indirect decompression from restoration of disc height
Adjacent segment disease
Revision for posterior pseudoarthrosis
Corpectomies for tumor or trauma can also be performed through the lateral approach with similar
reconstruction of the vertebral body and anterior column with a variety of static and expandable
cages or allograft struts (3,16).

CONTRAINDICATIONS

The iliac crest generally precludes performing an LLIF at L5–S1 and may make the approach to
L4–L5 challenging.
Variations in retroperitoneal anatomy, including prior surgery with scarring or abnormal location
of blood vessels (that may accompany rotational deformities of the spine), will make the lateral
approach more challenging. This anatomy should always be reviewed prior to the procedure.
In cases of severe central stenosis, the indirect decompression from LLIF alone will likely not be
enough to decompress the neural elements.
High-grade spondylolisthesis
Severe osteoporosis may predispose to greater subsidence; therefore, additional fixation is
recommended (1).

ADVANTAGES

LLIF is essentially a minimally invasive variation of anterior lumbar interbody fusion (ALIF). When
compared to ALIF, LLIF allows for interbody fusion without the need for an access surgeon and
without the potential disruption to peritoneal contents, the sympathetic hypogastric plexus, and
avoiding the need for mobilization of the great vessels (12,15).
When compared to posterior approaches for interbody fusion, LLIF spares the important posterior
paraspinal muscular-ligamentous structures. There is greater access to the disc space through a
larger portal for discectomy and interbody preparation without the need for retraction on the intracanal neural elements implicit to a transforaminal lumbar interbody fusion or posterior lumbar

interbody fusion. A larger implant can be placed after LLIF when compared to posterior interbody fusion.

The primary advantage is that the procedure is minimally disruptive, resulting in lower blood loss, shorter hospital stays, lower complication rates (REFs), and quicker return to function than traditional open approaches (2,6,14).

DISADVANTAGES

Approach-related challenges including potential direct or traction injury to the lumbar plexus or disruption of the psoas itself. These can be minimized with knowledge of the relevant anatomy and careful neurologic monitoring.

L5–S1 cannot be accessed through this approach.

No direct decompression of the neural elements can be performed.

The procedure is performed in the lateral decubitus position, and therefore, repositioning is typically required if additional posterior instrumentation or decompression is required.

PREOPERATIVE PREPARATION

Positioning

Patient positioning is critical in LLIF. The procedure is done in the lateral decubitus position. Either left- or right-sided approaches can be done. The relevant anatomy and the desired spinal deformity correction should be considered when deciding which side to approach from. In general, at L4–L5, we prefer to approach from the side with a more caudal iliac crest. Otherwise, right lateral decubitus position, allowing for a left-sided approach, is generally used, unless the spinal deformity dictates otherwise.

A radiolucent bendable surgical table is required. Portable C-arm fluoroscopy is used throughout the case and therefore must be able to pass freely under the table to obtain imaging.

Given these considerations, we prefer to use a regular operating room (OR) table, turned 180 degrees with the patient's head at the normal position of the feet. This allows for easier passage of the fluoroscopy machine under the table.

Neurophysiologic monitoring electrodes should be placed on the patient's lower extremities to allow for triggered and free-run electromyographic (EMG) testing during the procedure. The anesthesia provider should be informed to avoid using long-acting muscle relaxants, which may preclude accurate neurologic monitoring.

The patient should be positioned with the break in the bed at the level of the greater trochanter. The pelvis should be level, with the gluteal crease visualized from the bottom of the bed as a horizontal line, parallel to the table.

Appropriate padding is used over bony prominences and sites of nerve compression, particularly the peroneal and ulnar nerves. An axillary roll aids in positioning the trunk and arms, which can be draped over an arm board.

The patient is taped down in several places, which is again critical to success of the procedure. The trunk is secured to the table with one strip of tape over the rib cage, proximal to the field, and a second just below the iliac crest. The hips and knees should be flexed and taped with two individual strips. The first starts at the iliac crest and follows parallel to the femur, over the anterior knee, and to the table. This should provide some distal traction force to the iliac crest. The second follows the path of the tibia, crossing the other at 90 degrees and secured to the table at both ends (Fig. 29-1).

The table is flexed at the break, moving the pelvis caudally and the rib cage cranially away from the iliac crest, improving lateral access particularly at L4–L5, and opening up disc spaces in the lumbar spine (Fig. 29-2).

RADIOGRAPHIC LOCALIZATION

The surgeon stands posterior to the patient. Ideally, the C-arm is brought in from the anterior direction to be less obtrusive to the surgeon (Fig. 29-3).

An anteroposterior (AP) fluoroscopic image is obtained first. It is recommended to adjust the tilt of the table to get the desired true AP image and keep the C-arm in a fixed position. This allows for ease of transition between true AP and true lateral images throughout the case with only a 90-degree turn of the machine.

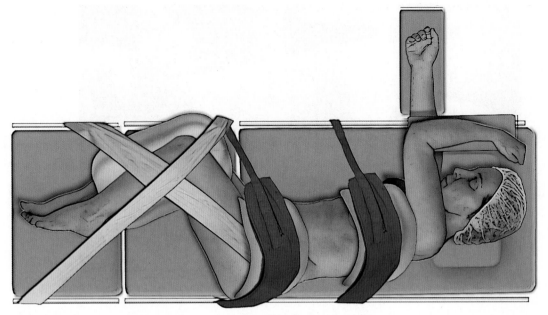

FIGURE 29-1
Taping configuration for patient positioning.

True AP and lateral images with centered spinous processes, symmetric pedicles, and distinct
   endplates should be obtained before prepping and draping (Fig. 29-4).

SKIN MARKING

A wide surgical field should be draped with the lateral border of the rectus abdominis as the anterior
   boundary and midline spinous processes posteriorly.
Before incision, localization of the disc space is performed on the lateral fluoroscopic image. For a
   single level, an incision from the anterior to posterior border of the disc can be used, in line with
   the disc space itself (Fig. 29-5). For multiple levels, it is possible to use a more oblique incision to
   access 2 or 3 discs. This should be angled with a trajectory from posterior superior to an anterior
   inferior to account for the lordosis.
If desired, a counterincision into the retroperitoneal space can be made to aid in the initial passage
   of instruments into the retroperitoneal space. This is a horizontal incision made posterolaterally
   (Fig. 29-6). Ideally, this is made just at the lateral border of the erector spinae muscle and also
   allows for palpation of the psoas, transverse processes, and even the disc space itself although this
   will vary in larger patients. The finger in the retroperitoneal space is used to escort instruments
   inserted laterally on to the psoas muscle.

TECHNIQUE

Initial Approach and Retroperitoneal Exposure

If the two-incision technique is used, the counterincision should be made first.
After dissection through subcutaneous tissue with electrocautery, Metzenbaum scissors are used for blunt
   dissection through the abdominal oblique musculature at a 45-degree angle. Once a loss of resistance
   is felt, the retroperitoneal space has been entered. Scissors are carefully spread to dilate the opening.
Scissors are removed, and the surgeon's finger is then passed through the plane created into the retroperitoneal space. Abdominal contents should have fallen sufficiently forward, but blunt finger dissection
   can be done additionally to better ensure the path is clear and any adhesions are disrupted (Fig. 29-7).
The undersurface of the direct lateral approach incision is then palpated. The incision is made,
   and dissection can be done with the Bovie down through the abdominal musculature toward the
   retroperitoneum and onto the surgeon's finger.
This approach can be done safely through a single incision as well. Care should be taken through the
   dissection. Distinct muscle layers of the external abdominal oblique, internal abdominal oblique,

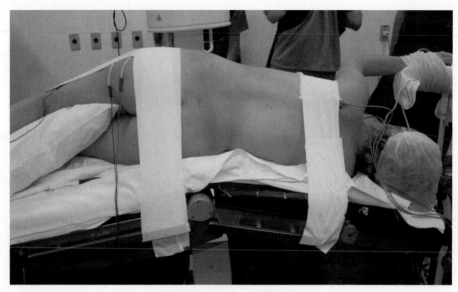

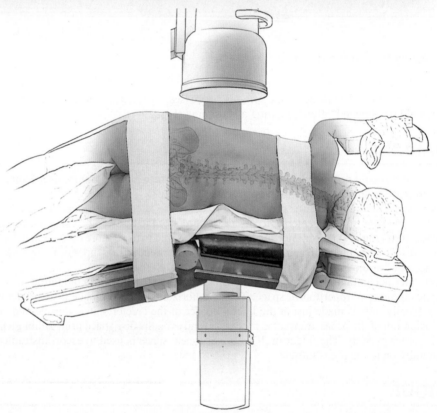

FIGURE 29-2

Photograph and illustration of table flexion improving lateral access and opening of disc spaces in the lumbar spine.

and transversalis abdominis can be identified to aid in knowledge of the depth of the approach. The transversalis fascia has a smooth, glistening appearance, which can be recognized and is the last layer to traverse before entering the retroperitoneal space.

Transpsoas Approach and Intervertebral Disc Access

A small cannulated initial dilator is passed into the wound. If the counterincision has been made, dilators can be guided into the retroperitoneum with the surgeon's finger and onto the psoas (Fig. 29-8A and B). This should be connected to the EMG system for neurologic monitoring while traversing the psoas. Lateral and AP fluoroscopy are used to reconfirm position of the dilator over the center of the intervertebral disc.

The transpsoas approach places the lumbar plexus in danger. It runs primarily within the posterior two-thirds of the psoas (Fig. 29-9). The genitofemoral nerve exits the psoas at L3 or L4 and then travels on the abdominal surface of the muscle and can be injured as well.

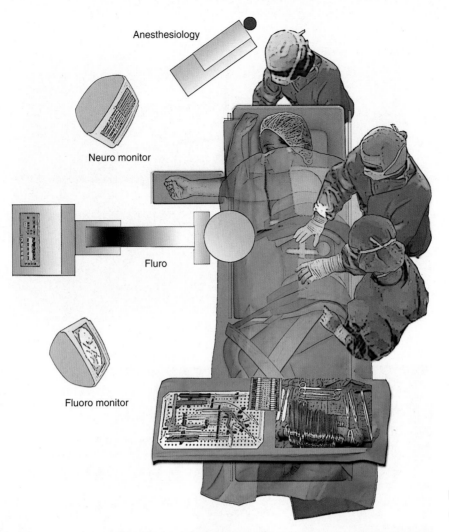

FIGURE 29-3
Operating room setup.

Anesthesiology

Neuro monitor

Fluro

Fluoro monitor

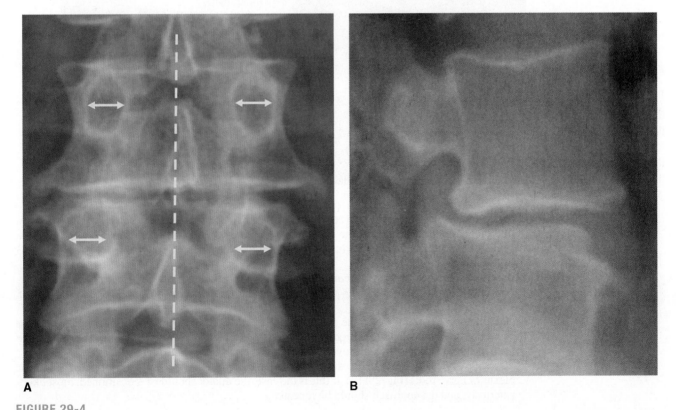

A

B

FIGURE 29-4
True radiographic AP **(A)** and lateral **(B)** images of the level in question, with centered spinous processes, symmetric pedicles, and distinct endplate.

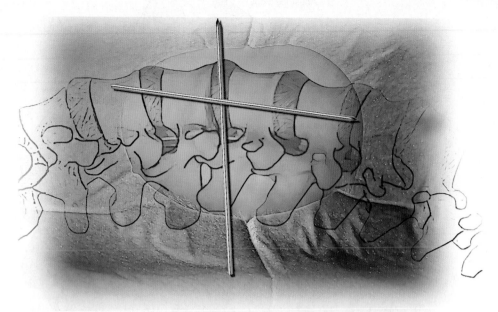

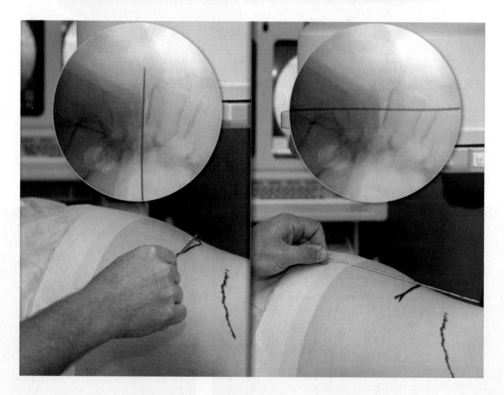

FIGURE 29-5

Illustration and photograph of technique to localize the center of the disc space in question before incision.

The nerve trunk has been shown to be a mean of 14 mm posterior to center of disc, which is a mean of 5 mm closer to the center of the disc than the exiting nerve root. Nerve trunks are closer to the center of the disc caudally in the lumbar spine with the distance ranging from 16.4 mm at L2–L3 to 10.6 mm at L4–L5 (11).

Therefore, the safe zone has been identified as the middle posterior quarter of the vertebral body from L1–L2 to L3–L4 and directly at the midpoint of the vertebral body at L4–L5 (Fig. 29-10) (18).

As the dilator is passed through the psoas, triggered EMG is performed (Fig. 29-11). The dilator should be oriented with the electrode directly posterior initially. As the dilator advances, it can be spun so the electrode stimulates over the entire posterior half of the approach path.

EMG activity typically lower than a threshold of 10 mA represents proximity too close to the lumbar plexus or nerve roots (Fig. 29-12). If this is the case, the dilator should be repositioned, most likely anteriorly, and the approach should be repeated.

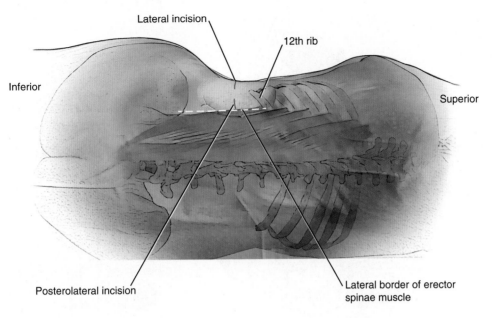

Lateral incision

12th rib

Inferior

Superior

Posterolateral incision

Lateral border of erector
spinae muscle

FIGURE 29-6

Preoperative position and
location of incisions.

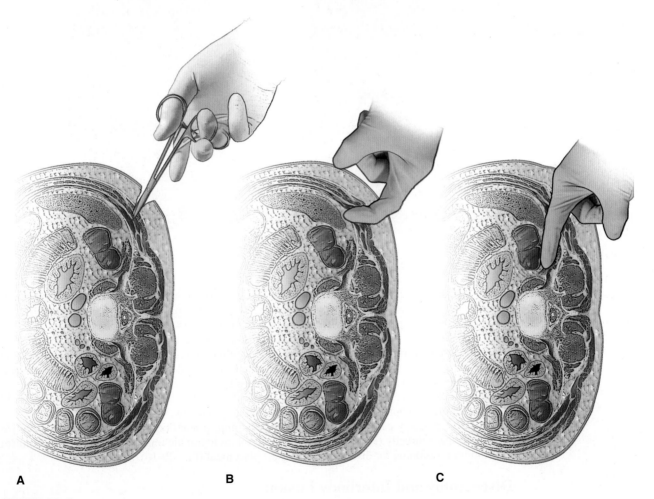

A

B

C

FIGURE 29-7

Retroperitoneal space is entered first with Metzenbaum scissors **(A)**. The surgeon's finger is then used to palpate the undersurface of the lateral incision **(B)** and the psoas **(C)**.

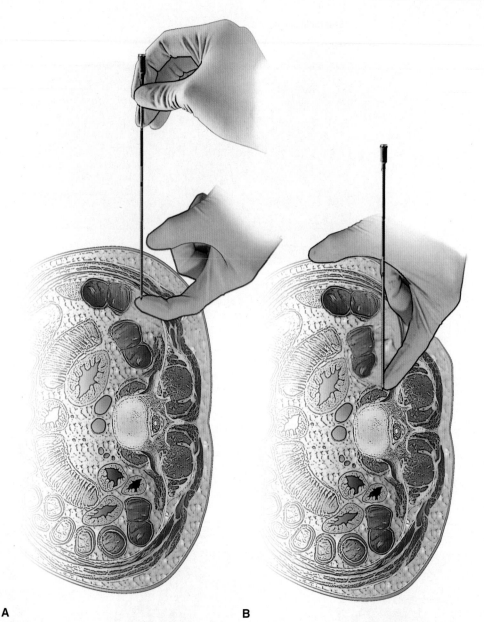

FIGURE 29-8

A: The surgeon's finger guides the dilators into the retroperitoneum. **B:** The surgeon's finger guides the dilators through the psoas.

A   **B**

Once the dilator passes safely, lateral fluoroscopy is used to confirm a position as close to the center of the disc space as possible (Fig. 29-13). A K-wire is then passed through the dilator into the center of the disc space to allow for stable docking (Fig. 29-14).

Sequential dilation is performed. Triggered EMG should be done as each dilator is passed through the psoas to confirm safety of the approach. Once dilation is safely completed, the expandable retractor or working cannula is passed and docked to the table. A light source can be attached. Lateral fluoroscopy confirms position over the disc space.

An EMG probe is then passed into the working portal, and the neurologic topography of the field can be carefully mapped out to ensure a safe operating window.

Bipolar electrocautery can be used to remove remaining psoas fibers and soft tissue to visualize the disc space directly (Fig. 29-15). AP and lateral radiographic images can be taken to confirm optimum positioning for discectomy and graft placement (Fig. 29-16).

Discectomy and Interbody Fusion

Annulotomy can be made with a long knife.

The disc space should be evacuated with pituitary rongeurs, shavers, and curettes (Fig. 29-17).

A contralateral annular release can be done by passing a small Cobb elevator along each endplate until contact is made with the contralateral annulus (Fig. 29-18). The Cobb can then be gently

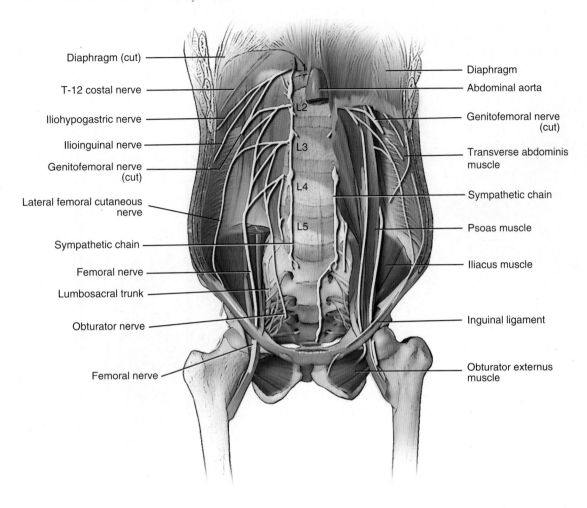

Diaphragm (cut)

T-12 costal nerve

Iliohypogastric nerve

Ilioinguinal nerve

Genitofemoral nerve
(cut)

Lateral femoral cutaneous
nerve

Sympathetic chain

Femoral nerve

Lumbosacral trunk

Obturator nerve

Femoral nerve

Diaphragm

Abdominal aorta

Genitofemoral nerve
(cut)

Transverse abdominis
muscle

Sympathetic chain

Psoas muscle

Iliacus muscle

Inguinal ligament

Obturator externus
muscle

FIGURE 29-9
Surgical anatomy of the lumbar plexus.

advanced through the annulus with care taken not to plunge into the contralateral psoas, which can cause hematoma or nerve injury. This release improves symmetric distraction of the disc space and is best done under AP fluoroscopy.

Kerrison rongeurs can be helpful to safely widen the annulotomy from inside the disc space to improve visualization.

Endplates should be prepared with complete removal or cartilage and disc material using various curettes. Care should be taken not to violate the osseous endplate, which can lead to increased bleeding and subsidence.

Once discectomy is complete, trials are placed, and sizing is performed (Fig. 29-19). AP fluoroscopy is used to check size and position. The implant should span the entire disc space and vertebral ring apophysis in the coronal plane to maximize surface area for fusion and stability. Implant height can be determined to appropriately improve lordosis and restore disc and foraminal height.

Implants or bone graft is placed (Fig. 29-20). Typically, this is a polyether ether ketone-type spacer with the surgeon's choice of osteobiologic or bone graft packed into the cage. Implant placement should be done under direct vision and AP and lateral fluoroscopy to ensure appropriate final positioning (Fig. 29-21).

Closure

Copious irrigation is performed.

Hemostasis is achieved with Floseal and bipolar electrocautery. The psoas is visualized to rebound with removal of the retractor.

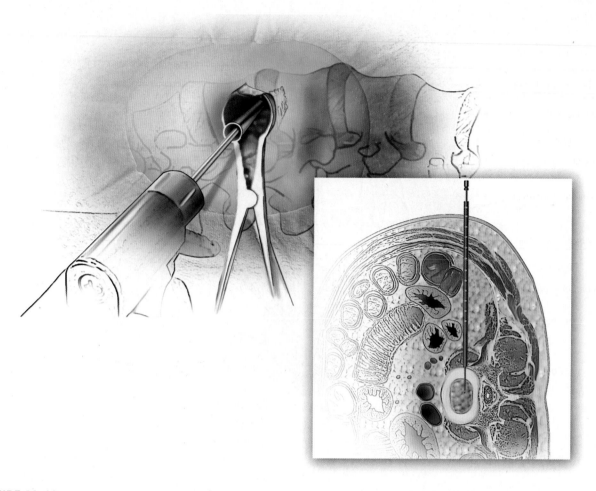

FIGURE 29-10

The dilator is passed through the psoas, and the guidewire is placed into the intervertebral disc.

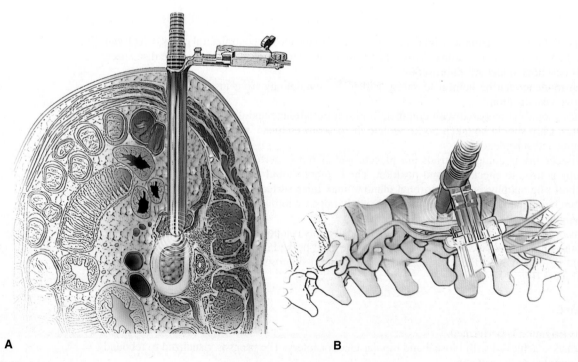

A

B

FIGURE 29-11

Free-run EMG is performed to assure a safe working window through the psoas muscle.

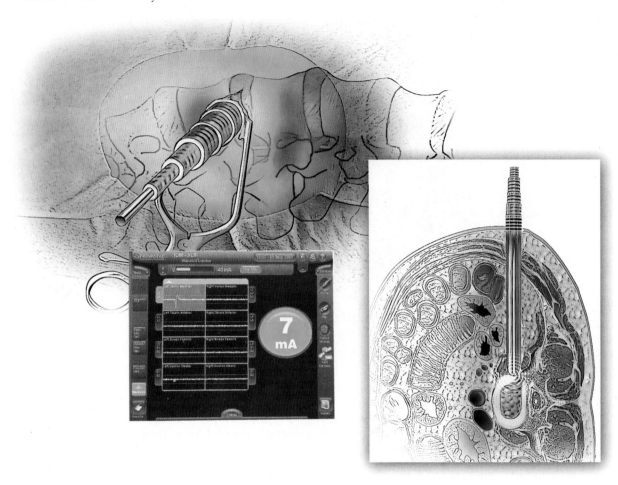

FIGURE 29-12

When the dilator is passed through the psoas, EMG activity typically lower than a threshold of 10 mA represents proximity too close to the lumbar plexus or nerve roots.

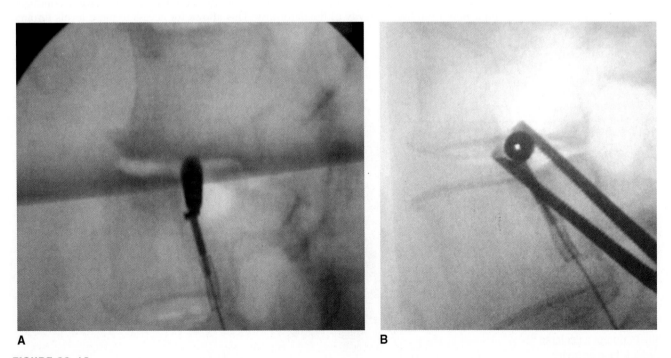

A   B

FIGURE 29-13

Lateral fluoroscopic images **(A and B)** showing appropriate position of the dilator in the center of the disc space.

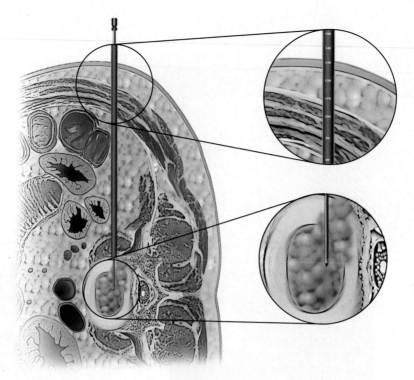

FIGURE 29-14

The guidewire is placed through the dilator and docked into the inter- vertebral disc.

The wound is closed in layers paying particular attention to closure of the transversalis fascia.
If open or percutaneous posterior approach is required for additional stability, then the patient is repositioned.

Pearls and Pitfalls (Special Advice for the Advanced Techniques)

Careful attention must be paid to preoperative imaging to ensure safety when approaching the spine and to determine the most efficacious approach. Intraoperative imaging including true lateral and AP radiographs is necessary to navigate a safe corridor between the nervous and vascular structures to the interspace (9).

When treating multiple levels in a patient with degenerative lumbar scoliosis, we recommend approaching from the concavity of the deformity. This allows for access to more levels through

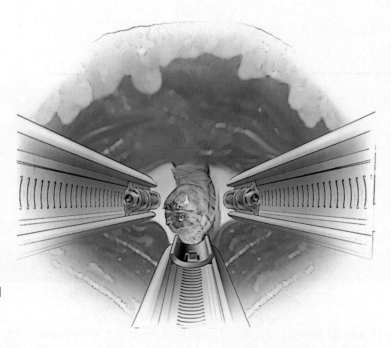

FIGURE 29-15

Illustration of a centered view of the disc space through the retractor.

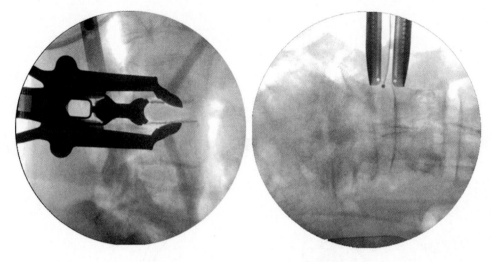

FIGURE 29-16

Lateral and AP fluoroscopic image showing appropriate working window and retractor position just prior to discectomy.

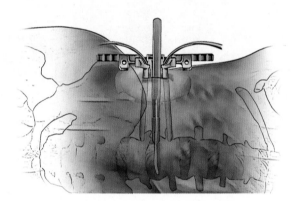

FIGURE 29-17

Illustration of contra-lateral release with small Cobb elevator.

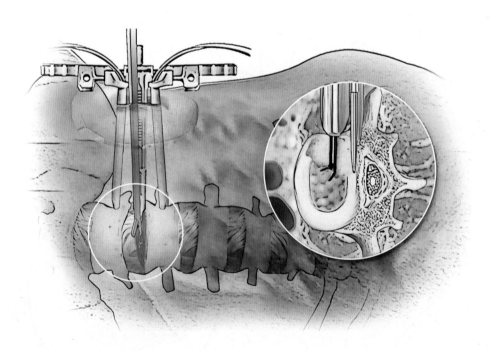

FIGURE 29-18

Illustration of removal of disc material with pituitary.

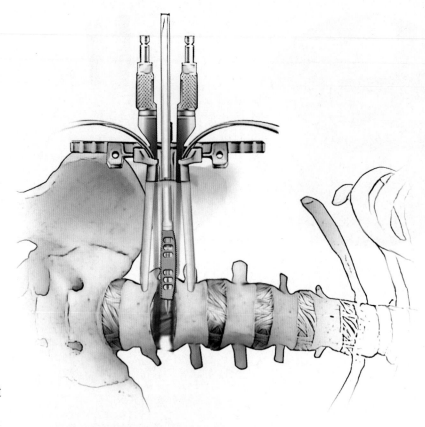

FIGURE 29-19

Illustration of placement of intervertebral trial.

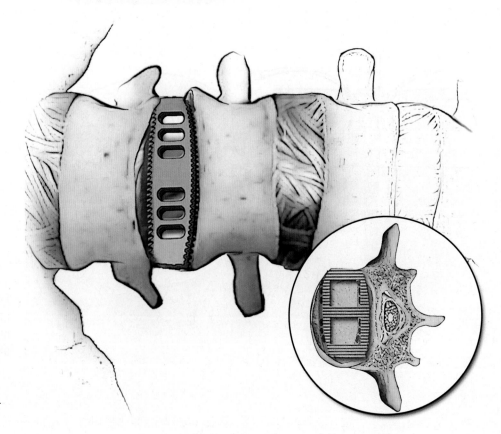

FIGURE 29-20

Illustration of intervertebral spacer placed.

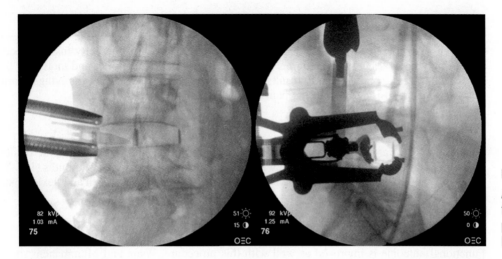

FIGURE 29-21

AP and lateral fluoroscopic image after placement of intervertebral spacer.

fewer incisions. The concavity is the side of greater soft tissue contracture, foraminal narrowing, and bony compression. Therefore, approach on this side of the spine allows for a more comprehensive soft tissue release at the site of greater pathology. Releasing the deformity here will allow for improved deformity correction and restoration of foraminal height and indirect neural decompression. In addition, this usually facilitates easier access to L4–L5 above the iliac crest. Also, by placing the concavity up, the table bend will help facilitate correction of the scoliosis (9).

When treating multiple levels, we recommend beginning at the most caudad level and continuing cephalad. Because of the segmental deformity in most degenerative scoliosis, the operating table and fluoroscopy may need to be adjusted at each level to ensure optimal radiographic imaging. Grafts should be wide enough to engage the stronger ring apophysis to minimize subsidence. Lordotic grafts are usually helpful as well as many of these patients have a flat or kyphotic back (9).

If L4–L5 is to be approached, careful preoperative consideration must be given to the position of the iliac crest. The anatomy of some patients will make this approach very difficult. Access is improved with maximum side bending of the table.

Flexion of the hips to 90 degrees allows for relaxation of the psoas. This may decrease postoperative psoas swelling and weakness and the potential for groin and anterior thigh pain.

Neurologic monitoring is key to the safety of the procedure. It is very important to use the EMG probe in and around the working field to define a safe working zone.

POSTOPERATIVE MANAGEMENT

Postoperative management is standard. The patient is usually allowed to ambulate as tolerated. Bracing can be done at the surgeon's discretion for additional stability.

In certain situations, the patient may return to the OR for additional posterior surgery if the procedure is staged.

COMPLICATIONS

The most common complications are postoperative groin or thigh pain, numbness and weakness related to the transpsoas approach, and irritation of the lumbar plexus. This is usually a sensory nerve injury resulting in paresthesias or transient post-op anterior thigh numbness, ipsilateral to the approach, occurring in about 10% to 12% of patients (2,7). Motor injury, resulting in lower extremity weakness, is less frequent, occurring about 0.7% to 3.4% of the time in larger series (6,7,13). Recovery of either motor or sensory deficits can be expected about 3 to 6 months after surgery (5).

In a large review of 600 cases (714 levels), the overall incidence of periop complications was 6.2%. Most were minor medical complications including urinary tract infection, myocardial infarction, pneumonia, postoperative ileus, and anemia requiring transfusion. These occur at a frequency less than open spine surgery with a reported incidence between 1.9% (6) and 3.7% (13). There were no wound infections, no vascular injuries, no intraoperative visceral injuries, and 4 (0.7%) transient postoperative neurologic deficits. Eleven events (1.8%) resulted in additional procedures/reoperation (13).

Other possible complications to be aware of are those to abdominal viscera including the bowel and kidney (6,17). This is extremely rare but can be of significant consequence.

RESULTS

The minimally invasive transpsoas lateral approach to the spine for interbody fusion is becoming increasingly popular because it requires significantly less soft tissue injury and morbidity than the traditional anterior approach. Early results have shown excellent efficacy in improving deformity in degenerative scoliosis and decreasing pain (6).

Arthrodesis

Fusion rates have also been promising. Wang and Mummaneni showed radiographic evidence of fusion in 84 out of 86 levels they treated with LLIF at mean follow-up of 13.4 months (19). Youssef et al. (20) showed fusion in 68 of 84 patients (81%) at 15 months by CT scan and flexion/extension radiographs.

Functional Outcome

Functional outcome is improved as well with this procedure. Wang and Mummaneni showed an improvement of 3.96 in the visual analog scale (VAS) for axial pain (19). A study of 25 patients receiving this treatment for degenerative scoliosis by Dakwar et al. (2) demonstrated an improvement of 5.7 points on VAS and 23.7% on oswestry disability index.

Lumbar Stenosis

Radiographic studies have shown significant indirect decompression of the neural elements with LLIF. In an MRI study of 21 patients (43 levels), increases of 41.9% in average disc height, 13.5% in foraminal height, 24.7% in foraminal area, and 33.1% in central canal diameter were noted on postoperative radiographs (10).

RECOMMENDED READING

1. Cappuccino A, et al.: Biomechanical analysis and review of lateral lumbar fusion constructs. *Spine (Phila Pa 1976)* 35(26 Suppl): S361–S367, 2010.
2. Dakwar E, et al.: Early outcomes and safety of the minimally invasive, lateral retroperitoneal transpsoas approach for adult degenerative scoliosis. *Neurosurg Focus* 28(3): E8, 2010.
3. Eck JC: Minimally invasive corpectomy and posterior stabilization for lumbar burst fracture. *Spine J* 11(9): 904–908, 2011.
4. Fraser RD: Interbody, posterior, and combined lumbar fusions. *Spine (Phila Pa 1976)* 20(24 Suppl): 167S–177S, 1995.
5. Houten JK, et al.: Nerve injury during the transpsoas approach for lumbar fusion. *J Neurosurg Spine* 15(3): 280–284, 2011.
6. Isaacs RE, et al.: A prospective, nonrandomized, multicenter evaluation of extreme lateral interbody fusion for the treatment of adult degenerative scoliosis: perioperative outcomes and complications. *Spine (Phila Pa 1976)* 35(26 Suppl): S322–S330, 2010.
7. Knight RQ, et al.: Direct lateral lumbar interbody fusion for degenerative conditions: early complication profile. *J Spinal Disord Tech* 22(1): 34–37, 2009.
8. Madan S, Boeree NR: Outcome of posterior lumbar interbody fusion versus posterolateral fusion for spondylolytic spondylolisthesis. *Spine (Phila Pa 1976)* 27(14): 1536–1542, 2002.
9. Mundis GM, Akbarnia BA, Phillips FM: Adult deformity correction through minimally invasive lateral approach techniques. *Spine (Phila Pa 1976)* 35(26 Suppl): S312–S321, 2010.
10. Oliveira L, et al.: A radiographic assessment of the ability of the extreme lateral interbody fusion procedure to indirectly decompress the neural elements. *Spine (Phila Pa 1976)* 35(26 Suppl): S331–S337, 2010.
11. Park DK, et al.: The relationship of intrapsoas nerves during a transpsoas approach to the lumbar spine: anatomic study. *J Spinal Disord Tech* 23(4): 223–228, 2010.
12. Rajaraman V, et al.: Visceral and vascular complications resulting from anterior lumbar interbody fusion. *J Neurosurg* 91(1 Suppl): 60–64, 1999.
13. Rodgers WB, Gerber EJ, Patterson J: Intraoperative and early postoperative complications in extreme lateral interbody fusion: an analysis of 600 cases. *Spine (Phila Pa 1976)* 36(1): 26–32, 2011.
14. Rodgers WB, Gerber EJ, Rodgers JA: Lumbar fusion in octogenarians: the promise of minimally invasive surgery. *Spine (Phila Pa 1976)* 35(26 Suppl): S355–S360, 2010.
15. Sasso RC, et al.: Analysis of operative complications in a series of 471 anterior lumbar interbody fusion procedures. *Spine (Phila Pa 1976)* 30(6): 670–674, 2005.
16. Smith ZA, et al.: Minimally invasive lateral extracavitary corpectomy: cadaveric evaluation model and report of 3 clinical cases. *J Neurosurg Spine* 16(5): 463–470, 2012.
17. Tormenti MJ, et al.: Complications and radiographic correction in adult scoliosis following combined transpsoas extreme lateral interbody fusion and posterior pedicle screw instrumentation. *Neurosurg Focus* 28(3): E7, 2010.
18. Uribe JS, et al.: Defining the safe working zones using the minimally invasive lateral retroperitoneal transpsoas approach: an anatomical study. *J Neurosurg Spine* 13(2): 260–266, 2010.
19. Wang MY, Mummaneni PV: Minimally invasive surgery for thoracolumbar spinal deformity: initial clinical experience with clinical and radiographic outcomes. *Neurosurg Focus* 28(3): E9, 2010.
20. Youssef JA, et al.: Minimally invasive surgery: lateral approach interbody fusion: results and review. *Spine (Phila Pa 1976)* 35(26 Suppl): S302–S311, 2010.

30 Sacropelvic Fixation

Han Jo Kim and Keith H. Bridwell

INDICATIONS/CONTRAINDICATIONS

Sacropelvic fixation involves the use of pelvic fixation methods for the purpose of protecting S1 screws in fusions performed to the sacrum. The reason for this is inherent to the anatomic characteristics of the S1 pedicle—which is patulous, cancellous, and usually comprised of thin cortical bone. Therefore, excessive stress on the S1 screw can result in screw loosening, pullout, loss of fixation, and pseudarthrosis. The indications for sacropelvic fixation therefore include (5)

Long fusions to the sacrum in adults (proximal fusion level L2 or above)
Short lumbosacral fusions under settings of severe osteoporosis
High-grade spondylolisthesis at L5–S1 (greater than 50% slip)
Flat-back deformity requiring three-column osteotomy
Correction of pelvic obliquity
Sacral fractures with spinopelvic dissociation
Tumor resection after sacrectomy

From a conceptual standpoint, constructs that will result in huge biomechanical stresses on the S1 screws will require use of sacropelvic fixation. This includes constructs that provide a substantial amount of coronal or sagittal plane corrections.

Contraindications for sacropelvic fixation are analogous to surgical contraindications for fusions involving the sacrum. If there is absolute certainty as to obviate the use of pelvic fixation for a fusion to the sacrum, sacropelvic fixation is not necessary and should not be performed since pelvic fixation does increase operative times and can increase total operative blood loss.

PREOPERATIVE PREPARATION

Decision making on fusing adult curves to the sacrum is based in part on the patient's complaints and where the principal pain seems to be (i.e., the thoracic spine, the thoracolumbar junction, or the distal lumbar spine). Appropriate bending films are helpful as well as upright films. It is most helpful that the upright films be long cassette to assess overall balance. 14 × 17 inches anteroposterior (AP) and laterals may be helpful to discern individual and regional segment pathology. Flexibility films that are helpful include a long cassette supine AP x-ray and right- and left-side benders. A supine hyperextension x-ray will help determine the flexibility in the sagittal plane. Also, what we have termed a "push-prone" x-ray may facilitate decision making as to the flexibility of the various curves in the coronal plane. What is usually assessed is the flexibility of the main lumbar curve from T10 or T11 down to L4 and then the fractional curve below, which extends from L3 to the sacrum. The flexibility of that curve from L3 to the sacrum and the degree of degeneration of those segments are part of the decision-making process on whether or not to extend to the sacrum.

MRI evaluation is helpful to determine the extent of disc degeneration at L4–L5 and L5–S1. The study also shows whether there is substantial central, lateral recess or foraminal stenosis at those segments. The parasagittal views are most helpful in assessing stenosis at L4–L5 and L5–S1 foramen. The MRI study is more helpful to evaluate the fractional curve from L4 to the sacrum than it is to evaluate the primary curve where extensive rotation makes visualization difficult. Extra attention to the orientation of the deformity is necessary by adjusting the gantry and allowing for in plane or perpendicular to plane visualization of the segments.

CASE 30-1

A 63-year-old female with complaints of progressive scoliosis and kyphosis. She lost 4 to 5 inches of height over last 30 years. There was no leg pain but increased back pain.
   A,B: 4 years post-op. Substantial improvement in lumbar back pain (**C**).

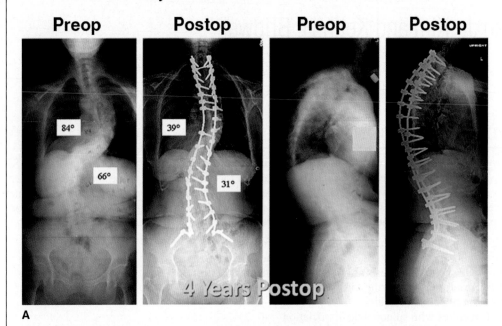

Patient 4 inches Taller Postop
Double Major Curve In a 63-Year-Old Female

A

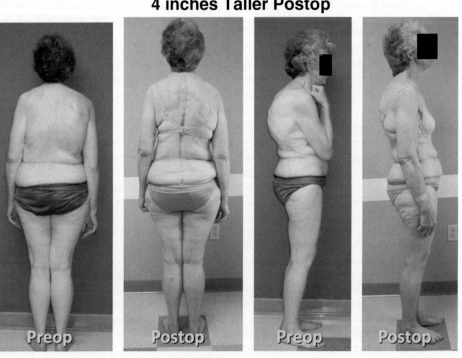

4 inches Taller Postop

B

CASE 30-1 (*Continued*)

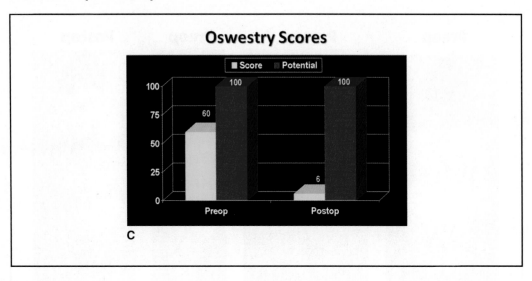

CASE 30-2

A 66-year-old female with progressive adult lumbar scoliosis and severe spinal stenosis at L2–L3 and L3–L4 with substantial spinal claudication symptoms and back pain.

   A,B: She underwent a T11-sacrum and pelvis posterior spinal fusion with segmental instrumentation with a decompression at L2–L4. Pre- and post-op clinical photo and radiographs at 5-year follow-up with significant improvement in outcome scores (**C,D**).

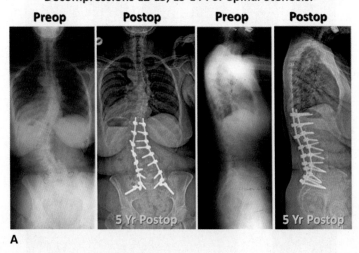

(*Continued*)

CASE 30-2 (*Continued*)

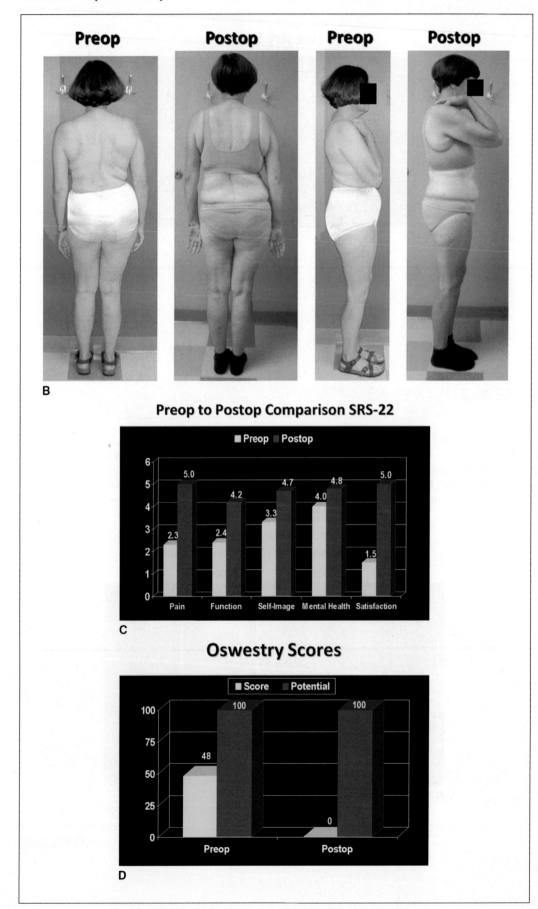

CASE 30-3

A 50-year-old female with progressive distal junctional degeneration and back pain. She had two surgeries: first a Harrington long fusion to L4 and then a revision for a pseudarthrosis at the thoracolumbar junction. She presented with a T4 to L4 fusion with a single Harrington compression rod around her thoracolumbar junction. **A:** She had a harvested left ilium from the first surgery and right ilium for the second surgery (see CT scan). **B:** She underwent a revision T11-sacrum and pelvis PSF/PSSI with a Smith-Peterson osteotomy at L3–L4. A S2 iliac screw was used in the left ilium due to altered anatomy from a prior iliac harvest. Pre- and post-op radiographs are shown.

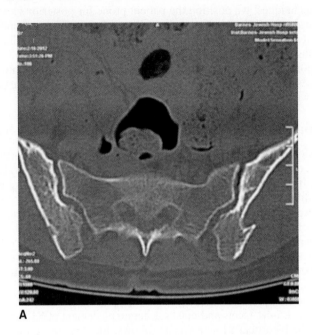

A

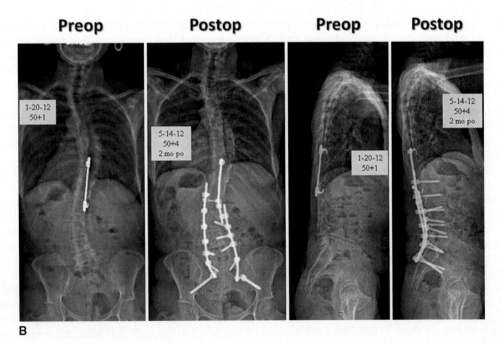

Preop   Postop   Preop   Postop

B

Under the setting of primary surgery, plain radiography is usually sufficient for visualizing the sacrum and pelvis to rule out any congenital anomalies of the sacrum and pelvis such as a bifid sacrum (see Case 30-1). Under the setting of revision surgery, visualization may be difficult due to obscurities from fusion masses and/or from extensive prior iliac crest harvest for bone graft (see Cases 30-2 and 30-3). It is helpful to have a MRI or CT scan study of the pelvis to delineate the anatomy and to demonstrate the extent of prior iliac harvesting to see whether iliac fixation is feasible on one or both sides.

TECHNIQUE

We currently utilize two methods for sacropelvic fixation: iliac screw fixation and S2 iliac screw fixation. With both techniques, we position the patient prone for posterior sacropelvic fixation. To maximize lordosis, use a frame in which the chest, ilium, and thighs are supported, but the thighs are in a relatively extended position. Keep the pads off the anterior superior iliac spine to avoid lateral femoral cutaneous nerve irritation, and flex the knees and feet to take tension off of peripheral nerves. If a long fusion to the sacrum is being performed, then do a wide draping of the patient to accomplish some assessment of spinal balance after the fusion and fixation are completed. So drape out the shoulders as well as the trunk and pelvis.

Surgical Approach for Sacropelvic Fixation with Iliac Screws

A midline skin incision is made to expose the spine from the midline. In particular at L5–S1, we expose out to the tips of the L5 transverse processes, out to the tips of the sacral ala, and then out to the ilium bilaterally. If we are planning to perform S2 iliac screw fixation, we usually do not need to expose out to the ilium.

In the process of exposing the sacrum, we perform more of an extraperiosteal rather than subperiosteal approach to avoid falling into the dorsal sacral foramina, which tend to have substantial veins. The use of Cobb elevators and Hibbs retractors is helpful to lift muscles off of the inner aspect of the ilium on both sides. In particular, the distal aspect of the ilium should be exposed and, to some extent, the lateral aspect of the ilium as well to establish the direction of the iliac screws.

Self-retaining retractors such as Adson-Beckman and deep Gelpi retractors are helpful but have to be placed just proximal to the ilium. Exposing out to the ilium on both sides facilitates the exposure of the sacral ala and the L5–S1 facets and makes accurate placement of S1 bicortical screws easier.

The placement of the bicortical S1 screw is as follows. Identify the confluence between the ala and the lateral facet of S1. Use a burr to find the starting point. Next, use a gear shift to find the way to the anterior cortex of the sacrum. Then check with a ball-tipped probe to be sure that there is still an anterior cortex. Mark the gear shift 5 mm longer, and then, using a mallet, gently tap the gear shift to perforate the anterior cortex of the sacrum. Verify the perforation carefully, and place a bicortical screw. Most commonly, the length of this bicortical screw is 45 mm. The diameter of the sacral screw (if it is going to be protected with an iliac screw) is usually satisfactory at 6.5 mm. It is important to angle in enough lordosis to hit the sacral promontory rather than the sacral endplate if the plan is to place cages or femoral rings in the L5–S1 disc space. Also, it is important to angle medially. If the ilium is in the way or there is insufficient lateral exposure, there is a tendency to not angle the sacral screw medially enough. If the S1 screw comes out laterally rather than medially, there is potential to irritate the L5 root as it is passing underneath the ala.

The entry point for the iliac screw is the very distal ilium. Use a Leksell rongeur or a burr to find cancellous bone. Use a gear shift, and very carefully, develop the interval between the inner and outer cortex. If this interval does not come easily, then check the direction under fluoroscopy, or accomplish a more lateral exposure of the ilium. Then check with a sounder to be sure the dissection is entirely within bone. Once it is verified that there is a bottom of 60 to 70 mm in length, then place a K-wire, and tap over this K-wire about halfway. Then place the ultimate iliac screw. It is ideal to accomplish an iliac screw of 60 or 70 mm in length. After placing the iliac screw, try to bury it so that it is not dorsally prominent. Take a lateral connecting rod, cut it somewhat short, and place it in the iliac screw. Connecting the iliac screw to the sacral screw usually involves bending quite a bit of lordosis into the rod. Start off bending as much lordosis as possible with the French bender, but often, this is not enough lordosis. Then, rotate the rod a full 180 degrees, take the kyphosing in situ benders, and use them to bend the extra amount of lordosis into the rods. It is often not feasible to bend enough lordosis with the lordosing benders because they bump into each other. Fasten down, but do not tighten the set screws on the connecting rod and the iliac screw until the rod is engaged into both these fixation points and the sacral screw. Use a sacral screw that is top opening. The most common diameter iliac screw to use is 7.5 mm. See Figures 30-1 to 30-9, step-by-step sacroiliac fixation.

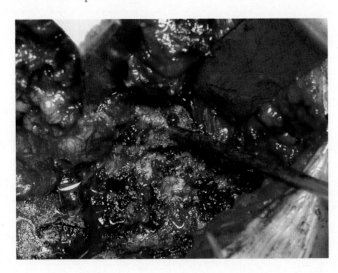

FIGURE 30-1
The iliac starting point.

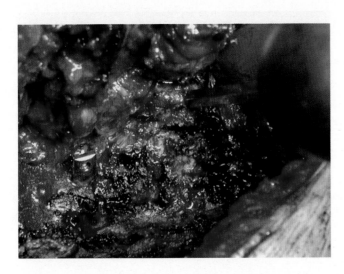

FIGURE 30-2
Finding the iliac interval.

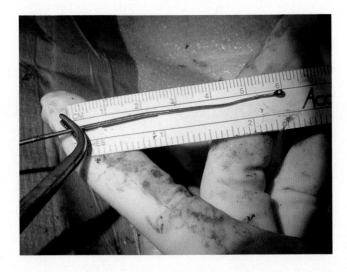

FIGURE 30-3
Measuring screw length.

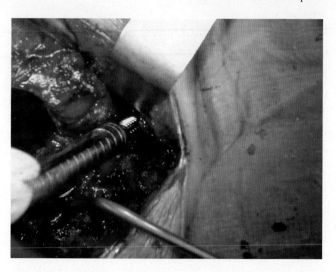

FIGURE 30-4
Tapping the track over a K-wire.

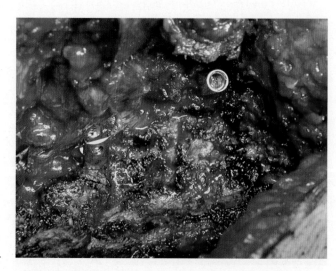

FIGURE 30-5
The iliac screw placed.

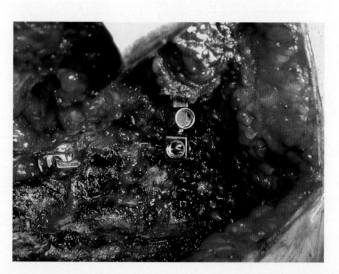

FIGURE 30-6
The lateral connecting rod.

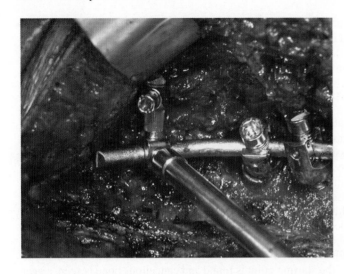

FIGURE 30-7
Lining up the screws.

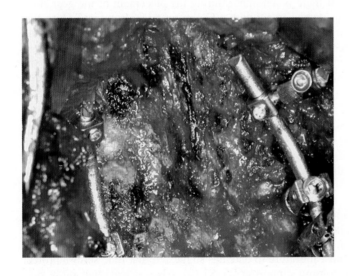

FIGURE 30-8
Need a lot of lordosis from the S1
screw to the iliac screw.

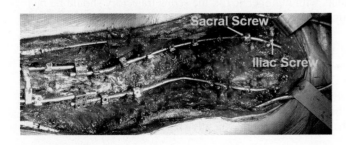

FIGURE 30-9
The construct.

Consider using this technique for paralytic/neuromuscular scoliosis in teenage patients and young adults. Here, also use bilateral S1 and iliac screws. In the teenage paralytic group, more commonly, use an iliac screw that is 6.5 mm in diameter and 60 mm in length because the ilium is generally smaller in such patients than it is in an ambulatory adult patient.

Surgical Approach for S2 Iliac Fixation

It is the senior author's preference that S2 iliac fixation be used more for revision settings or under conditions where the proximal aspect of the ilium is so distorted from prior iliac crest harvest that placement of an iliac screw is not possible (see Case 30-3).

Exposure does not need to be quite as extensive laterally as in the exposure used for iliac screw fixation. However, the S2 dorsal foramen should be exposed to allow of visualization of the foramen as well as a moderate lateral dissection, which allows for palpation of the distal border of the ilium since this will guide how far of a caudal trajectory we can have with screw placement. Once exposure is achieved in the manner described above, the starting point is exposed using the 5-mm acorn-tipped burr. The bony lamina between the S1 and S2 foramen is exposed, and the starting point is found in line with the S1 pedicle screw, usually 2 to 4 mm lateral and 4 to 8 mm distal to the S1 dorsal sacral foramen (5). Once the starting point is found and cancellous bone is seen, a gear shift is used with a trajectory of 40 degrees in the horizontal plane and 20 to 30 degrees caudal until the feel of the cancellous bone stops and cortical bone is encountered. At this point, you should be 25 to 35 mm deep, and the feel of cortical bone is an indication that you are at the sacroiliac joint. The gear shift is taken out, and a ball-tipped probe is used to confirm you are in bone. Then, the gear shift is replaced and continued in the same trajectory, or if the bone is particularly hard, the use of a mallet may be helpful for piercing the sacroiliac joint. Once the sacroiliac joint is pierced, the gear shift is removed, and a ball-tipped probe is used again to ensure you are in bone and to palpate the bony floor another time. Once confirmed, the gear shift is replaced and pushed along the same trajectory to a depth of 70 to 80 mm. If there is resistance during the placement of the gear shift, there is a low threshold for confirming its placement with a C-arm on a teardrop view. Once this depth is reached, the ball-tipped probe is used one more time to confirm you are within bone, and once a bony floor is also felt, a long K-wire is used and placed down the hole. The cannulated tap is used to a depth of approximately 40 mm so that a few threads also engage the ilium, and then, the ultimate screw is placed. Use of the S2 iliac screw obviates the use of a cross connector although the rod must still be contoured.

PEARLS AND PITFALLS

If the ilium has been harvested before, then it will be more difficult to place an iliac screw, but not necessarily impossible (3,5). Often, the very distal ilium will be preserved. At times, it may not be possible to accomplish a 60- to 70-mm screw, and a 50-mm screw on one side may have to be accepted. If this is not possible, an S2 iliac screw can be used with good fixation.

Placing a crosslink distally between the S1 and iliac fixation points may protect a somewhat weaker iliac screw on one side. Also, accomplishing anterior column support at L5–S1 with the use of either a trapezoidal mesh cage or a trapezoidal fresh-frozen femoral ring will also protect the S1 screws somewhat. However, most literature to date has suggested that iliac screws protect the sacral screws more than anterior column support at L5–S1 (2). Also, at least one study suggests that additional sacral fixation points (7) are not quite as beneficial at protecting the S1 screws as are iliac screws (6).

When placing the iliac screws, it is important not to perforate the iliac cortex. A very small perforation may be acceptable, but it is unacceptable to have more than a thread or two of the iliac screw outside of the iliac cortex distally because of the proximity of other crucial structures. So strive to keep the iliac screws entirely within bone distally. The most common angle of the iliac screw is approximately 20 degrees from medial to lateral and 15 degrees cranial to caudal. But this varies quite a bit from patient to patient and should be individualized according to the angle of that particular patient's ilium. For those patients with high pelvic tilt, the screw trajectory should be more vertical vice versa for patients with low pelvic tilt.

POSTOPERATIVE MANAGEMENT

If you can accomplish two bicortical sacral and iliac screws of 60 mm or longer, stand the patient the day after surgery and have them at least walk in place. We have a fairly extensive experience of doing this without putting patients in braces with thighs incorporated. If the iliac fixation is reduced on one side because of previous iliac harvesting, then it may be advisable to put the patient in a brace with one thigh incorporated for a period of time. In that circumstance, it becomes more important to provide adequate anterior structural support at L5–S1. If iliac fixation on one side is not possible, then an alternative is iliac fixation on the opposite side but then on the ipsilateral side to previous iliac graft harvesting to place one or two hooks into the dorsal sacral foramen.

One of the problems with long fusions in the adult population is the tendency for the distal fixation points to loosen and for one or two of the most distal motion segments to kyphose. If this happens, it often recreates a sagittal imbalance problem for the patient. We have seen this commonly with long fusions to L5 and to the sacrum without iliac protection. But in the patients that have had fusion to the sacrum with iliac protection, we do not see gradual kyphosing of the distal segments and therein seem to be able to prevent and even salvage previous sagittal imbalance problems that have occurred with previous fixations to L5 or S1 without protection of the sacral screws.

How quickly the patient's activity should be advanced, postoperatively, is something that has to be individualized. There is a potential difference between mobilizing a patient with a 2- or 3-segment fusion to the sacrum versus a 13- to 15-segment fusion to the sacrum. In most cases, a primary patient will rehabilitate and mobilize quicker than a revision patient.

But some basic guidelines are the following. Try to have the patient stand and walk the day after surgery. On discharge, the patient should be able to ambulate with a walker and have some experience walking up and down stairs. Suggest lots of walking for the first 4 months post-op. Discourage running, jumping, and bending over. Encourage the patient to keep the spine vertical, extended, and lordotic. Tell the patient to avoid putting the spine in a flexed or more horizontal position. Teach the patient to bend at the knees to pick things up, rather than bending at the waist.

Advance the activities of an older adult patient slower than a young adult patient and, obviously, a young adult patient slower than a teenage patient. Remind the patients that a definitive statement about a "solid fusion" with a multilevel fusion to the sacrum is often not possible until the patient is 5 years post-op.

Most of the biologic process of fusion will occur in the first year after surgery. So, most of the protection of the spinal arthrodesis should occur in that first year. After the first year, suggest liberalizing the patient's activity. Most patients, who have long fusions to the sacrum, starting at T3 or T4, will not go back to activities such as highly competitive sports and running and jumping. However, it is quite possible that they will be able to go back to sports such as bicycling, tennis or golf, or, in some circumstances, light jogging as well.

Also discourage the use of nonsteroidal inflammatory medicines for at least the first few months postoperatively. Many patients having a long fusion to the sacrum will have arthritis of other joints. It is known that nonsteroidal anti-inflammatory drugs (NSAIDs) block the inflammatory phase of the spine fusion. We do not really know how long the inflammatory phase of the spine fusion takes in a human. So there is no definitive answer for whether patients should be off their NSAIDs for 4 months or 6 months or 1 year after surgery. But it is advisable to, at least, have the patients off of those medicines for the first 4 months after surgery.

COMPLICATIONS

To date, we have not seen a substantial problem with sacroiliac joint pain and arthritis. There have been some minor issues with posterior prominence of those iliac screws.

These iliac screws all loosen with time as motion continues to occur through the sacroiliac joint. So ultimately, all these iliac screws will develop a halo. We have found it is not common that this is symptomatic. However, if it does become symptomatic for the patient, then the iliac screws can be removed. However, we would not encourage doing this unless there is unquestionably a solid fusion at L5–S1 and that the patient has good enough bone quality that stress fracture through the proximal sacrum is not likely to occur.

To date, we have not had any substantial injuries to nerves, vessels, or viscera around the ilium or the sacrum with this technique. Often, when we do our secondary anterior exposure of L5–S1, we will see the tips of the sacral screws out the anterior sacrum. But this has not posed any problem to date.

The advantages of this technique over the Galveston technique (1) include the following. Placing a threaded screw into the ilium is somewhat more precise and provides a more interdigitated connection with the ilium. Extensive three-plane bending of the rod is not required. The iliac fixation is somewhat protected by the sacral fixation and vice versa.

RESULTS

With this technique to date, we have not yet seen failure of the sacral screws (6). We do have a few cases of nonunion at L5–S1, and what has happened here is that the rods have broken at that segment. But in terms of loosening, pullout, or fracture of the sacral screws, we have not seen this in any circumstance where we have been able to accomplish bilateral bicortical S1 screw fixation and bilateral iliac screw fixation where the iliac screws have been at least 60 mm in length. Also, we have not seen problems with fracture through the proximal sacrum or sacral fixation points as have been described (3) in older patients having long circumferential fusions to the sacrum in which there is not protection of the sacral screws with iliac screws. We have used sacropelvic fixation of this nature to salvage fractures through the sacrum. In those cases, we have not only used sacroiliac fixation but also a fibular strut graft of a dowel nature across the sacral fracture (4,8).

RECOMMENDED READING

1. Allen BL, Ferguson RL: The Galveston technique of pelvic fixation with L-rod instrumentation of the spine. *Spine* 9: 388–394, 1984.
2. Cunningham BW, Lewis SJ, Long J, et al.: Biomechanical evaluation of lumbosacral reconstruction techniques for spondylolisthesis: an in-vitro porcine model. *Spine (Phila PA 1976)* 27(21): 2321–2327, 2002.
3. Dwyer TF, O'Brien MF, Dewald C, et al.: Traumatic sacral spondylolisthesis following instrumentation for spinal deformity. Paper no. 55 presented at the annual meeting of the Scoliosis Research Society, Cleveland, Ohio, September 19–22, 2001.
4. Hanson DS, Bridwell KH, Rhee JM, et al.: Dowel fibular strut grafts for high-grade dysplastic isthmic spondylolisthesis. *Spine (Phila Pa 1976)* 27(18): 1982–1988, 2002.
5. Kebaish KM: Sacropelvic fixation: techniques and complications. *Spine (Phila Pa 1976)* 35(25): 2245–2251, 2010.
6. Kuklo TR, Bridwell KH, Lewis SJ, et al.: Minimum 2-year analysis of sacropelvic fixation and L5-S1 fusion using S1 and iliac screws. *Spine* 26(18): 1976–1983, 2001.
7. Mirkovic S, Abitbol JJ, Steinman J, et al.: Anatomic consideration for sacral screw placement. *Spine* 16(16): S289–S294, 1991.
8. Smith MD, Bohlman HH: Spondylolisthesis treated by a single-stage operation combining decompression with in situ posterolateral and anterior fusion. *J Bone Joint Surg Am* 72: 415–420, 1990.

31 Techniques for Intradural Tumor Resection

Christine L. Hammer, Sanjay Yadla, and James S. Harrop

P rimary spinal cord tumors (SCTs) or neoplasms represent approximately 2% to 4.5% of all central nervous system (CNS) neoplasms (4,10). They are significantly less common, 10 to 15 times fewer, than primary intracranial tumors (10). These SCTs are classified or categorized based on their anatomical location such as extradural, intradural extramedullary, or intradural intramedullary (10,42). Other clinical features and factors that are significant in their diagnosis include clinical presentation, age, genetic disorders, and gender of the patient (2).

The focus of this chapter is the diagnosis and management of primary intradural SCTs. In general, intradural intramedullary tumors are more common in children, and intradural extramedullary tumors are more common in adults (42). In adults, these are compressive rather than invasive and primarily treated surgically. Postoperative outcome depends on preoperative neurologic status, histology, grade, and location of the tumor (10). Patients typically present with a pain syndrome with either localized back pain or radicular pain, and then symptoms will eventually progress to myelopathy if not treated (2). The clinical presentation and imaging studies are important in the diagnosis since there is a large differential diagnosis of other abnormalities that may present with similar features (2).

INTRADURAL EXTRAMEDULLARY

Intradural extramedullary tumors represent about 80% of adult SCTs and approximately 65% of SCTs in children (2,22). They can be further classified by histology or cell-type origin. Examples include meningiomas that arise from arachnoid cap cells of the leptomeninges or benign peripheral nerve sheath tumors (PNSTs) such as schwannomas and neurofibromas that arise from the cells covering the nerve roots (42). Other less common tumors include paragangliomas, hamartomas, metastases, peripheral nerve sheath myxomas, lipomas, sarcomas, and vascular tumors (10,42). About 50% of intradural extramedullary tumors and 77% of PNSTs have extradural extension (32). Meningiomas, hamartomas, and sarcomas are other intradural extramedullary tumors that are not limited by the dura. About 10% to 15% of meningiomas occupy both intra- and extradural space (22,42).

Spinal meningiomas are characteristically benign (WHO grade 1) tumors located in the thoracic spine of middle-aged women (2,46,49). Most lesions are solitary and located lateral to the spinal cord. Clinically, these lesions present with local or radicular pain and motor dysfunction greater than long tract or radicular sensory disturbances or sphincter deficits (10,22,43).

About 25% of intradural extramedullary tumors are PNSTs (42). However, these tumors are rarely simply intradural or extramedullary in location. About 10% to 15% are dumbbell shaped with extension beyond the dura into the vertebral foramen (28). These tumors are usually located at the anterior lateral aspect of the cord. While most intradural PNSTs are benign, about 2.5% are malignant with about half of those cases occurring in patients with neurofibromatosis type 1 (NF-1) (10,42) (Fig. 31-1).

Neurofibromas may be classified as solitary, multiple, or plexiform with a network of neurofibroma tissue bundles extending over nerve roots often involving multiple branches and plexi (10). These tumors contain Schwann cells, collagen, and reticulin fibers and encase rather than displace nerve roots (2). While most neurofibromas are benign (WHO grade 1), malignant forms usually arise from solitary or plexiform neurofibromas, and irradiation has been implicated in malignant transformation of neurofibromas (2,16,17,25). Approximately 90% of spinal cord neurofibromas are solitary tumors; however, multiple neurofibromas, as well as multiple schwannomas and meningiomas, may be found in patients with neurofibromatosis type two (NF-2) (2,4,17,47). Clinically, neurofibromas present often with pain and sensory dysesthesias (10).

Schwannomas, the most common spinal nerve tumor, usually arise from the dorsal (sensory) nerve root compared with neurofibromas, which usually arise from the ventral (motor) root (10,42). These tumors are typically benign (WHO grade 1), solitary, slowly growing PNSTs (2). When associated with NF-2, there may be multiple tumors, and they may precede the development of vestibular tumor and may also have a higher risk of malignant transformation (2,19). These are usually found incidentally secondary to their frequent involvement of nonfunctional nerve roots with one study showing just 23% with postoperative motor or sensory deficits (31). When symptomatic, a schwannoma may present with shooting pain or paresthesias associated with contact and rarely present with pain (10). These tumors grow along the nerve unlike neurofibromas which tend to infiltrate the neural elements. Surgically, this is important since schwannomas typically can be dissected off the nerve, thus preserving function, as opposed to the neurofibromas, in whose case complete resection often results in loss of function.

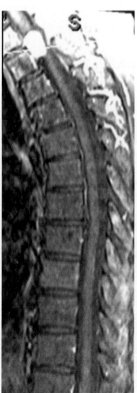

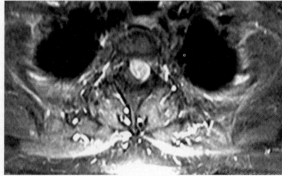

FIGURE 31-1

Intradural extra-medullary thoracic meningioma (T1W gadolinium-enhanced MRI). **A:** Saggital. **B:** Axial.

A   B

INTRADURAL INTRAMEDULLARY

Intradural intramedullary spinal tumors are the rarest spinal tumors and account for just 5% to 10% of CNS tumors, 20% of all SCTs in adults, and about 30% of all SCTs in children (2,22,42). Intramedullary spinal tumors may be of glial origin, such as ependymomas and astrocytomas, or of nonglial origin, such as hemangioblastomas, cavernomas, metastases, or lymphomas (2). In adults, approximately 60% to 70% are ependymomas and 30% to 40% are astrocytomas (10,24).

Patients typically present with back pain localized to the spine (24). Patients with glial SCTs typically have pain that is worse at night or upon awakening. This is believed to be secondary to tumor-induced disturbances in venous outflow in the valveless spinal canal venous system, referred to as the Batson plexus, causing venous engorgement in the supine position (24). Intramedullary tumors may present with "central cord syndrome" features of disassociation between pain/temperature sensation and proprioception as well as symmetric motor neuron dysfunction and myelopathy (10,47).

Spinal ependymomas can present throughout a patient's life but are more common in middle-aged adults. This is compared to spinal astrocytomas, which are more commonly found in children (10,47). These spinal tumors account for about 35% of all CNS tumors in adults and about 60% of all intramedullary tumors (2). Unlike meningiomas, which are more common in women, these tumors exhibit a gender preference for men (39,42).

Approximately 65% of patients with ependymomas have intraspinal syrinxes (47). Forty percent of intradural ependymomas are of the subclassification of myxopapillary. These tumors are believed to arise from the filum terminale and occur at the conus medullaris or in the filum terminale (10,42). Ependymomas usually present with sensory disturbances, particularly dysesthesias initially, and progress to pain in a distribution related to tumor location.

Spinal cord astrocytomas are the second most common spinal tumor type in adults with a prevalence in the first three decades of life and account for 80% of intramedullary tumors in children (42,47). Most pediatric cases are benign, while malignant astrocytomas and glioblastomas account for about 10% of intramedullary spinal cord astrocytomas in children (43). In adults, the malignant fibrillary astrocytomas are more common but may have pilocytic features (42,44). Low-grade, WHO grade 1 to 2, fibrillary astrocytomas typically have excellent surgical outcomes. However, higher-grade spinal tumors are associated with a poor outcome secondary to high incidence of dissemination via spinal fluid and rapidly progressive course (11,45). Radiographically, these tumors' radiographic features usually illustrate a fusiform expansion of the spinal cord. As with most spinal intramedullary cord tumors, weakness usually follows pain and sensory symptoms (22). Sensory symptoms tend to be paresthesias rather than dysesthetic pain (burning pain) as with ependymomas (24). Prior to diagnosis, symptom onset may occur over years in cases of low-grade astrocytomas or over months for high-grade gliomas (24).

Hemangioblastomas are the third most common intramedullary SCT. While most lesions are sporadic, about one-quarter of patients will have von Hippel-Lindau (VHL) syndrome, which accounts for about one-third of patients with VHL (13,24,42). These tumors tend to be engorged with blood vessels and are commonly embolized prior to surgical resection. Their location is often dorsal with subsequent predominance of sensory symptoms such as proprioception deficits (10,15,53).

INDICATIONS AND CONTRAINDICATIONS

The patient's neurologic function at presentation has been shown to be among the greatest factors affecting outcome. Thus, surgical goals should be preservation of neurologic function through resection or diagnosis through biopsy rather than restoration of neurologic function (8,10,42,47). In general, early and aggressive surgical treatment is indicated for patients with symptoms of weakness, sensory deficits, and/or pain (23). If symptoms are not significant and have no neurologic deficit, patients may be followed with serial imaging. However, simple observation does risk spontaneous hemorrhage. Progression of size, cysts, or syringomyelia over serial imaging should be evaluated for surgical intervention given the likelihood of future neurologic function loss.

Schwannomas and meningiomas should be surgically resected when they become symptomatic or serial images show a progress in their size (10). Stereotactic radiosurgery has arisen as a potential treatment for patient with subtotal resection or patient with multiple medical conditions prohibiting surgical options (19). The plexiform neurofibroma may be considered a malignant peripheral nerve sheath tumor, and postoperative radiotherapy and, possibly, chemotherapy are often used in their treatment (10).

Surgical outcome of the resection of intramedullary tumors has been improved through advanced operative techniques and the use of intraoperative monitoring. Spinal ependymomas and hemangioblastomas usually have well-defined margins, which can afford for gross total resection, while spinal astrocytomas tend to be infiltrative and full resection should not be expected or, in some cases, attempted (10).

Intraoperative open biopsy may be useful to either encourage the surgeon to avoid aggressive resection if a malignant tumor is identified or continue searching for the spinal cord/tumor interface in cases of ependymoma (47).

PREOPERATIVE PREPARATION

Magnetic resonance imaging (MRI) is the preferred diagnostic modality for patients with SCTs since it is noninvasive and gives excellent anatomic detail of the spinal canal and spinal cord (42). An MRI with gadolinium (contrast agent) with sagittal and axial T1- and T2-weighted sequences is an essential element for preoperative planning (2). The contrast agent aids in distinguishing cysts or syrinx from neoplasms and can aid in distinguishing the neoplasm's margins (2). When an MRI may have limited visualization due to metallic hardware artifacts, CT myelography is the next modality of choice. Myelography may show fusiform cord widening and syrinxes and identify tumors causing incomplete or complete block.

A digital subtraction angiography may provide relevant information about the relationship of feeding and draining vessels and may guide presurgical planning for interventions such as embolization (2,6,34,51). Angiograms are most helpful with very vascular tumors such as hemangioblastomas (Figs. 31-2 to 31-4).

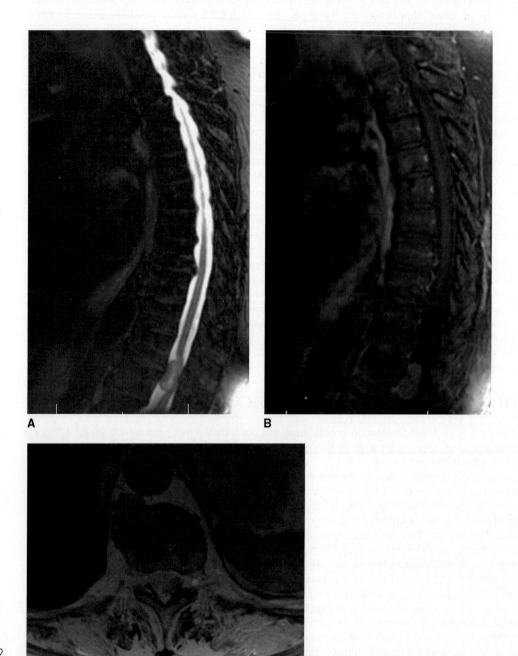

A   **B**

C

FIGURE 31-2

Intradural extramedullary meningioma with posterior and lateral displacement of the spinal cord at T11–T12. **A,C:** T2W MRI. **B:** T1W gadolinium-enhanced MRI.

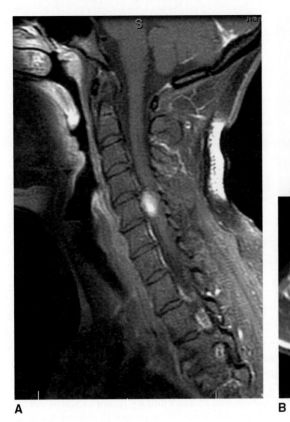

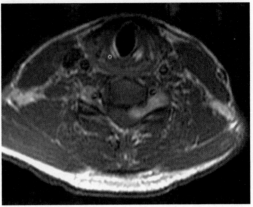

A   **B**

FIGURE 31-3

Intradural extramedullary PNST, schwannoma, with extension into a widened left C56 neural foramen (T1W gadolinium-enhanced MRI). **A:** Saggital. **B:** Axial.

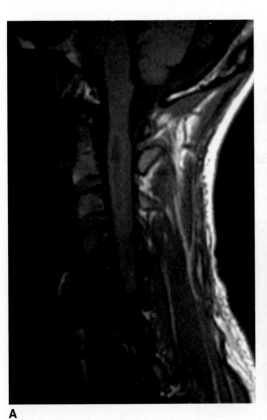

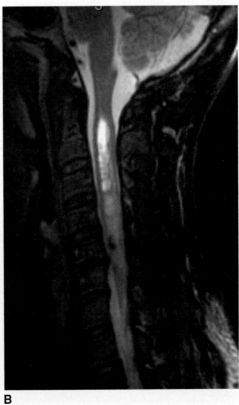

A   **B**

FIGURE 31-4

Intradural intramedullary ependymoma with a syrinx: **A,C:** T1W MRI, **B:** T2W MRI, and **D:** T1W gadolinium-enhanced MRI.

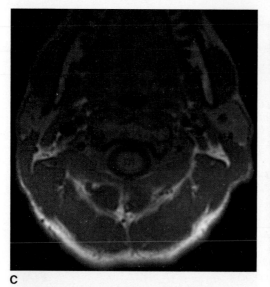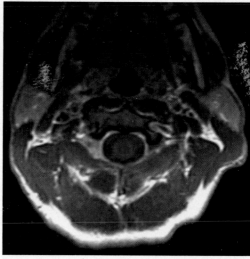

C   D

FIGURE 31-4
(*Continued*)

GENERAL APPROACH

A thorough and comprehensive review of preoperative imaging is necessary to plan the surgical approach for these spinal tumors. The ideal approach should have a surgical corridor that completely exposes the tumor while minimizing disruption of surrounding normal neurovascular anatomy (23,35,52,54,55). In general, intramedullary tumors and extramedullary tumors located dorsal to the spinal cord are approached via a midline posterior corridor with the patient in a prone position (3,30,50). Extramedullary tumors located ventral or lateral to the spinal cord are approached via a posterolateral or lateral corridor. Often, these tumors compress the spinal cord eccentrically to one side. Therefore, a window of exposure can often be afforded through which internal decompression and debulking can be performed with bipolar cauterization and suction or ultrasonic aspiration. The portions of the tumor that were not initially accessible can then be delivered and rolled away from the neural elements for further resection. However, a clear plane of dissection between tumor and spinal cord must be developed prior to performing such maneuvers. Rarely, ventral tumors or ventrolateral tumors can be approached via an anterior corridor (7,9,20,21,29,37,41,48).

In our practice, we routinely use intraoperative neurophysiologic monitoring including somatosensory evoked potentials (SSEPs), motor evoked potentials (MEPs), and corticospinal MEPs (D wave) (18,26,33,38). As part of this protocol, the intraoperative blood pressure is monitored with a radial arterial line, and mean arterial pressures (MAPs) are maintained greater than 85mm Hg throughout the procedure after induction of anesthesia (Fig. 31-5).

TECHNIQUES: INTRADURAL EXTRAMEDULLARY

These tumors are comprised primarily of meningiomas and PNSTs that can be addressed via a posterior approach as described above for intramedullary tumors. For cervical and cervicothoracic pathology, the patients are positioned prone on chest rolls with a Mayfield head holder

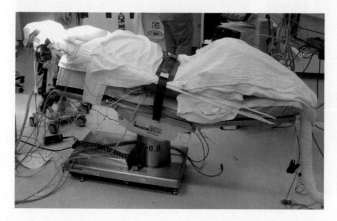

FIGURE 31-5
Preoperative setup.

(OMI Inc.; Cincinnati, OH). For thoracic and lumbar pathology, we prefer the prone position on a Jackson table (Mizuho OSI; Union City, CA). The exact spinal level of pathology is confirmed by fluoroscopy for midthoracic tumors or a lateral cross-table x-ray for other levels.

A laminectomy is performed over the spinal neoplasm exposing the dura mater, and hemostasis is achieved. If the tumor is located ventral or lateral to the spinal cord, a posterolateral approach may be chosen. This may include facetectomy in the cervical spine or a transpedicular approach or costotransversectomy in the thoracic spine. The durotomy is routinely made in the midline. However, some meningiomas or intradural schwannomas may compress the spinal cord eccentrically, and in these cases, it may be more prudent to open the dura along a paramedian tract on the side where the tumor is located. The dura is retracted with 4-0 Nurolon suture, which can be secured with hemostats or tacked to the fascia. The arachnoid can be opened with microscissors.

With meningiomas, an arachnoid cleavage plane can be found between tumor and spinal cord and should be developed to the surgeon's advantage. The dentate ligaments may tether the spinal cord and can be sectioned to assist with lateral exposure. The tumor with significant mass effect should be internally debulked and folded in upon itself. This allows the surgeon to minimize retraction on the spinal cord. A plane often can be developed between the tumor and normal dura. If it cannot be developed, the involved dura should be coagulated with bipolar cautery or resected completely.

Schwannomas typically involve the dorsal sensory root. They may reach a large size in which the spinal cord is compressed to the contralateral side. An arachnoid plane can be developed between the spinal cord and tumor similar to meningiomas. The nerve rootlets entering and exiting the tumor can be tested for motor involvement with neurophysiologic monitoring prior to sectioning. The nerve root is cauterized with the bipolar and cut halfway. It is cauterized again and cut with microscissors. Dumbbell extension of tumors involves the root sleeve and may require resection of the entire spinal nerve (42) (Fig. 31-6).

TECHNIQUES: INTRADURAL INTRAMEDULLARY TUMORS

Intramedullary tumors are routinely approached via a midline posterior incision with the patient in prone position (5,23). For midthoracic tumors, we localize the level of pathology by fluoroscopy prior to incision and again once the bony anatomy is exposed. Other thoracic, cervical, and lumbar tumors are localized with a lateral x-ray after the bony anatomy is exposed. For the majority of these tumors, a traditional midline laminectomy performed at the level of pathology as well as one spinal level above and below provides adequate exposure.

The pars interarticularis is used to judge the lateral extent of the laminectomy. Troughs are created bilaterally with a high-speed drill and matchstick bit. Spinous processes are carefully lifted upward and gently dissected off the thecal sac using a 2-0 Kerrison rongeur (Medetz Surgical Instruments, Inc; Dallas, PA) and nerve hook.

Prior to opening the dura, an intraoperative Doppler ultrasound is utilized to confirm that both the cranial and caudal apices of the tumor are visualized. The craniocaudal extent of the laminectomy should be larger than the durotomy, which should be larger than the tumor. The wound is irrigated and inspected for hemostasis prior to proceeding with the intradural portion of the procedure.

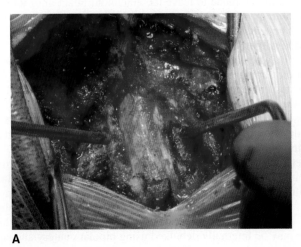
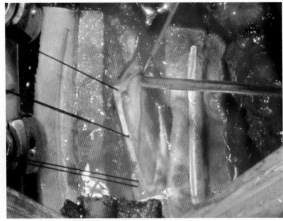

A   **B**

FIGURE 31-6

A–E: Resection of an intradural extramedullary meningioma: **A:** Laminectomy, **B:** Dural tack ups.

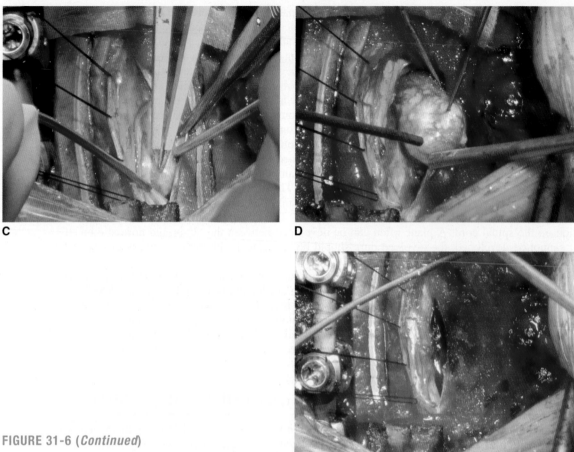

FIGURE 31-6 (*Continued*)

C: Exposure, **D:** Removing the tumor, and **E:** Postresection.

Bony bleeding can be stopped with bone wax, and epidural bleeding can be controlled with bipolar cautery and hemostatic matrix sealants. Cotton patties are placed on either side of the laminectomy defect to absorb any residual rundown and provide a surface for suctioning during the remainder of the surgery.

Once dura is exposed, the durotomy can be performed under loupe magnification, or the operating microscope can be brought into the operative field. The durotomy is initiated with a no. 15 blade down the midline. The footplate of a Woodson dura elevator (Blacksmith Surgical, Ltd; Karachi, Pakistan) can then be placed just under the dural leaflets and advanced along with a no. 15 blade to extend the durotomy. An attempt should be made to leave the arachnoid intact until the dura is completely opened. The dura is tacked up by 4-0 Nurolon stitches (Ethicon, Inc.; San Angelo, TX), which can be secured using hemostats beyond the edge of the wound or sutured to fascia at the side of the wound. The arachnoid is divided with microscissors.

The spinal cord is then inspected; it may be deformed or enlarged by the tumor, and occasionally, a portion of the tumor may crown at the subpial surface causing discoloration. The midline should be identified as this is generally the safest route to the tumor except in cases of eccentrically located lesions. Vessels along the pial surface should be preserved and dissected carefully. In a midline approach, they may need to be retracted laterally to expose the dorsal median sulcus. The plane between the posterior columns should be microdissected and the pia divided. The pia can then be tacked up using 6-0 sutures, which are then sutured laterally to the dura.

A plane must then be developed between normal spinal cord and the tumor. This can be extremely difficult with astrocytomas and may alter the goals of surgery from total resection to subtotal resection or open biopsy. It may be helpful to dissect above or below the apices of the tumor in order to find a clear cord-tumor interface, particularly if there is an apical syrinx or cyst. The plane is developed using microdissectors in the craniocaudal direction and then carefully around the circumference of the tumor. The tumor may be internally debulked using bipolar cautery and suction or ultrasonic aspiration. It can then be folded in upon itself to allow for further exposure around the periphery. Both frozen and permanent specimens should be sent to the pathology lab for diagnosis after the tumor is initially encountered.

Once resection is completed, we achieve hemostasis with hemostatic matrix sealants and cotton micropatties. The dura is closed using a running 4-0 Nurolon or 6-0 Gore-tex (Goretex) suture in a watertight fashion. A Valsalva maneuver is performed to confirm that no cerebrospinal fluid leaks are present. If a small leak is present, a simple suture using 4-0 Nurolon or 6-0 Gore-tex is usually sufficient to buttress the closure. A small piece of muscle may be tacked down at the site of the leak as well. Finally, a thin layer of either fibrin or cyanoacrylate glue is applied along the suture line. The wound is irrigated, hemostasis is confirmed, and the wound is closed in the normal watertight fashion.

PEARLS AND PITFALLS

- Vertebral Artery Anatomy: Preoperative imaging should be studied extensively including the course of the vertebral artery in cervical cases. Any aberrancy in the course of the vertebral artery may make a routine procedure (i.e., facetectomy for dumbbell tumor) treacherous.
- Use of Intraoperative Monitoring: We use continuous intraoperative monitoring in all intradural tumor cases, particularly in cases of myelopathy.
- Craniocaudal Extent of Laminectomy: To facilitate opening and watertight closure of the dura, the laminectomy should be performed well beyond the planned durotomy. This prevents needing to extend the laminectomy while the dura is open and spinal cord exposed.
- We continuously monitor MAP and recommend maintaining if greater than 85mm Hg through the procedure and induction of anesthesia.
- Frozen specimens should be sent as soon as possible as they may alter the extent or aggressiveness of resection particularly with intramedullary tumors.

POSTOPERATIVE MANAGEMENT

Patients with well-maintained dural closures postoperatively are encouraged to ambulate in order to prevent postoperative vascular or respiratory complications such as deep vein thrombosis and pneumonia (47). Orthostatic hypotension may occur after spinal cord injury secondary to tumor growth. This is thought to be secondary to the disruption of sympathetic activity control (12,47). This is seen more often after the resection of cervical or high thoracic intramedullary lesions and is thought to be due to reduction of plasma adrenaline and noradrenaline levels (12). These situations may be managed with fluids and gradual mobilization. Steroid therapy may be utilized after resection of spinal tumors although these should be limited to a short duration such to avoid the complications. High cervical spine lesions have been reported to cause a posterior fossa syndrome characterized by neuropsychological symptoms including akinetic mutism and behavioral changes, which are believed to respond to steroid therapy (36,47). Bacterial meningitis should not be discounted and should be evaluated with a spinal tap in patients with suspicious clinical findings (47).

The most common postoperative complaint after resection of an intramedullary tumor is posterior column dysfunction and motor deficits beyond baseline, which tend to improve with time (14,42). This is usually secondary to midline myelotomy required for tumor access as well as traction and manipulation of the posterior columns during surgery (24). This typically is manifested when the patients are ambulating such that they have difficulty navigating their feet due to a loss of proprioception.

Surgical resection outcome depends on the neural/tumor plane, and the tumor histology influences the rate of recurrence. In general, the primary operation affords the highest likelihood of a gross total resection. Postoperative radiotherapy indications are controversial (10). Spinal tumors in general have a slow growth rate, and therefore, radiation surgery is not usually effective in deterring growth. In addition, there is the potential for neurologic injury due to the radiation. In some tumor types, due to their high rate of recurrence, external beam radiotherapy has been employed. For example, partially resected WHO grade 2 ependymomas, malignant WHO grade 3 ependymomas, (10,27), and malignant schwannomas may be treated with postoperative radiotherapy (10). Studies have shown that patients with pilocytic astrocytomas respond better to postoperative radiotherapy only in cases with clinical or radiologic progression compared with the majority of patients with infiltrative astrocytomas who have been found not to respond well to postoperative radiotherapy (1,10).

Chemotherapy for spinal tumors has limited clinical use, and the primary treatment method is surgical resection. However, chemotherapy has been utilized for unresectable ependymomas and hemangioblastomas (10,47). Thus, it is reserved for patients with ependymomas who have not been able to have surgery, for whom radiotherapy has already been administered, for those with progressive disease, or for those with high-grade histology (40).

Patients are followed with an early postoperative MRI and subsequent annual gadolinium-enhanced MRIs to monitor for progression (47). This practice provides for the identification of tumor progression prior to clinical symptoms and will likely allow early intervention before neurologic deficits are present (42). Since the degree of progression or recurrences is based on histology, patient follow-up may be tailored accordingly.

COMPLICATIONS/ADVERSE EVENTS

As with any spinal surgery, the most concerning adverse event is neurologic loss. With surgical treatment of spinal tumors in general, the patients retain their degree of neurologic function. In other words, patients that are ambulating prior to surgical intervention will continue to ambulate. Unfortunately, though, patients can neurologically deteriorate with surgery due to manipulation of the neural elements. As noted previously with intramedullary tumors, a patient has an almost 100% chance of sensory alterations due to dividing the posterior columns during exposure of the tumor.

Other adverse events include spinal fluid leak, pseudomeningocele, and wound dehiscence or infections. These events are particularly more common in patients who have had prior surgery or prior radiation therapy (47). Patients with wound dehiscence or infections typically require a revision closure and possibly the assistance of plastic surgeons (47). In patients with persistent spinal leaks, this risk of nonhealing is decreased by a fascial closure that is watertight and without tension and consideration of the use of a lumbar drain (42).

Facet or ligamentous disruption and loss of neuromuscular control may increase the risk for postoperative kyphosis. This is particularly prevalent in patients with surgery over the cervical and cervicothoracic junction. Other complications include bacterial and chemical meningitis, instability, chronic pain, and nerve dysfunctions such as bladder or bowel dysfunction and sexual dysfunction (24).

RESULTS

The majority of surgical series on spinal tumors indicate that the strongest predictor of postoperative neurologic functional outcome is preoperative functional ability (47). Significant improvements in neurologic deficits should not be expected since atrophy, scarring, and chronic cord compression are poor predictors of functional outcome (47). The anatomic location of the tumor also affects outcome (8,47). For example, patients with thoracic lesions are more likely to have postoperative function decline secondary to the tenuous blood supply, and intradural tumors have a higher potential morbidity than extradural lesions (47).

OUTCOMES: INTRADURAL EXTRAMEDULLARY

Complications with resection of intradural extramedullary tumors are potentially less severe or common since there is limited manipulation of the spinal cord, nerve roots, or/and cauda equina. However, nerve root manipulation is usually well tolerated by the patient (42). Gross total resection of PNSTs (schwannoma and neurofibromas) is generally curative unless the tumor is extensive or associated with neurofibromatosis. On the contrary, malignant PNSTs carry an overall poor prognosis with survival only about 1 year (42).

The recurrence rate of spinal cord meningiomas is greater and has been reported to be 7% over 6 years or more follow-up after complete resection (22). The histologic subtype, psammomatous meningioma, is associated with an even less favorable outcome (46). In addition, the extradural extension of meningiomas is also indicative of a greater likelihood to recur (42). Anterior or lateral tumor position, a location below C4, and good preoperative neurologic function have been found to be associated with a good outcome (46).

OUTCOMES: INTRADURAL INTRAMEDULLARY

In symptomatic patients with intramedullary SCTs, microsurgical removal is the optimal treatment since it can lead to complete elimination of the tumor and no need for further treatment (42). Recurrence is rare, and morbidity is, as in all intramedullary tumors, associated with preoperative condition, particularly with spinal ependymomas. However, spinal astrocytomas have a different prognosis since gross total resection is uncommon. Several series have suggested that age is the most significant prognostic factor with the best outcomes in those presenting at age less than 21 (42). Spinal hemangioblastomas also have an excellent prognosis with surgical treatment, similar to ependymomas, and recurrence is rare.

RECOMMENDED READING

1. Abdel-Wahab M, et al.: Spinal cord gliomas: a multi-institutional retrospective analysis. *Int J Radiat Oncol Biol Phys* 64: 1060–1071, 2006.
2. Abul-Kasim K, et al.: Intradural spinal tumor: current classification and MRI features. *Neuroradiology* 50: 301–314, 2008.
3. Acosta FL Jr, et al.: Modified paramedian transpedicular approach and spinal reconstruction for intradural tumors of the cervical and cervicothoracic spine: clinical experience. *Spine (Phila Pa 1976)* 32(6): E203–E210, 2007.
4. Aghayev K, Vrionis F, Chamberlain MC: Adult intradural primary spinal cord tumors. *J Natl Compr Canc Netw* 9(4): 434–447, 2011.
5. Angevine PD, et al.: Surgical management of ventral intradural spinal lesions. *J Neurosurg Spine* 15(1): 28–37, 2011.
6. Baleriaux D, Gultasli N, eds.: Intradural spinal tumors. In: Van Goethem JWM, van den Hauwe L, Parizel PM, eds. *Spinal imaging.* Berlin, Germany: Springer Verlag, 2007: 417–460.
7. Banczerowski P, et al.: Surgery of ventral intradural midline cervical spinal pathologies via anterior cervical approach: our experience. *Ideggyogy Sz* 56(3–4): 115–118, 2003.
8. Bowers DC, Weprin BE: Intramedullary spinal cord tumors. *Curr Treat Options Neurol* 5: 207–212, 2003.
9. Casha S, Xie JC, Hurlbert RJ: Anterior corpectomy approach for removal of a cervical intradural schwannoma. *Can J Neurol Sci* 35(1): 106–110, 2008.
10. Chamberlain MC, Tredway TL: Adult primary intradural spinal cord tumors: a review. *Curr Neurol Neurosci Rep* 11: 320–328, 2011.
11. Ciappetta P, et al.: Spinal glioblastomas: report of seven cases and review of the literature. *Neurosurgery* 28: 302–306, 1991.
12. Claydon VE, Steeves JD, Krassioukov A: Orthostatic hypotension following spinal cord injury: understanding clinical pathophysiology. *Spinal Cord* 44: 341–351, 2006.
13. Couch V, et al.: von Hippel Lindau disease. *Mayo Clin Proc* 75: 265–272, 2000.
14. Cristante L, Herrmann HD: Surgical management of intramedullary spinal cord tumors: functional outcome and sources of morbidity. *Neurosurgery* 35(1): 74–76, 1994.
15. Eskridge JM, et al.: Preoperative endovascular embolization of craniospinal hemangioblastomas. *AJNR Am J Neuroradiol* 17(3): 525–531, 1996.
16. Evans DG, et al.: Malignant transformation and new primary tumours after therapeutic radiation for benign disease: substantial risks in certain tumour prone syndromes. *J Med Genet* 43: 289–294, 2006.
17. Ferner RE: Neurofibromatosis 1 and neurofibromatosis 2: a twenty first century perspective. *Lancet Neurol* 6(4): 340–351, 2007.
18. Forster MT, et al.: Spinal cord tumor surgery—importance of continuous intraoperative neurophysiological monitoring after tumor resection. *Spine (Phila Pa 1976)* 37(16): E1001–1008, 2012.
19. Gerszten PC, et al.: Radiosurgery for benign intradural spinal tumors. *Neurosurgery* 62: 887–895, 2008.
20. Gilsbach JM: Extreme lateral approach to intradural lesions of the cervical spine and foramen magnum. *Neurosurgery* 28(5): 779, 1991.
21. Giroux JC, Nohra C: Anterior approach for removal of a cervical intradural tumor: case report and technical note. *Neurosurgery* 2(2): 128–130, 1978.
22. Greenberg MS: *Handbook of neurosurgery.* 7th ed. New York: Thieme Publishers, 2010.
23. Harrop JS, et al.: Primary intramedullary tumors of the spinal cord. *Spine (Phila Pa 1976)* 34(22 Suppl): S69–S77, 2009.
24. Harrop JS, Sharan AD, Senders ZJ: Spinal cord tumors—management of intradural intramedullary neoplasms. Medscape. July 2012; Available from: http://emedicine.medscape.com.
25. Hottinger AF, Khakoo Y: Neurooncology of familial cancer syndromes. *J Child Neurol* 24: 1526–1535, 2009.
26. Hsu W, Bettegowda C, Jallo GI: Intramedullary spinal cord tumor surgery: can we do it without intraoperative neurophysiological monitoring? *Childs Nerv Syst* 26(2): 241–245, 2010.
27. Isaacson SR: Radiation therapy and the management of intramedullary spinal cord tumors. *J Neurooncol* 47: 231–238, 2000.
28. Isu T, et al.: Intraoperative monitoring for spinal cord tumor by spinal cord evoked potential following unilateral spinal cord stimulation. *No Shinkei Geka* 21(6): 519–526, 1993.
29. Iwasaki Y, et al.: Anterior approach to intramedullary hemangioblastoma: case report. *Neurosurgery* 44(3): 655–657, 1999.
30. Kim CH, Chung CK: Surgical outcome of a posterior approach for large ventral intradural extramedullary spinal cord tumors. *Spine (Phila Pa 1976)* 36(8): E531–E537, 2011.
31. Kim T, Foust RJ, Mojtahedi S: MR imaging of asymptomatic brainstem and spinal cord lesions in sisters with neurofibromatosis. *AJNR Am J Neuroradiol* 10(5 suppl): S71–S2, 1989.
32. Klekamp J, Samii M, eds.: Extramedullary tumors. In: Klekamp J, Samii M, eds. *Surgery of spinal tumors.* Berlin, Germany: Springer, 2007: 143–320.
33. Kothbauer KF: Intraoperative neurophysiologic monitoring for intramedullary spinal-cord tumor surgery. *Neurophysiol Clin* 37(6): 407–414, 2007.
34. Lee DK, et al.: Spinal cord hemangioblastoma: surgical strategy and clinical outcome. *J Neurooncol* 61: 27–34, 2003.
35. Manzano G, et al.: Contemporary management of adult intramedullary spinal tumors-pathology and neurological outcomes related to surgical resection. *Spinal Cord* 46(8): 540–546, 2008.
36. Marien P, et al.: Posterior fossa syndrome in adults: a new case and comprehensive survey of the literature. *Cortex* 49(1): 284–300, 2011.
37. Markert JM, et al.: Use of the extreme lateral approach in the surgical treatment of an intradural ventral cervical spinal cord vascular malformation: technical case report. *Neurosurgery* 38(2): 412–415, 1996.
38. McCormick PC: Surgical management of dumbbell and paraspinal tumors of the thoracic and lumbar spine. *Neurosurgery* 38: 67–74, 1996.
39. McCormick PC, Stein BM: Intramedullary tumors in adults. *Neurosurg Clin N Am* 1: 609–630, 1990.
40. Minehan KJ, et al.: Prognosis and treatment of spinal cord astrocytoma. *Int J Radiat Oncol Biol Phys* 73(3): 727–733, 2009.
41. Ogden AT, Feldstein NA, McCormick PC: Anterior approach to cervical intramedullary pilocytic astrocytoma. Case report. *J Neurosurg Spine* 9(3): 253–257, 2008.

42. Parsa AT, et al.: Spinal cord and intradural extraparenchyma spinal tumors: current best care practices and strategies. *J Neurooncol* 69: 291–318, 2004.
43. Raco A, et al.: Long-term follow-up of intramedullary spinal cord tumors: a series of 202 cases. *Neurosurgery* 56(5): 972–981, 2005.
44. Rauhul F, et al.: Intramedullary pilocytic astrocytomas: a clinical and morphological study after combined surgical and photon or neutron therapy. *Neurosurg Rev* 12: 309–313, 1989.
45. Sarabia M, et al.: Intracranial seeding from an intramedullary malignant astrocytoma. *Surg Neurol* 26: 573–576, 1986.
46. Schaller B: Spinal meningioma: relationship between histological subtypes and surgical outcomes. *J Neurooncol* 75: 157–161, 2005.
47. Schwartz TH, McCormick PC: Intramedullary ependymomas: clinical presentation, surgical treatment strategies and prognosis. *J Neurooncol* 47: 211–218, 2000.
48. Sen CN, Sekhar LN: An extreme lateral approach to intradural lesions of the cervical spine and foramen magnum. *Neurosurgery* 27(2): 197–204, 1990.
49. Solero CL, et al.: Spinal meningiomas: review of 174 operated cases. *Neurosurgery* 25(2): 153–160, 1989.
50. Steck JC, Dietze DD, Fessler RG: Posterolateral approach to intradural extramedullary thoracic tumors. *J Neurosurg* 81(2): 202–205, 1994.
51. Sun B, et al.: MRI features of intramedullary spinal cord ependymomas. *J Neuroimaging* 13: 346–351, 2003.
52. Sun J, et al.: Microsurgical treatment and functional outcomes of multi-segment intramedullary spinal cord tumors. *J Clin Neurosci* 16(5): 666–671, 2009.
53. Sutter B, et al.: Treatment options and time course for intramedullary spinal cord metastasis. Report of three cases and review of the literature. *Neurosurg Focus* 4(5): e3, 1998.
54. Taricco MA, et al.: Surgical treatment of primary intramedullary spinal cord tumors in adult patients. *Arq Neuropsiquiatr* 66(1): 59–63, 2008.
55. Yang S, Yang X, Hong G: Surgical treatment of one hundred seventy-four intramedullary spinal cord tumors. *Spine (Phila Pa 1976)* 34(24): 2705–2710, 2009.

Index

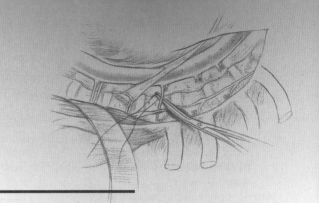

Note: Page numbers followed by "f" indicate figures and those followed by "t" indicate tables.